CW01373754

Springer

*Berlin
Heidelberg
New York
Barcelona
Budapest
Hong Kong
London
Milan
Paris
Santa Clara
Singapore
Tokyo*

P. Malfertheiner · J. E. Domínguez-Muñoz
U. Schulz · H. Lippert (Eds.)

Diagnostic Procedures in Pancreatic Disease

With 149 Figures and 70 Tables

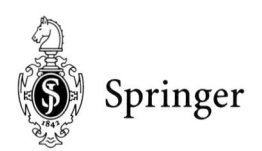

Springer

Professor Dr. P. Malfertheiner
Klinik für Gastroenterologie, Hepatologie und Infektiologie

Dr. med. J. E. Domínguez-Muñoz
Klinik für Gastroenterologie, Hepatologie und Infektiologie

Dr. med. H.-U. Schulz
Allgemeinchirurgie

Professor Dr. H. Lippert
Chirurgische Klinik

Otto-von-Guericke-Universität
Leipziger Straße 44
D-39120 Magdeburg, Germany

```
Library of Congress Cataloging-in-Publication Data

Diagnostic procedures in pancreatic diseases / P. Malfertheiner ...
   [et al.] (eds).
        p.   cm.
   Includes bibliographical references and index.
   ISBN 3-540-61821-X
   1. Pancreas--Diseases--Diagnosis.  I. Malfertheiner, P. (Peter),
1950-   .
   [DNLM: 1. Pancreatic Diseases--diagnosis--congresses.  WI 800
D536 1997]
   RC857.5.D53  1997
   616.3'7075--dc21
   DNLM/DLC
   for Library of Congress                                     97-5281
                                                                   CIP
```

ISBN 3-540-61821-X Springer-Verlag Berlin Heidelberg New York

This work is subject to copyright. All rights are reserved, whether the whole or part of the material is concerned, specifically the rights of translation, reprinting, reuse of illustrations, recitation, broadcasting, reproduction on microfilms or in any other way, and storage in data banks. Duplication of this publication or parts thereof is permitted only under the provisions of the German Copyright Law of September 9, 1965, in its current version, and permission for use must always be obtained from Springer-Verlag. Violations are liable for prosecution under the German Copyright Law.

© Springer-Verlag Berlin Heidelberg 1997
Printed in Germany

The use of general descriptive names, registered names, trademarks, etc. in this publication does not imply, even in the absence of a specific statement, that such names are exempt from the relevant protective laws and regulations and therefore free for general use.

Product liability: The publishers cannot guarantee the accuracy of any information about dosage and application contained in this book. In every individual case the user must check such information by consulting the relevant literature.

Book production: PRO EDIT GmbH, 69216 Heidelberg, Germany
Coverdesign: Design & Production GmbH, 69121 Heidelberg, Germany
Typesetting: Mitterweger Werksatz GmbH, 68723 Plankstadt, Germany

SPIN: 10539174 23/3134 - 5 4 3 2 1 0 - Printed on acid-free paper

Preface

"A decade of diagnostic efforts in pancreatic diseases (1985–1995)"

The diagnostic access to the pancreas was revolutionized two decades ago by the advent of endoscopic retrograde pancreatography, ultrasound, and computed tomography. The "hidden" organ was made visible by these diagnostic milestones. In a process of slow but continuous evolution, these imaging techniques have been further refined and complemented by nuclear magnetic resonance imaging, and together they provide the standards on which therapeutic decisions depend. Progress has also been made in the functional assessment of the pancreas in various conditions of disease such as acute pancreatitis, chronic pancreatitis, and cancer. New developments in molecular biology also promise more significant achievements in the near future.

Ten years ago we gathered a panel of international specialists dedicated to the study and management of pancreatic diseases and invited them to share their experiences with the available diagnostic methods. We have now repeated this process in order to review the past decade of progress in diagnostic procedures in pancreatic disease and to update the current state of expertise and stimulate further developments. The concept of the meeting, held in Magdeburg in December 1995, was to individually analyze the different diagnostic procedures and their specific use in the different disease conditions. The rationale for the interpretation of diagnostic findings is derived from the understanding of basic physiological and pathophysiological events and the resultant morphological alterations.

The purpose of this book is to share the updated knowledge about diagnostic progress in pancreatic diseases with those interested in the field. Our deep thanks go to everyone who has kindly contributed their expertise and time to the meeting and to this book. The augury is for this group to meet again in ten years for the next update of a decades advances in diagnostic procedures in pancreatic disease.

Magdeburg, 1996   The Editors

List of Contributors

Prof. Dr. Guido Adler
Medizinische Universitätsklinik und Poliklinik
Abteilung Innere Medizin I
Robert-Koch-Straße 8
D-89081 Ulm, Germany

Åke Andrén-Sandberg MD PhD
Department of Surgery
Lund University Hospital
S-22185 Lund, Sweden

C. Assmus
Medizinische Abteilung
Städtisches Krankenhaus
Bögelstraße 1
D-21339 Lüneburg, Germany

C. Bassi, M.D.
Surgical Department
Borgo Roma University Hospital
University of Verona
I-37134 Verona, Italy

Prof. Dr. H. Beger
Chirurgische Klinik
Klinikum der Universität
Steinhövelstraße 9
D-89075 Ulm, Germany

Prof. Dr. C. Beglinger
Abteilung für Gastroenterologie
Katonsspital Basel, Universitätskliniken
Petersgraben 4
CH-4031 Basel, Switzerland

Dr. med. Stefan Benz
Chirurgische Universitätsklinik Rostock
Schillingallee 35
D-18057 Rostock, Germany

P. Berberat, M.D.
Department of Visceral and Transplantation Surgery
University of Bern, Inselspital
CH-3010 Bern, Switzerland

Dr. W. Beyer
Abteilung für Nuklearmedizin
Radiologische Universitätsklinik
Universitätskrankenhaus Eppendorf
Martinistraße 52
D-20246 Hamburg, Germany

Dale E. Bockman
Department of Cellular Biology and Anatomy
Medical College of Georgia
Augusta, GA 30912-2000, U.S.A.

Dr. H. K. Bohuslavizki
Christian-Albrechts-Universität
Klinik für Nuklearmedizin
Arnold-Heller-Straße 9
D-24105 Kiel, Germany

A. Bonora, M.D.
Surgical Department
Borgo Roma University Hospital
University of Verona
I-37134 Verona, Italy

Prof. Dr. O. Bordalo
Hospital Universitario de Santa Maria
Rua da Estrela, 29 – 1° Dto.
1200 Lisboa, Portugal

Prof. Dr. Hans Bosseckert
Klinikum der Friedrich-Schiller-Universität Jena
Innere Medizin I – Gastroenterologie-Hepatologie-Infektiologie
Erlanger Allee 101
D-07740 Jena, Germany

Prof. Dr. M.W. Büchler
Klinik für Viszerale und Transplantationschirurgie
Universitätsklinik Bern (Inselspital)
CH-3010 Bern, Switzerland

E. Caldiron, M.D.
Surgical Department
Borgo Roma University Hospital
University of Verona
I-37134 Verona, Italy

List of Contributors

Prof. Dr. F. Carballo
Servicio de Medicina Interna
Hospital Universitario General
c/Donante de Sangre s/n
E-19002 Guadalajara, Spain

Suresh, T. Chari, M.D.
Department of Gastroenterology
Mayo Clinic Scottsdale
13400 E-Shea Boulevard
Scotsdale, AZ 85259, U.S.A.

Prof. Dr. M. Clausen
Abteilung für Nuklearmedizin
Radiologische Universitätsklinik
Universitätskrankenhaus Eppendorf
Martinistraße 52
D-20246 Hamburg, Germany

Prof. Dr. M. Cremer
Université Libre de Bruxelles – Hôpital Erasme
Service Médico-Chirurgical de Gastroentérologie
et d'Hépato-Pancréatologie
Route de Lennik 808
B-1070 Brussels, Belgium

Myriam Delhaye, M.D.
Université Libre de Bruxelles – Hôpital Erasme
Serice Médico-Chirurgical de Gastroentérologie
et d'Hépato-Pancréatologie
Route de Lennik 808
B-1070 Brussels, Belgium

Prof. Dr. E. P. DiMagno
Gastroenterology Research Unit
Mayo Clinic and Mayo Foundation
200, First Street S.W.
Rochester, MN 55905, U.S.A.

Dr. P. di Sebastiano
Unitá de Chirurgia
Universitá G. D'Annunzio
c/o Clinica Pierangeli
I-65124 Pescara, Italy

Prof. Dr. W. Döhring
Klinik für Diagnostische Radiologie
Otto-von Guericke-Universität
Leipziger Straße 44
D-39120 Magdeburg, Germany

Dr. J. E. Domínguez-Muñoz
Klinik für Gastroenterologie
Otto-von-Guericke-Universität
Leipziger Straße 44
D-39120 Magdeburg, Germany

Dr. M. Ebert
Klinik für Gastroenterologie
Otto-von-Guericke-Universität
Leipziger Straße 44
D-39120 Magdeburg, Germany

J. D. Evans. M.D.
University of Liverpool
Royal Liverpool University Hospital
P. O. Box 147
Liverpool L69 3BT, England

Prof. Massimo Falconi, M.D.
Surgical Department
Borgo Roma University Hospital
University of Verona
I-37134 Verona, Italy

Prof. Dr. L. Fernández-Cruz
Department of Surgery
Hospital Clinic
University of Barcelona
C/Villarroel, 170
E-8036 Barcelona, Spain

P. C. Freeny, M.D.
Professor of Radiology
Department of Radiology, Box 357115
University of Washington School of Medicine
1959 Pacific Avenue
Seattle, WA 98195, U.S.A.

H. Friebel, M.D.
Klinik für Gastroenterologie
Zentrum für Innere Medizin
Otto-von-Guericke-Universität
Leipziger Straße 44
D-39120 Magdeburg, Germany

Prof. Dr. med. J. M. Friedrich
Radiologisches Institut
Gustav-Adolf-Straße 10
D-97422 Schweinfurt, Germany

List of Contributors

Helmut Friess, M.D.
Dept. of Visceral and Transplantation Surgery
University of Bern, Inselspital
CH-3010 Bern, Switzerland

R. Girelli, M.D.
Surgical Department
Borgo Roma University Hospital
University of Verona
I-37134 Verona, Italy

Bernhard Glasbrenner, M.D.
Department of Internal Medicine I
University of Ulm
Robert-Koch-Straße 8
D-89081 Ulm, Germany

K. S. Glaser
Department of Surgery II
University of Innsbruck
Anichstraße 35
A-6020 Innsbruck, Austria

Dr. med. T.M. Gress
Abteilung Innere Medizin I
Universität Ulm
Robert-Koch-Straße 8
D-89081 Ulm, Germany

Prof. Dr. Lucio Gullo
Istituto di Clinica Medica e Gastroenterologia
Policlinico S. Orsola
Via Massarenti, 9
I-40138 Bologna, Italy

Dr. med. A. Hackelsberger
Klinik für Gastroenterologie
Zentrum für Innere Medizin
Otto-von-Guericke-Universität
Leipziger Straße 44
D-39120 Magdeburg, Germany

P. Hannesson
Department of Diagnostic Radiology
Lund University Hospital
S-22185 Lund, Sweden

Prof. Dr. E. Henze
Christian-Albrechts-Universität
Klinik für Nuklearmedizin
Arnold-Heller-Straße 9
D-24105 Kiel, Germany

Prof. Dr. U. T. Hopt
Klinikdirektor
Chirurgische Universitätsklinik Rostock
Schillingallee 35
D-18057 Rostock, Germany

I. Ihse
Department of Surgery
Lund University Hospital
S-22185 Lund, Sweden

Dr. H. U. Kasper
Institut für Pathologie
Universitätsklinikum
Otto-von-Guericke-Universität
Leipziger Straße 44
D-39120 Magdeburg, Germany

K. Kazakoff
University of Nebraska Medical Center
Eppley Institute
600 South 42nd Street
Omaha, NE 68198-6805

J. Kleeff, M.D.
Department of Visceral and Transplantation Surgery
University of Bern, Inselspital
CH-3010 Bern, Switzerland

Anton Klingler, Ph.D.
Division of Theoretical Surgery
Department of Surgery II
University of Innsbruck
Schoepfstraße 41
A-6020 Innsbruck, Austria

Prof. Dr. med. Günter Klöppel
Institut für Allgemeine Pathologie
und Pathologische Anatomie
Christian-Albrechts-Universität zu Kiel
Michaelistraße 11
D-24105 Kiel, Germany

List of Contributors

Prof. Dr. P. G. Lankisch
Medizinische Abteilung
Städtisches Krankenhaus
Bögelstraße 1
D-21339 Lüneburg, Germany

Professor René Laugier
Service de Gastroentérologie
Hôpital de la Conception
147, boulevard Baille
F-13385 Marseille Cedex 5, France

Prof. Dr. Peter Layer
Abteilung Innere Medizin
Israelitisches Krankenhaus
Orchideenstieg 14
D-22297 Hamburg, Germany

Prof. Dr. Bernhard Lembcke
Medizinische Klinik II
Klinikum der J.W. Goethe-Universität
Theodor-Stern-Kai 7
D-60590 Frankfurt am Main, Germany

Prof. Dr. H. Lippert
Chirurgische Klinik
Otto-von-Guericke-Universität
Leipziger Straße 44
D-39120 Magdeburg, Germany

G. Liu
University of Nebraska Medical Center
Eppley Institute
600 South 42nd Street
Omaha, NE 68198-6805

Dr. med. R. Lüthen
Medizinische Klinik und Poliklinik
Klinik für Gastroenterologie und Hepatologie
Heinrich-Heine-Universität
Moorenstraße 5
D-40225 Düsseldorf, Germany

C. Lundstedt
Department of Diagnostic Radiology
Lund University Hospital
S-22185 Lund, Schweden

Dr. Reiner Mahlke
Medizinische Abteilung
Städtisches Krankenhaus
Bögelstraße 1
D-21339 Lüneburg, Germany

Prof. Dr. Peter Malfertheiner
Department of Gastroenterology, Hepatology, and Infectious Diseases
Otto-von-Guericke-University
Leipziger Straße 44
D-39120 Magdeburg, Germany

Dr. med. G. Manes
Klinik für Gastroenterologie
Zentrum für Innere Medizin
Otto-von-Guericke-Universität
Leipziger Straße 44
D-39120 Magdeburg, Germany

Dr. med. H. Meier
Klinik für Gastroenterologie
Zentrum für Innere Medizin
Otto-von-Guericke-Universität
Leipziger Straße 44
D-39120 Magdeburg, Germany

Dr. Janos Mester
Abteilung für Nuklearmedizin
Radiologische Universitätsklinik, UKE
Martinistraße 52
D-20246 Hamburg, Germany

M. Möschel
Department of Surgery II
University of Innsbruck
Anichstraße 35
A-6020 Innsbruck, Austria

Professor Joachim Mössner, M.D.
Medizinische Klinik und Poliklinik II
Zentrum für Innere Medizin
Philipp-Rosenthal-Straße 27
D-04103 Leipzig, Germany

Carlos Morán, M.D.
Hospital de Gastroenterologia Bonorino Odaondo
C/Caseros, 2061
1264 Buenos Aires, Republic of Argentina

Dr. Friederike Müller-Pillasch
Abteilung Innere Medizin I
Universität Ulm
Robert-Koch-Straße 8
D-89081 Ulm, Germany

Dr. S. Navarro
Department of Gastroenterology
Hospital Clinic
University of Barcelona
C/Villarroel, 170
E-8036 Barcelona, Spain

Daniel K. Nelson
Director of Research
Assistant Professor of Medicine
Isaac Gordon Center for Digestive Diseases and Nutrition
The Genesee Hospital
University of Rochester
224 Alexander Street
Rochester, NY 14607, U.S.A.

Prof. J. P. Neoptolemos, MA MD FRCS
University of Liverpool
Royal Liverpool University Hospital
P.O. Box 147
Liverpool L69 3BT, England

Prof. Dr. C. Niederau
Medizinische Klinik und Poliklinik
Klinik für Gastroenterologie und Hepatologie
Heinrich-Heine-Universität
Moorenstraße 5
D-40225 Düsseldorf, Germany

R. F. Palma
Hospital Universitario de Santa Maria
1200 Lisboa, Portugal

Dr. C. Parada
Department of Surgery
Hospital Clinic
University of Barcelona
C/ Villarroel, 170
E-8036 Barcelona, Spain

Prof. Paolo Pederzoli, M.D.
Surgical Department
Borgo Roma University Hospital
University of Verona
I-37134 Verona, Italy

Dr. Miguel Pérez-Mateo
Servicio de Medicina Interna
Hospital General Universitario de Alicante
Maestro Alonso 109
E-03004 Alicante, Spain

Parviz M. Pour, M.D.
The Eppley Institute
University of Nebraska Medical Center
600 South 42nd Street
Omaha, NE 68198-6805, U.S.A.

P. G. Rabitti, M.D.
Pancreas Unit
Department of Gastroenterology
Cardarelli Hospital
Via Cardarelli 9
I-80131 Napoli, Italy

Prof. Dr. Th. Rösch
Medizinische Klinik II, TU München
Klinikum rechts der Isar
Ismaningerstraße 22
D-81675 München, Germany

Prof. Dr. med. A. Roessner
Institut für Pathologie
Universitätsklinikum
Otto-von-Guericke-Universität
Leipziger Straße 44
D-39120 Magdeburg, Germany

Priv.-Doz. Dr. Michael Rünzi
Abteilung für Gastroenterologie
Medizinische Klinik
Universitätsklinikum Essen
Hufelandstraße 55
D-45122 Essen, Germany

Dr. L. Sabater
Department of Surgery
Hospital Clinic
University of Barcelona
C/ Villarroel, 170
E-8036 Barcelona, Spain

List of Contributors

R. Salvia M.D.
Surgical Department
Università di Verona
Via della Menegone
I-37134 Verona, Italy

W. Sanger
University of Nebraska Medical Center
Department of Pathology & Microbiology
600 South 42nd Street
Omaha, NE 68198-6805

N. Sartori, M.D.
Surgical Department
University of Verona
Via della Menegona
I-3714 Verona, Italy

M. Scheetz
University of Nebraska Medical Center
Eppley Institute of Research in Cancer &
Department of Internal Medicine
600 South 42nd Street
Omaha, NE 68198-6805

Dr. Hans-Ulrich Schulz
Klinik für Chirurgie
Universitätsklinikum
Leipziger Straße 44
D-39120 Magdeburg, Germany

Dr. M. Siech
Chirurgische Klinik und Poliklinik I
Klinikum der Universität
Steinhövelstraße 9
D-89075 Ulm, Germany

Manfred V. Singer, M.D.
Professor of Medicine & Chairman
Department of Medicine IV
University Hospital of Heidelberg at Mannheim
Theodor-Kutzer-Ufer 1
D-68167 Mannheim, Germany

J. Stein, M.D. Ph.D.
Division of Gastroenterology
2nd Department of Internal Medicine
Johann-Wolfgang-Goethe-University
Theodor-Stern-Kai 7
D-60950 Frankfurt, Germany

H. Stridbeck
Department of Diagnostic Radiology
Lund University Hospital
S-22185 Lund, Sweden

I. Toshkov
University of Nebraska Medical Center
Eppley Institute
600 South 42nd Street
Omaha, NE 68198-6805

J. Tschmelitsch
Department of Surgery II
University of Innsbruck
Anichstraße 35
A-6020 Innsbruck, Austria

Dr. W. Uhl
Klinik für Viszerale und Transplantationschirurgie
Universitätsklinik Bern (Inselspital)
CH-3010 Bern, Switzerland

G. Uomo, M.D.
Pancreas Unit
Department of Gastroenterology
Cardarelli Hospital
Via Cardarelli 9
I-80131 Napoli, Italy

Dr. R. Vogel
Klinik für Viszerale und Transplantationschirurgie
Universitätsklinik Bern (Inselspital)
CH-3010 Bern, Switzerland

C. von Tirpitz, M.D.
Department of Internal Medicine I
University of Ulm
Robert-Koch-Straße 8
D-89081 Ulm, Germany

L. Weide
University of Nebraska Medical Center
Eppley Institute for Research in Cancer &
Department of Internal Medicine
600 South 42nd Street
Omaha, NE 68198-6805

List of Contributors

Dr. Paul Wilson, MRCP
University Department of Surgery
Clinical Research Block
Queen Elizabeth Hospital
Edgbaston
Birmingham B15 2TH, England

Contents

Introduction 1

Classification of Pancreatitis: Problems and Prospects
S. T. Chari, and M.V. Singer 3

A. Acute Pancreatitis 11

Morphology of Acute Pancreatitis in Relation to Etiology and Pathogenesis
G. Klöppel 13

Clinical Presentation and Course of Acute Pancreatitis
O. R. Bordalo, and R.F. Palma 21

I. Imaging Procedures 27

Ultrasound in the Diagnosis and Grading of Acute Pancreatitis
R. Mahlke, C. Assmus, and P. G. Lankisch 29

Computed Tomography in Acute Pancreatitis:
Diagnosis, Staging, and Detection of Complications
P. C. Freeny 37

Diagnosis of Infected Pancreatic Necrosis
C. Bassi, M. Falconi, A. Bonora, N. Sartori, E. Caldiron,
R. Salvia, R. Girelli, and P. Pederzoli 49

Endoscopic Retrograde Cholangiopancreatography in Acute Pancreatitis:
Indications and Limitations
P. G. Wilson, J. D. Evans, and J. P. Neoptolemos 57

II. Functional Methods 67

Appropriate Use of Serum Pancreatic Enzymes
for the Diagnosis of Acute Pancreatitis
F. Carballo, and J. E. Domínguez-Muñoz 69

Identification of the Etiological Factor in Acute Pancreatitis
H.-U. Schulz 73

Exocrine Pancreatic Function During and Following Acute Pancreatitis
J. E. Domínguez-Muñoz, and P. Malfertheiner 81

Endocrine Pancreatic Function During and Following Acute Pancreatitis
J. E. Domínguez-Muñoz, P. DiSebastiano, and P. Malfertheiner 87

III. Prognostic Evaluation 91

Pathophysiological Determinants of Severity of Acute Pancreatitis
R. Lüthen, and C. Niederau 93

Clinical Value of Multifactorial Classification
in the Prognostic Evaluation of Acute Pancreatitis
G. Uomo, G. Manes, and P. G. Rabitti 97

Biochemical Markers in the Early Prognostic Evaluation
of Acute Pancreatitis
J. E. Domínguez-Muñoz, and P. Malfertheiner 109

Prognostic Evaluation of Acute Pancreatitis:
When- and How-Consequences for Clinical Management
W. Uhl, R. Vogel, and M. W. Büchler 119

Diagnostic and Prognostic Evaluation of Graft Pancreatitis
S. Benz, and U. T. Hopt 131

IV. Guidelines 139

Acute Pancreatitis: Diagnostic Guidelines for General Practitioners,
Clinicians in Community Hospitals and in Specialized Centers
M. Pérez-Mateo 141

B. Chronic Pancreatitis

I. Chronic Pancreatitis: Clinical Features 149

Pathomorphological Feature of Chronic Pancreatitis
D. E. Bockmann 151

Pathophysiological Events in Chronic Pancreatitis: The Current Concept
C. Beglinger 161

Clinical Presentation and Course of Chronic Pancreatitis
G. Manes, J. E. Domínguez-Muñoz, M. Büchler,
H. G. Beger, and P. Malfertheiner 165

Painless Versus Painful Chronic Pancreatitis
C. Moran 173

II. Imaging Procedures 181

Role of Ultrasonography in the Diagnosis, Staging and Detection
of Complications of Chronic Pancreatitis
R. Laugier 183

Diagnosis and Staging of Chronic Pancreatitis by Computed Tomography
W. Döhring 189

Diagnosis and Staging of Chronic Pancreatitis
by Endoscopic Retrograde Cholangiopancreatography
H. Bosseckert 195

Radiologic Imaging of Chronic Pancreatitis
P. C. Freeny 203

Role of Pancreatic Duct Drainage for Evaluation of Pancreatic Pain
M. Delhaye, and M. Cremer 215

What Does the Surgeon Need in the Preoperative Evaluation
of Chronic Pancreatitis?
H. Lippert, and H.-U. Schulz 223

III. Function Tests 231

Neuroendocrine Abnormalities of Upper Gut Function
in Chronic Pancreatitis: Lessons for Physiology and Pathophysiology
D. K. Nelson 233

Direct Pancreatic Function Tests in the Diagnosis
and Staging of Chronic Pancreatitis
L. Gullo 249

Oral Pancreatic Function Tests in the Diagnosis
and Staging of Chronic Pancreatitis
M. Rünzi, and P. Layer 253

Present and Future of Breath Tests in the Diagnosis
of Pancreatic Insufficiency
B. Lembcke 261

Value of Serum Pancreatic Enzymes in the Diagnosis
of Chronic Pancreatitis
J. Mössner 271

New Fecal Tests in the Diagnosis of Exocrine Pancreatic Insufficiency
J. Stein 277

Extracellular Matrix in Pancreatic Diseases
F. Müller-Pillasch, T. Gress, and G. Adler 291

Endocrine Pancreatic Function in the Diagnosis
and Staging of Chronic Pancreatitis
B. Glasbrenner, C. von Tirpitz, P. Malfertheiner, and G. Adler 303

IV. Chronic Pancreatitis: Guidelines 311

Diagnostic Standards for Chronic Pancreatitis
E. P. DiMagno 313

Standards in Surgical Treatment of Chronic Pancreatitis
M. Siech, and H. G. Beger 321

C. Pancreatic Cancer 331

Langerhans Islets Are the Origin of Ductal-Type Adenocarcinoma
P. M. Pour, L. Weide, G. Liu, K. Kazakoff, M. Scheetz,
I. Toshkov, and W. Sanger 333

I. Imaging Procedures 341

Ultrasound and Endoscopic Ultrasound in the Diagnosis
of Pancreatic Tumors
H. Meier, and H. Friebel 343

Computed Tomography and Magnetic Resonance
Imaging in Pancreatic Cancer
J.-M. Friedrich 349

Endoscopic Retrograde Cholangiopancreatography in the Diagnosis
of Pancreatic Tumors
A. Hackelsberger, and G. Manes 359

Role of Laparoscopy and Laparoscopic Ultrasound in Pancreatic Cancer
A. Klingler, M. Möschel, J. Tschmelitsch, and K. S. Glaser 371

Intraportal Ultrasonography for Evaluation of Resectability
in Pancreatic Cancer
Å. Andrén-Sandberg, C. Lundstedt, P. Hannesson,
H. Stridbeck, and I. Ihse 379

II. Other Diagnostic Procedures 387

Serological Diagnosis of Pancreatic Cancer
M. Ebert, and P. Malfertheiner 389

Role of Cytology in the Diagnosis of Pancreatic Tumors
H. U. Kasper, and A. Roessner 395

Scintigraphic Procedures in the Detection of Pancreatic Tumors:
Role of Fluorodeoxyglucose Positron Emission Tomography
J. Mester, K. H. Bohuslawizki, W. Beyer, M. Clausen, and E. Henze 401

III. Molecular Biology 409

Clinical Applicability of Molecular Procedures in the Diagnosis
of Pancreatic Cancer
H. Friess, J. Kleeff, P. Berberat, and M.W. Büchler 411

IV. Guidelines 425

Pancreatic Cancer: Diagnostic Guidelines for General Practitioners
and Clinicians in Community Hospitals and Specialized Centers
L. Fernández-Cruz, L. Sabater, S. Navarro, and C. Parada 427

Subject Index 437

Introduction

Classification of Pancreatitis: Problems and Prospects

S.T. Chari · M.V. Singer

Introduction

The first international meeting on classification of pancreatitis was held in Marseilles, France in 1963. This meeting classified pancreatic inflammatory diseases into two mutually distinct categories – acute pancreatitis and chronic pancreatitis. In acute pancreatitis the pancreas returns to morphologic and functional normalcy after withdrawal of the acute insult. In chronic pancreatitis the pathologic lesions persist and progress in spite of withdrawal of the etiologic agent. In subsequent years three more international meetings have striven to improve and expand on this classification. The salient features of each of the four classifications are presented in tabular form (Tables 1–4). Even today, however, the classification of pancreatitis is far from perfect. This is to a large extent because of our inability in the early stages of the disease to differentiate acute from chronic pancreatitis. In this review, we analyse the drawbacks of the present classification and look and ahead to the possible improvements in the future.

Problems with Classification of Pancreatitis

Problem of Histologic Proof for Chronic Pancreatitis

The two Marseille classifications [1, 3, 4] and the Marseille-Rome classification [5] are based on histology of the pancreas. However, even today pancreatic tissue is not easy to obtain. Therefore, the difficulty in differentiating at the bedside an acute pancreatitis from an exacerbation of chronic pancreatitis (CP) in the absence of obvious features like pancreatic calculi still remains to be resolved.

Table 1. Marseille classification of pancreatitis (1963) [1, 21]

Type	Clinical characteristics	Morphologic characteristics	Course
Acute pancreatitis	Single episode	Not defined	Functional and morphologic restitution if the cause is removed
Acute relapsing pancreatitis	Multiple episodes	–	
Chronic relapsing pancreatitis	Multiple episodes	Irregular sclerosis with destruction and focal segmental or diffuse loss of parenchyma	Functional and morphologic lesions persist or even progress after the cause is removed
Chronic pancreatitis	No acute exacerbations	Varying dilatation of ductal system; strictures, intracanalicular stones (calcifications), cysts, pseudocysts; islets of Langerhans involved much later in the course of the disease; morphologic picture similar independent of cause	–

Table 2. Cambridge classification of pancreatitis (1983) [2, 21]

Type	Clinical characteristics	Morphologic characteristics	Course
Acute pancreatitis	Clinically defined as an acute illness that typically presents with acute abdominal pain; in general associated with an increase in pancreatic enzymes in blood or urine; the abdominal pain and the increase in pancreatic enzymes in blood or urine are secondary to pancreatic inflammation	Not defined	Acute pancreatitis can relapse
Chronic pancreatitis	Defined as a progressive inflammatory disease of the pancreas; patients typically present with abdominal pain and/or features of pancreatic insufficiency, can also remain painless; the only sign of an inflammatory process may be fibrosis indicating earlier pancreatic inflammation	Not clearly defined; characterised by irreversible morphologic changes; classification based on results of imaging studies	Many patients have acute exacerbations of pain

Table 3. Revised Marseille classification of pancreatitis (1984) [3, 4, 21]

Type	Clinical characteristics	Morphologic characteristics	Course
Acute pancreatitis	Acute onset of abdominal pain; increase in pancreatic enzymes in blood/urine	*Mild form:* peripancreatic fat necrosis interstitial oedema; as a rule pancreatic necrosis absent. *Severe form:* extensive peri- and intra-pancreatic fat necrosis, parenchymal necrosis, and haemorrhages; lesions may be either localized or diffuse	Usually benign; severe forms may be fatal; single episode or recurrent; exocrine and endocrine functions impaired to various extents for a variable duration; functional and morphologic restitution to normal occurs if primary cause and complications (such as pseudocysts) removed; acute pancreatitis may rarely lead to chronic pancreatitis
Chronic pancreatitis	Relapsing or persistent abdominal pain; Occasionally painless. Evidence of pancreatic insufficiency, such as steatorrhoea or diabetes, may be present	Irregular sclerosis with focal, segmental, or diffuse destruction and permanent loss of exocrine parenchyma; various extents of dilatation of segments of the ductal system; protein plugs, intraductal calculi, oedema, focal necrosis, inflammatory cells, and also cysts and pseudocysts observed to various extents; islets of Langerhans relatively well preserved; following descriptive terms can be used: (a) chronic pancreatitis with focal necrosis; (b) chronic pancreatitis with segmental or diffuse fibrosis; (c) chronic pancreatitis with or without calculi	Morphologic changes may lead to progressive and permanent loss of pancreatic exocrine and endocrine function; however, whether chronic pancreatitis is always progressive or may regress after removal of primary cause or causes should be investigated
Special form: obstructive chronic pancreatitis		Dilatation of the ductal system proximal to the occlusion of one of the main ducts (e.g. by tumour or scar)	Structural and functional changes tend to improve when the obstruction is removed

Table 4. Marseille-Rome classification of pancreatitis (1988) [5, 21]

Type	Clinical characteristics	Morphologic characteristics	Aetiology	Course
Acute pancreatitis	Not defined	Spectrum of inflammatory pancreatic and peripancreatic lesions: oedema, necrosis, haemorrhagic necrosis, fatty necrosis; in most confined to oedema and fatty necrosis	*Extrapancreatic*: gallstones, trauma, drugs, surgery, ERCP, hyperlipoproteinaemia, etc. *Intrapancreatic*: tumours, chronic pancreatitis? Pancreas divisum? Alcohol	Lesions generally considered reversible; necrosis may be infected; fluid collection progressing into peripancreatic space and filled with pancreatic juice, blood, and necrotic fragments may follow; these may become infected, disappear spontaneously or persist, forming *necrotic pseudocysts*; if necrosis involves a segment of the main pancreatic duct, stenosis may result, leading to obstructive chronic pancreatitis distal to the stenosis
Chronic pancreatitis	Initial stages: attacks of acute pancreatitis responsible for recurrent pain which may be the only clinical symptom; generally, after some years exocrine and endocrine insufficiency develop, and acute attacks decrease and disappear	*Chronic calcifying pancreatitis*: irregular fibrosis, lobular spotty distribution of lesions of different density in between neighbouring lobules; intraductal protein precipitates or plugs always found and, at least in late stages, calcified precipitates (calculi); atrophy and stenosis of ducts frequent and more often than in obstructive form; structural and functional changes may progress even if primary cause removed. *Chronic obstructive pancreatitis*: as described in Revised Marseille Classification (Table 3)	Chronic alcohol consumption, high-protein diet, abnormally low or high lipid diets, frequently associated with disease and probably represents aetiologic factors, such as hypercalcaemia; other clinical forms: non-alcoholic tropical and hereditary	Progresses in general from painful to painless disease; may progress in spite of removal of cause; *intrapancreatic retention cyst* may form distal to an obstruction due to dilatation of ducts; *retention pseudocysts* form when these cysts expand into peripancreatic tissues; *necrotic pseudocysts* form after an acute exacerbation; infected cysts or pseudocysts called abscesses
Chronic inflammatory pancreatitis		Loss of exocrine parenchyma replaced by a dense fibrosis infiltrated by mononuclear cells		

ERCP, endoscopic retrograde cholangiopancreatography.

Difficulty in Clinically Distinguishing Acute Pancreatitis from Acute Exacerbation of Chronic Pancreatitis

In the early stages of chronic pancreatitis (especially alcohol-induced) it can be very difficult to clinically distinguish an acute exacerbation of chronic pancreatitis from true acute pancreatitis. Often the possible etiology (e.g., presence of gallstones or history of heavy alcohol abuse) is used to make a tentative diagnosis. However, Ammann's study [6] has shown that not all alcoholic patients presenting with clinically acute pancreatitis will go on to develop chronic pancreatitis. In such patients only long-term follow-up will confirm the nature of the underlying pancreatic disease.

Lack of Correlation Between Histology and Results of Imaging and Function Studies

While in advanced CP function and imaging studies easily detect the disease, this is not always so in the early stages. Attempts to classify pancreatitis based on results of imaging and function studies, such as the Cambridge classification [2], therefore, have serious drawbacks. After an episode of acute pancreatitis pancreatic exocrine and endocrine dysfunction, which gradually tends to return normal, is seen in the majority of patients [3, 7, 8]. On the other hand, persistent detectable pancreatic dysfunction in CP is seen only after 90% of pancreatic parenchyma has been destroyed [9], and so these tests may be normal in the early stages of CP. Changes in duct morphology as seen on imaging studies may be observed before the function tests are abnormal. However, a normal endoscopic retrograde cholangiopancreatography (ERCP) may be present in patients with etablished CP on histology. Thus, in the early stages of the disease, a definite diagnosis of CP may not be immediately possible without pancreatic histology and its confirmation may have to await the appearance of detectable abnormalities in structure and function.

ERCP Changes in Chronic Pancreatitis Are Not Diagnostic

"Mild" changes seen in ERCP are not often correlated with presence of pancreatic disease. Apart from being subject to considerable observer variation [10], these changes are also attributable to the ageing process [11]. Wherever histology has been available in patients with mild pancreatographic abnormalities, only about 50% have had histological evidence of CP [12, 13].

Pancreatic duct changes are observed after acute pancreatitis [7, 8, 14]. Severe pancreatic duct damage sustained during an acute attack is known to lead to the development of pancreatic duct stricture. This was recognised in the second Marseille meeting [3, 4] as the only circumstance when acute pancreatitis could subsequently lead to development of obstructive chronic pancreatitis. However, less severe duct changes which may persist after resolution of morphological and functional changes can create diagnostic problems. In a recent study [15] 48% of patients with gallstones had an abnormal ERCP; 16% being labelled as severe chronic pancreatitis. In another study [7] 13 of 16 patients (81%) had abnormal ERCP 4–12 months after an episode of biliary pancreatitis; 58% still had abnormal ERCPs 13–40 months after the attack. In the study by Lankisch's group [14] ERCP abnormalities were seen to persist without any other evidence of chronic pancreatitis in a significant number of patients presenting with clinically acute pancreatitis followed for a mean duration of 104 + 46 months. Thus, postinflammatory ERCP changes can be due to acute or chronic pancreatitis, and cannot by themselves be used to diagnose CP.

ERCP changes changes classifiable as those of CP have been described in a number of autoimmune disorders such as primary biliary cirrhosis [16] and Sjogren's syndrome [17]. The pancreatic duct changes observed in sclerosing cholangitis [18, 19] have been seen to disappear spontaneously [18] or with ursodeoxycholic acid treatment [19]. Though these changes are often associated with pancreatic function abnormalities, the patients almost never experience pain and the pathology is not compatible with that classically described in Marseille classifications [20]. We have suggested the term autoimmune CP for this group of patients to differentiate it from the more common chronic calcifying pancreatitis [21].

While in most of these conditions the clincal picture would suggest an alternative diagnosis, it appears that in a number of circumstances ERCP changes *per se* cannot be accepted as evidence of CP.

Future Prospects

In the future, diagnosis and classification of pancreatitis would be improved if pancreatic tissue could be safely and routinely obtained. Since in the arly stages the histological changes of CP may be segmental, ability to take tissue from multiple sites could prove to be vital for accurate diagnosis. Presently used techniques for obtaining pancreatic tissue of echo- or computer tomography (CT)-guided fine needle aspiration cytology using Chiba needles and microhistology using Menghini- and TruCut-type needles [22], are more suited for diagnosing the malignant nature of ultrasonographically detectable pancreatic masses than for making positive diagnosis of inflammatory and fibrotic conditions such as pancreatitis. Endoscopic ultrasound (EUS) may prove to be superior in this respect. Preliminary studies [23, 24] suggest that EUS can reliably detect inflammatory changes in the pancreas. When associated with CP this has often been detected in the absence of ERCP changes. It remains to be seen whether changes of CP can be differentiated from changes following an episode of acute pancreatitis. The ability to take biopsies with newer versions of the EUS machines may prove valuable in differentiating acute from chronic pancreatitis.

Another important step would be to identify specific markers of acute or chronic pancreatitis in body fluids and tissues. For example, a deficiency or abnormal synthesis or secretion of pancreatic stone protein (lithostathine), which could be congenital [25], has been hypothesized to be the reason why only some alcoholics develop ACP. However, decreased lithostathine levels in pancreatic juice of CP patients have not been demonstrated by investigators other than the Sarles group [26].

Precipitation of protein plugs in the pancreatic juice has been described as an important early pathogenetic step in the development of CP [25]. In one study these were observed in normal controls (10%), alcoholics without clinical CP (20%) as well as those with etablished CP (65%) [27]. Further studies are needed to see if the detection of protein plugs in pancreatic juice and their chemical analyses will be help to establish the diagnosis of chronic pancreatitis.

Another test which shows promise is pancreatic juice lactoferrin levels. These assays have shown that there is an excellent separation of chronic pancreatitis patients from patients with other pancreatic or gastrointestinal diseases [28, 29]. In an interesting study Brugge et al. [30] studied duodenal juice lactoferrin levels in the basal state in healthy controls, asymptomatic alcoholics, alcoholics with acute pancreatitis, and alcoholics with established CP. While concentrations of lactoferrin were significantly elevated above those in controls in all three alcoholic groups, the lactoferrin output in mg/kg per h clearly differentiated asymptomatic from symptomatic alcoholics. The study appears to be certainly worth pursuing further.

References

1. Sarles H Pancreatitis Symposium, Marseille (1963) S. Karger, Basel, NY 1965
2. Sarner M, Cotton PB (1984) Classification of Pancreatitis. Gut 25: 756–9
3. Gyr K, Singer MV, Sarles H (1984) Pancreatitis: Concepts and Classifications. Proceedings of the Second International Symposium on the Classification of Pancreatitis in Marseille, France, March 28–30, 1984 Amsterdam, Excerpta Medica, pp 403–408
4. Singer MV, Gyr K, Sarles H (1985) Revised classification of pancreatitis: Report of the Second International Symposium on the Classification of Pancreatitis in Marseille, France, March 28–30, 1984. Gastroenterology 89: 683–90
5. Sarles H, Adler G, Dani R et al. (1989) The classification of pancreatitis and definition of pancreatic diseases. Digestion 43: 234–6
6. Ammann RW, Buehler H, Bruehlmann W, Kehl O, Muench R, Stamm B (1986) Acute (nonprogressive) alcoholic pancreatitis: prospective longitudinal study of 144 patients with recurrent alcoholic pancreatitis. Pancreas 1: 195–203
7. Büchler M, Hauke A, Malfertheiner P (1987) Follow-up after acute pancreatitis – Morphology and function. In: Beger HG, Büchler M (Eds) Acute Pancreatitis-research and clinical management. Springer-Verlag, Berlin: pp. 367–374
8. Sucro AL, Angelini G, Cavallini G (1984) Late outcome of acute pancreatitis. In: Gyr K, Singer MV, Sarles H (Eds) Pancreatitis: Concepts and Classifications. Proceedings of the Second International Symposium on Classification of Pancreatitis in Marseille, France, March 28–30, 1984, Amsterdam, Excerpta Medica
9. DiMagno EP, Go VLW, Summerskill WHJ (1973) Relations between pancreatic enzyme outputs and malabsorption in severe pancreatic insufficiency. N. Engl. J. Med. 288: 813
10. O'Malley VP, Cannon JP (1985) Pancreatic pseudocysts: Cause; therapy and results. Am J Surg 150: 680–2
11. Bockmann DE, Boydston WR, Parsa I (1983) Architecture of the human pancreas: Implications for early changes in pancreatic disease. Gastroenterology 85: 55–61
12. Kizu M, Newmann J, Cotton PB, Kasugai T (1977) Histological correlation with pancreatography in necropsy specimens. Gut 18: 399–400
13. Trapnell JE (1979) Chronic relapsing pancreatitis: A review of 64 cases. Br J Surg 66: 471–5
14. Seidensticker F, Otto J, Lankisch PG (1995) Recovery of the pancreas after acute pancreatitis is not necessarily complete. Int. J. Pancreatol. 17: 225–9
15. Misra SP, Gulati P, Choudhary V, Anand BS (1990) Pancreatic duct abnormalities in gallstone disease: an endoscopic retrograde cholangiopancreatography. Gut 31: 1073–5
16. Epstein O, Chapman RW, Lake-Bakaar G, Rosalki SB, Sherlock S (1982) The pancreas in primary biliary cirrhosis and primary sclerosing cholangitis. Gastroenterology 83: 1177–82
17. Lindstrom E, Lindstrom F, von Schenck H, Ihse I (1991) Pancreatic ductal morphology and function in Sjogren's syndrome. Int J Pancreatol 8: 141–9

18. Bastid C, Sahel J, Sarles H (1990) Spontaneous healing of sclerosing cholangitis associated with stricture of the main pancreatic duct. Pancreas 4: 489–82
19. Lebovics E, Salama M, Elhosseiny A, Rosenthal WS (1992) Resolution of radiographic abnormalities with ursodeoxycholic acid treatment of primary sclerosing cholangitis. Gastroenterology 102: 2143–7
20. Kawaguchi K, Koike M, Tsuruta K, Okambo A, Tabata I, Fujita N (1991) Lymphoplasmacytic sclerosing pancreatitis with cholangitis: a variant of primary sclerosing cholangitis extensively involving the pancreas. Human Pathol 22: 387–95
21. Chari ST, Singer MV (1994) The problems of classification and staging of chronic pancreatitis – Proposals based on current knowlege of its natural history. Scand J Gastroenterol 29: 949–960
22. Glenthoj A, Sehested M, Torp-Pederson S (1990) Ultrasonically guided histological and cytological fine needle biopsis of the pancreas. Reliability and reproducibility of diagnosis. Gut 31: 930–933
23. Wiersema MJ, Hawes RH, Lehman GA, Kochman ML, Sherman S, Kopecky KK (1993) Prospective evaluation of endoscopic ultrasonography and endoscopic retrograde cholangiopancreatography in patients with chronic abdominal pain of suspected pancreatic origin. Endoscopy 25: 555–564
24. Nattermann C, Goldschmidt AJW, Dancygier H (1993) Endosonography in chronic pancreatitis – A comparison between endoscopic retrograde pancreatography and endoscopic ultrasonography. Endoscopy 25: 565–570
25. Sarles H, Bernard JP, Johnson M (1989) Pathogenesis and epidemiology of chronic pancreatitis. Ann Rev Med 40: 453–68
26. Hayakawa T, Naruse S, Kitagawa M, Nakae Y, Harade H, Ochi K, Kuno N, Kurimoto K, Hayakawa S (1995) Pancreatic stone protein and lactoferrin in human pancreatic juice in chronic pancreatitis. Pancreas 10: 137–42
27. Guy O, Robles-Diaz G, Adrich Z, Sahel J, Sarles H (1983) Protein content of precipitates present in pancreatic juice of alcoholic subjects and patients with chronic calcifying pancreatitis. Gastroenterology 84: 102–7
28. Multigner L, Figarella C, Sahel J, Sarles H (1980) Lactoferrin and albumin in human pancreatic juice: a valuable test for diagnosis of pancreatic disease. Dig Dis Sci 25: 173–8
29. Multigner L, Figarella C, Sarles H (1981) Diagnosis of chronic pancreatitis by measurement of lactoferrin in duodenal juice. Gut 22: 350–4
30. Brugge WR, Burke CA (1988) Lactoferrin secretion in alcoholic pancreatic disease. Dig Dis Sci 33: 178–84

A
Acute Pancreatitis

Morphology of Acute Pancreatitis in Relation to Etiology and Pathogenesis

G. Klöppel

Introduction

The classification system for acute pancreatitis that was developed in Atlanta in 1991 [1–3] distinguishes a mild form of acute pancreatitis from a severe form on the basis of both clinical and morphological criteria. The mild form is largely comparable to the type of pancreatitis that has been described as acute edematous pancreatitis, while the severe form corresponds to acute hemorrhagic-necrotizing pancreatitis. Clinically, mild acute pancreatitis is associated with minimal organ dysfunction and an uneventful recovery. Severe acute pancreatitis, however, leads to organ failure and/or local complications such as necrosis, abscess, or pseudocyst. This classification is clinically oriented and based on the hypothesis that various etiological factors lead to the same morphological changes in the pancreas. Although this assumption seems to be true in most cases of acute pancreatitis, notably those caused by gallstones or alcohol, there is morphological evidence that in a few cases the pattern of pancreatic changes is specific to etiology and pathogenesis.

Etiology Related to Morphology

Chronic alcohol abuse [4–6] and gallstone disease [7, 8] are responsible for 60%–80% of cases of acute pancreatitis. Among the less common causal factors are shock, pancreatic tumors, drugs, lipid abnormalities, and trauma. In a considerable number of patients there is no obvious cause.

It appears that all the etiological factors just mentioned result in similar pancreatic changes characterized by autodigestive tissue necrosis in and around the pancreas. The gross and histopathological features of biliary pancreatitis therefore do not differ in principle from alcoholic pancreatitis. However, they often differ in severity since biliary pancreatitis is usually mild, whereas alcoholic pancreatitis is severe. The only types of pancreatitis that exhibit a "specific" pattern of morphological lesions are cases of acute pancreatitis occurring during the terminal stages of severe extrapancreatic disease and infectious pancreatitis [9–12] (see "Pathogenesis and Necrosis Pattern").

Pathogenesis and Necrosis Pattern

Although the etiological factors are known in most patients with acute pancreatitis, pathogenesis of the disease remains obscure. Thus, we do not know how alcohol abuse [13] and biliary disease [14, 15] induce autodigestive tissue necrosis in and around the pancreas. The two working hypotheses most commonly discussed at present postulate either primary damage to the acinar cells or ductal obstruction combined with reflux of bile [16].

The acinar-cell-damage theory focuses on a complex disturbance of acinar cell function culminating in deranged intracellular compartmentation and uncontrolled liberation of enzymes. These alterations could lead to intracellular enzyme activation by lysosomal hydrolases [16, 17] and/or sudden effusion of enzymes into interstitial space and adipose tissue [18]. Because these changes appear to occur predominantly in the peripheral acinar cells of lobules and because these cells are furthest away from the artery supplying a lobule, it is possible that the effects of the different etiologic factors are mediated by microcirculatory changes.

The "duct-obstruction-bile reflux" theory (based on Opie's common channel theory) [19] postulates that temporary obstruction of the common bile duct and the main pancreatic duct by gallstones causes increased intraductal pressure and/or ampullary incontinence, with duodenopancreatic and bile reflux. This activates pancreatic proenzymes, which leak from small ducts into interstitial space. Although there is no doubt that migration of gallstones is associated with the induction of pancreatitis, it has not been possible so far to obtain definite functional and morphological proof that the pathogenesis of human acute pancreatitis is due to ductal obstruction.

Whatever the postulated pathogenetic mechanisms are that lead to acute pancreatitis, the resulting damage pattern is the same for most ($>95\%$) patients. The pancreatitis in these patients is usually associated with alcoholism and gallstone disease. The common damage pattern ("type 1 necrosis pattern") is characterized by interstitial fatty-tissue necrosis and its sequelae, i.e., necrosis of adjacent vessels (with hemorrhage), acinar cells, and ducts (Fig. 1). Fatty tissue necrosis is probably caused by lipase (one of the few pancreatic enzymes that need no activation) after an abrupt effusion of zymogens from peripheral acinar cells into interstitial space [18, 20]. Whether fat necrosis depends on the action of lipase alone or the combined action of lipase and other enzymes such as phospholipase A_2 and trypsin is still unknown, but it seems that proenzymes that leave the acinar cells together with lipase become activated during this process and may help to destroy surrounding tissues.

Necrosis patterns that are distinct from the one described above are rare, but may occur. The "type 2 necrosis pattern" seems to occur in patients with prolonged circulatory failure as a consequence of major extrapancreatic disease. It is characterized by ductal necrosis and is followed by periductal inflammation [21]. It is possible that this lesion is initiated by the activation of trypsinogen via autocatalyzation in ductal precipitates of pancreatic secretions after all secretory processes in the exocrine pancreas have been impaired due to severe extrapancreatic disease (Fig. 1).

Normal pancreas

Lobule
Duct
Enzymes

Acute pancreatitis

Causes
Alcohol gallstones — Prolonged circulatory failure — Infectious disease

Necrosis pattern
Type 1 — Type 2 — Type 3

Enzymes — Enzymes (Auto Activation) — Enzymes

Lesion
Autodigestive fat necrosis due to enzyme effusion and activation — Ductal and periductal necrosis — Disseminated acinar necrosis

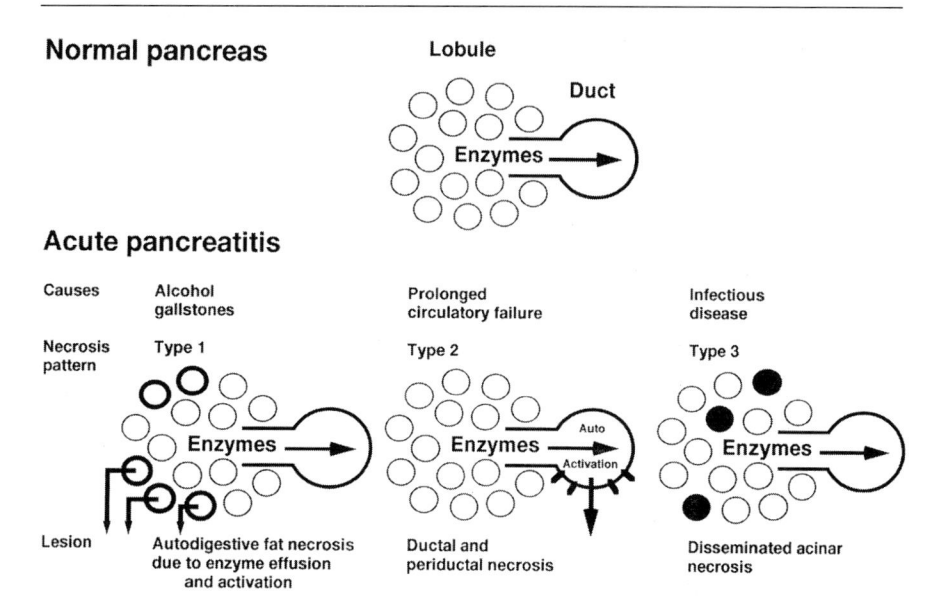

Fig. 1. Pathogenetic mechanisms and necrosis patterns found in acute pancreatitis

Another infrequent necrosis pattern, the "type 3 necrosis pattern", is seen in infectious pancreatitis. It is related to the direct cytotoxic effect of microorganisms on acinar cells [22]. This causes acinar cell necrosis, but surprisingly no autodigestion of fatty tissue (Fig. 1).

Gross Pathology

The gross changes in a pancreas with a type 1 necrosis pattern may be divided into mild and severe ones. In mild pancreatitis the gland is usually edematous and its surface shows spotty-fatty-tissue necrosis. The gland may be hard and enlarged, but without hemorrhage and intraparenchymal necrosis.

In severe acute pancreatitis with the type 1 necrosis pattern, there are usually extensive necrotic changes in peripancreatic fatty tissue, while, as a rule, the parenchyma of the gland appears to be affected less. This implies that the external appearance of the surface of the pancreas is not a reliable indicator of the extent of parenchymal necrosis within the pancreas. Characteristically, necrosis on the surface of the pancreas shows an extremely variegated pattern, with large areas of chalky-white-fat necrosis alternating with hemorrhages. Disseminated foci of fat necrosis may also be present in the bursa omentalis, omentum, and mesentery, as well as in the deep retroperitoneum. The peritoneal cavity contains turbid or hemorrhagic fluid. The cut surface of the pancreas usually displays only few hemorrhagic foci associated with a network of fat necrosis between the pancreatic lobuli. In the most severe cases, however, necrosis also involves parts of the lobular parenchyma, often transforming these areas into firm hemorrhagic-necrotic masses. In these cases, necrosis also affects the main pancreatic duct or the large tributaries, causing rupture. The pattern and distribution of necrosis differ from patient to patient, and in some patients necrosis may be present in only a portion of the gland.

The gross changes in a pancreas with a type 2 necrosis pattern seem to differ from those described above in that the gland, although distinctly swollen, shows no or only few definite areas of fat necrosis. Similar changes may be encountered in infectious pancreatitis with a type 3 necrosis pattern lacking autodigestive changes.

Histopathology

Type 1 Necrosis Pattern

In patients with mild pancreatitis, disseminated small spots of peripancreatic fat necrosis, with or without interstitial edema, are usually the only changes found [23]. In severe pancreatitis, peripancreatic tissue shows numerous large areas of fat necrosis. In addition, pancreatic parenchyma displays areas of necrosis, usually alternating with regions in which only interstitial edema is present. Intrapancreatic necrosis develops in the interlobular fatty tissue and is therefore dependent upon the amount of fat in the pancreas. In patients with a lot of intrapancreatic fat, for instance obese or elderly subjects, necrosis may be so severe that the lobuli are embraced by cords of confluent fat necrosis (Fig. 2). Intrapancreatic fat necrosis usually merges with the necrotic areas outside the pancreas. Fat necrosis that involves blood vessels leads to swelling of vessel walls, infiltration by granulocytes, thrombosis, and eventually necrosis, rupture, and hemorrhage. Arterial thrombosis is much less frequent than venous thrombosis, but may result in panlobular ischemic necrosis. Focal destruction of single interlobular ducts and peripheral acinar cells are further sequelae of

Fig. 2. Severe acute pancreatitis. Interlobular fatty-tissue necrosis (type 1 necrosis pattern) affecting the peripheral regions of the bordering lobules (*arrows*). H&E, × 40

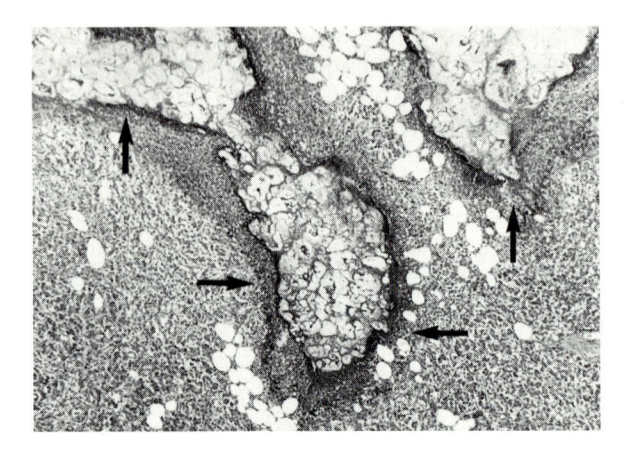

Fig. 3. Acute pancreatitis. Ductal necrosis (type 2 necrosis pattern) with protein precipitate (*P*), rupture of duct wall (*arrows*), and leukocytes infiltrating interstitial space. H&E, ×250

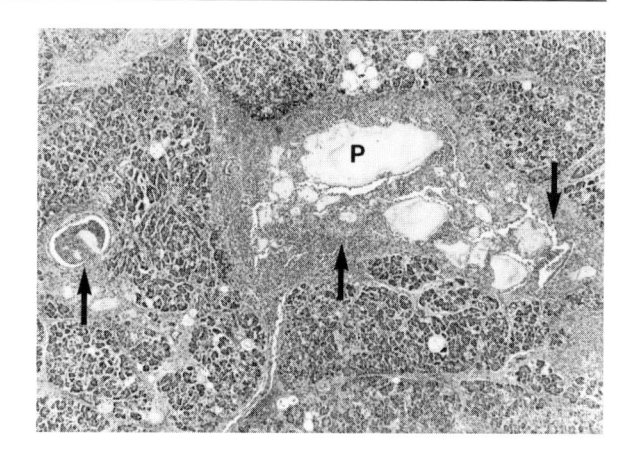

expanding fat necrosis, but it is often striking how well preserved these structures are despite their proximity to areas of fat necrosis. Nonnecrotic acinar cells at the margin of areas of fat necrosis usually form so-called tubular complexes, i.e., acini with widened lumina which may be filled with PAS-positive secretions. Islets are affected only in lobuli that are largely or entirely necrotic. Necrotic areas are demarcated by granulocytes and macrophages.

Type 2 Necrosis Pattern

Type 2 necrosis is characterized by disseminated ductal and periductal necrotic foci that outnumber the foci of fat necrosis and, more importantly, may even be present without any fat necrosis [21, 24]. Ductal necrosis appears to start with precipitation of eosinophilic secretions in small and medium-sized interlobular ducts, which then become infiltrated by granulocytes although still lined by intact epithelium. The next step is necrosis of part of the duct epithelium and rupture of the duct wall (Fig. 3). This leads to periductal necrosis, with an extensive acute inflammatory infiltrate extending through interstitial spaces. In advanced periductal necrosis, the duct is replaced by necrotic material. Despite this severe inflammatory process, acinar tissue remains largely unaffected. Bacteria have not yet been identified in the lumina of the affected ducts. It seems, however, that these patients may easily develop purulent peritonitis [24].

Type 3 Necrosis Pattern

Type 3 necrosis is characterized by scattered acinar cell necrosis with an acute inflammatory infiltrate, but no concomitant fat necrosis or ductal necrosis (Fig. 4). It appears that these changes are indicative of pancreatitis due to infection, either by certain viruses (e.g., mumps, Coxsackie B, measles, cytomegalovirus) [25–28] or bacteria (e.g., *Leptospira icterohaemorrhagica* [22]). In the

Fig. 4. Acute pancreatitis. Acinar cell necrosis (type 3 necrosis pattern; *arrows*) with inflammatory infiltrate. H&E, × 250

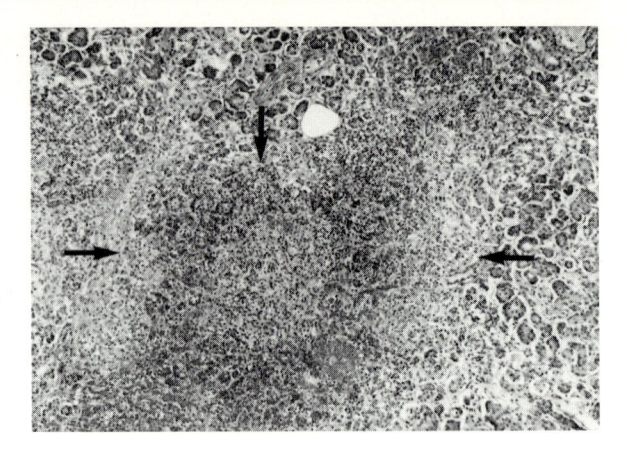

rare cases of pancreas involvement in generalized tuberculosis, syphilis, *Mycobacterium avium-intracellulare* infection, or sarcoidosis, pancreatic parenchyma displays the granulomatous changes typical of these diseases [28–30], but also lacks autodigestive lesions.

Immunocytochemical and Ultrastructural Findings

Immunostaining of the normal human pancreas for such enzymes as amylase, lipase, phospholipase A_2, trypsin, and chymotrypsin strongly labels the acinar cells [18, 31–35]. In severe acute pancreatitis with the type 1 necrosis pattern, staining intensity differs from cell to cell, with some acinar cells being entirely negative for enzymes and others having normal enzyme content (Fig. 5). Most enzyme-negative acinar cells are found at the periphery of lobuli adjoining areas of fat necrosis [18]. The acinar lumina lined by hese cells may contain enzyme-positive secretions. Electron-microscopically, the acinar cells adjacent to areas of necrosis are small and severely degranulated [18, 34, 36], with the remaining zymogen granules irregularly distributed in the cytoplasm and along the cell membrane. Some acinar cells display large autophagic vacuoles containing floccular material and remnants of membranes and zymogen granules [35]. Acinar lumina may be filled with fine fibrillar material probably representing secreted pancreatic enzymes. The same material may also be observed in interstitial spaces [37]. Occasionally, acinar lumina contain lethally damaged acinar cells and cellular debris. The epithelial lining of the duct system appears to be preserved, even in those regions where most of the acinar cells are damaged and infiltrated by granulocytes. Some of the duct cells display large lysosomes containing debris from membranes and zymogen granules.

Fig. 5. Acute pancreatitis. Pancreatic lobule adjacent to fat necrosis (*N*) with severe degranulation of numerous acinar cells (*arrows*). Immunostaining for trypsin, × 250

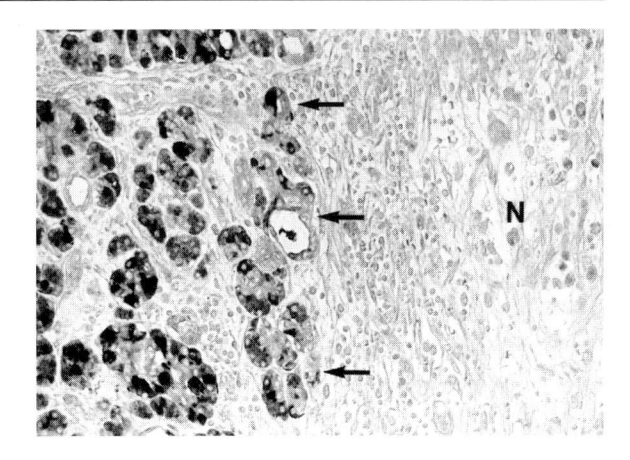

Conclusion

The common form of pancreatitis particularly associated with biliary disease and alcohol abuse starts with necrosis of fatty tissue in and around the pancreas (type 1 necrosis pattern). If this remains the only change, pancreatitis may be classified as mild. In severe acute pancreatitis, fat necrosis involves and damages adjacent vessels, acinar cells, and ducts, leading to thrombosis, hemorrhage, necrotic parenchyma, and duct leakage. Uncommon types of acute pancreatitis are associated with prolonged circulatory failure or infections. While the former type is characterized by ductal necrosis (type 2 necrosis pattern) as the initial injury, the latter type shows disseminated acinar cell necrosis (type 3 necrosis pattern).

References

1. Klöppel G, Maillet B (1993) Pathology of acute and chronic pancreatitis. Pancreas 8: 659–670
2. Bradley EL III (1993) A clinically based classification system for acute pancreatitis. Arch Surg 128: 586–590
3. Bradley EL III (1994) The necessity for a clinical classification of acute pancreatitis: The Atlanta system. In: Bradley EL III (ed.) Acute Pancreatitis: Diagnosis and Therapy, New York: Raven Press, chapter 4: 27–32
4. Marks IN, Bornman PC (1994) Acute alcoholic pancreatitis: A South African viewpoint. In: Bradley EL III (ed.) Acute Pancreatitis: Diagnosis and Therapy, New York: Raven Press, chapter 36: 271–277
5. Storck G, Petterson G, Edlund Y (1976) A study of autopsies upon 116 patients with acute pancreatitis. Surg Gynecol Obstet 143: 241–245
6. Renner IG, Savage WT, Pantoja JL, Renner VJ (1985) Death due to acute pancreatitis. A retrospective analysis of 405 autopsy cases. Dig Dis & Sci 30: 1005–1018
7. Ammann R (1976) Acute pancreatitis; In: Bockus HL (ed.) Gastroenterology, Volume 3, Third Edition. Philadelphia, London, Toronto: Saunders, 1020–1039
8. Creutzfeldt W, Schmidt H (1976) Etiology and pathogenesis of pancreatitis; In: Bockus HL ed. Gastroenterology, Volume 3, Third Edition. Philadelphia, London, Toronto: Saunders, 1005–1019
9. Naficy K, Nategh R, Ghadimi (1973) Mumps pancreatitis without parotitis. Brit Med J i: 529

10. Witte CL, Schanzer CB (1968) Pancreatitis due to mumps. AMA 203: 1068–1069
11. Capner P, Lendrum R, Jeffries DJ, Walker G (1975) Viral antibody studies in pancreatic disease. Gut 16: 866–870
12. Imrie CW, Ferguson JC, Sommerville RG (1985) Coxsackie and mumps virus infection in a prospective study of acute pancreatitis. Gut 18: 53–56
13. Malagelada JR (1986) The pathophysiology of alcoholic pancreatitis. Pancreas 1: 270–278
14. Acosta JM, Ledesma CL (1974) Gall stone migration as a cause of acute pancreatitis. N Engl J Med 290: 484–487
15. Acosta JM, Pellegrini CA, Skinner DB (1980) Etiology and pathogenesis of acute biliary pancreatitis. Surgery 88: 118–125
16. Steer ML (1989) Classification and pathogenesis of pancreatitis. Surg Clin North Am 69: 467–480
17. Scheele GA, Adler G, Kern HF (1984) Role of lysosomes in the development of acute pancreatitis. In: Gyr KE, Singer MV, Sarles H (eds.) Pancreatitis – Concepts and classification, Amsterdam – New York – Oxford: Excerpta Medica, 17–23
18. Klöppel G., Dreyer T, Willemer S, Kern HF, Adler G (1986) Human acute pancreatitis: its pathogenesis in the light of immunocytochemical and ultrastructural findings in acinar cells. Virchows Arch [A] 409: 791–803
19. Opie EL (1981) The etiology of acute hemorrhagic pancreatitis. Bull Johns Hopkins Hosp 12: 182–192
20. Schmitz-Moormann P (1981) Comparative radiological and morphological study of the human pancreas. IV. Acute necrotizing pancreatitis in man. Path Res Pract 171: 325–335
21. Foulis AK (1980) Histological evidence of initiating factors in acute necrotising pancreatitis in man. J Clin Pathol 33: 1125–1131
22. Rickaert F, Klöppel G: Acute pancreatitis in lethal leptospirosis: a special type of pancreatitis with disseminated acinar cell necrosis. (unpublished observation)
23. Klöppel G, von Gerkan R, Dreyer T (1984) Pathomorphology of acute pancreatitis. Analysis of 367 autopsy cases and 3 surgical specimens. In: Gyr KE, Singer MV, Sarles H (eds.) Pancreatitis – Concepts and classification. Amsterdam – New York – Oxford: Excerpta Medica, Elsevier Science Publishers BV, 29–35
24. Kimura W, Ohtsubo K (1989) Clinical and pathological features of acute interstitial pancreatitis in the aged. Int J Pancreat 5: 1–9
25. Sibert JR (1975) Pancreatitis in children. A study in the north of England. Arch Dis Child 50: 443
26. Jensen AB, Rosenberg HS, Notkins AL (1980) Pancreatic islet-cell damage in children with fatal viral infections. Lancet 2: 354
27. Nguyen T, Abramowsky C, Ashenburg C, Rothstein F (1988) Clinicopathologic studies in childhood pancreatitis. Hum Pathol 19: 343–349
28. Bonacini M (1991) Pancreatic involvement in human immunodeficiency virus infection. J Clin Gastroenterol 13: 58–64
29. del Castello CF, Gonzalez-Ojeda A, Reyes E, Quiroz-Ferrari F, Uribe M, Robles-Diaz G (1990) Tuberculosis of the pancreas. Case report. Pancreas 5: 693–696
30. Stürmer J, Becker V (1987) Granulomatous pancreatitis – granulomas in chronic pancreatitis. Virchows Arch [A] 410: 327–338
31. Aho HJ, Putzke HP, Nevalainen TJ, Löbel D, Pelliniemi LJ, Dummler W, Suonpää AK, Tessenow W (1983) Immunohistochemical localization of trypsinogen and trypsin in acute and chronic pancreatitis. Digestion 27: 21–28
32. Nevalainen TJ, Aho HJ, Eskola JU, Suonpää AK (1983) Immunohistochemical localization of phospholipase A2 in human pancreas in acute and chronic pancreatitis. Acta Path Microbiol Immunol Scand Sect A 91: 97–102
33. Aho HJ, Sternby B, Kallajoki M, Nevalainen TJ (1989) Carboxyl ester lipase in human tissues and in acute pancreatitis. Int J Pancreat 5: 123–134
34. Willemer S, Adler G (1989) Histochemical and ultrastructural characteristics of tubular complexes in human acute pancreatitis. Dig Dis & Sci 34: 46–55
35. Willemer S, Klöppel G, Kern HF, Adler G (1989) Immunocytochemical and morphometric analysis of acinar zymogen granules in human acute pancreatitis. Virchows Archiv [A] 415: 115–123
36. Bockman DE, Büchler M, Beger HG (1987) Ultrastructure of human acute pancreatitis. Int J Pancreatol 1: 141–153
37. Aho HJ, Nevalainen TJ, Havia VT, Heinomen RJ, Aho AJ (1982) Human acute pancreatitis. A light and electron microscopic study. Acta Path Microbiol Immunol Scand Sect A 90: 367–373.

Clinical Presentation and Course of Acute Pancreatitis

O. R. Bordalo · R. F. Palma

Acute pancreatitis is a common disorder the incidence of which is increasing in emergency units and which is still associated with high mortality.

The main pathophysiological event that characterises acute pancreatitis consists in the positive feedback of auto-digestive activation of pancreatic pro-enyzmes within the gland along with the systemic extension of the inflammatory process.

Some years ago in a necropsy survey of 2000 cases of gastroenterologycal diseases at the University Hospital of Santa Maria, among pancreatic disorders almost all chronic pancreatitis patients were alcoholic and biliary lithiasis accounted for approximately 1 % of acute pancreatitis as primary cause of death and today the same is true [1].

Iatrogenic factors, viruses, hypertriglyceridemia and microlithiasis of the gallbladder play an important role as causative factors although in Western countries are much less frequent than the two major causes of pancreatitis: alcohol and macroscopic lithiasis.

Clinically, the vast majority of patiens with acute pancreatitis present a mild episode of abdominal pain requiring only analgesia and monitoring of vital parameters in order to assess early complications.

The "pancreatic drama of Dieulafois", corresponding to both the fulminant disease and severe forms (10 %–15 %), is fortunately not a frequent pattern of presentation [2].

However, a smaller percentage of patients (around 20 % in some series) requires intensive care treatment since they are at risk of developing serious complications.

The clinical diagnosis usually relies in simple criteria, such as a former history of pancreatitis or likely epidemiological risk factors and the typical history of upper abdominal pain together with serum elevations of pancreatic enzymes. However, these parameters can not predict the course of the disease.

Both the clinical presentation and some complications (Table 1) may be reversible, regardless of initial symptoms and enzymatic determinations. Consequently, the course cannot be predicted based on this data alone.

Therefore, to evaluate the severity of the disease and the likelihood of progression with life-threatening complications and to adopt the most appropriate management of the patient, the objective must be the accurate distinction between a mild edematous pancreatitis and a severe necrotizing pancreatitis as early as possible, because the staging of the disease is life-saving for the patient (Table 2).

Table 1. Acute pancreatitis: clinical picture and main complications

Clinical picture	Systemic complications	Local complications

Classical form
  "Dieulafois drama"
    Pain
      Vomiting
        Shock
Ileus
Cholecystitis like
Perfuration like
Mild forms
	Hypovolemia
	Renal dysfunction
	Respiratory distress
	syndrome
	Hypocalcemia
	Hyperglycemia
	Coagulopathy
	Distant fat necrosis
		Acute fluid collections
		Necrosis
		Abscess
		Peudocysts
		Haemorrhage
		Intestinal obstruction
		Perforation

Table 2. Acute pancreatitis: clinical staging and pathomorphology

Clinical/echo/CT/Biochemical staging	Pathomorphologic features
MILD ⇅ Moderate ⇅ SEVERE ↓ ICU	Edema Steatonecrosis ↓ Necrosis / Haemorrhage → Medical care → Surgical strategy

ICU, intensive cave unit.

Imaging techniques and recently developed enzymatic determinations are the golden standards to better evaluate the course and hence the best therapeutic procedures to be applied.

Contrast-enhanced computed tomography (CT) is now considered the best imaging method for the staging of acute pancreatitis. However, it is pertinent to remember that around 80% of patients presenting with mild forms of disease do not need to be submitted to this technique, thus avoiding some of its drawbacks, i.e. high cost and exposure to radiation. Recent trials denoted the difficulties involved in identifying small necrotic areas and peripancreatic necrosis [2]. Nuclear magnetic resonance is virtually radiation free and has to be considered a promising alternative technique needing further evaluation to be introduced in clinical routine, in spite of being more expensive and time consuming than CT.

To evaluate the severity and to detect complications, some biochemical and enzymatic determinations have been grouped together in multifactorial score systems, on a combination of various diagnostic criteria (Ranson, Imrie, APACHE II, [3–5]). However the predictive value for severe attacks is limited, requiring a 48-h evaluation and therefore its accuracy is lacking for earlier prognosis.

Simple and easy methods are required to select patients at risk of developing complications.

Based on the better knowledge of molecular biology and on the early pathophysiological events occurring in acute pancreatitis, the inflammatory activity in the pancreas was recently introduced in the diagnostic strategy.

According to recent studies conducted to evaluate the clinical usefulness of several circulating and inflammatory mediators it was shown that determinations of plasma levels of polymorphonuclear (PMN) elastase in the first hours, followed by the determination of C-reactive protein levels are the most accurate markers to assess the severity of acute pancreatitis [6]. A positive correlation was also found between the following parameters: interleukin-6, C-reactive protein, phospholipase A_2 and the clinical severity of the disease [7, 8]. Some studies have been conducted at our laboratory and the results agree with previous data. The best results are obtained with C-reactive protein (Fig. 1) (Antunes and Bordalo 1992, unpublished data).

Therefore, enhanced computed tomography and the biological markers for severity criteria are essential to predict the course and to guide a therapeutic approach: (a) conservative treatment; (b) prophylaxis of the infection in necrotizing disease; (c) surgical management in case of established necrotic tissue infection and sepsis [9].

Based on our experience we have hypothesised and published in previous work that acute pancreatitis may progress to death in severe forms, to cure with "restitutio ad integrum" once the cause is removed, or may run in a cycle of recurrences and remissions, being the final outcome the chronic inflammatory disease of the pancreas (Fig. 2).

Fig. 1. Discriminative value of C-reactive protein in acute pancreatitis. *Top trace,* necrotizing pancreatitis; *bottom trace,* edematous pancreatitis

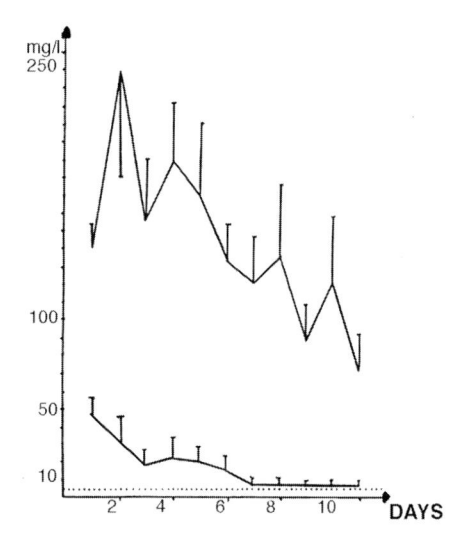

```
                    EVOLUTION
                  Acute Pancreatitis
        ↓               ↓                    ↓
     Death       Clinical or subclinical    "Restitutio
                    recurrencies            ad integrum"
                        ↓
                   Inflammation
                        ↓
                 Periacinar fibrosis
                        ↓
                   Cell necrosis
                        ↓
              Peri- and intralobular fibrosis
                        ↓
                ┌──────────────────────┐
                │ CHRONIC PANCREATITIS │
                └──────────────────────┘
```

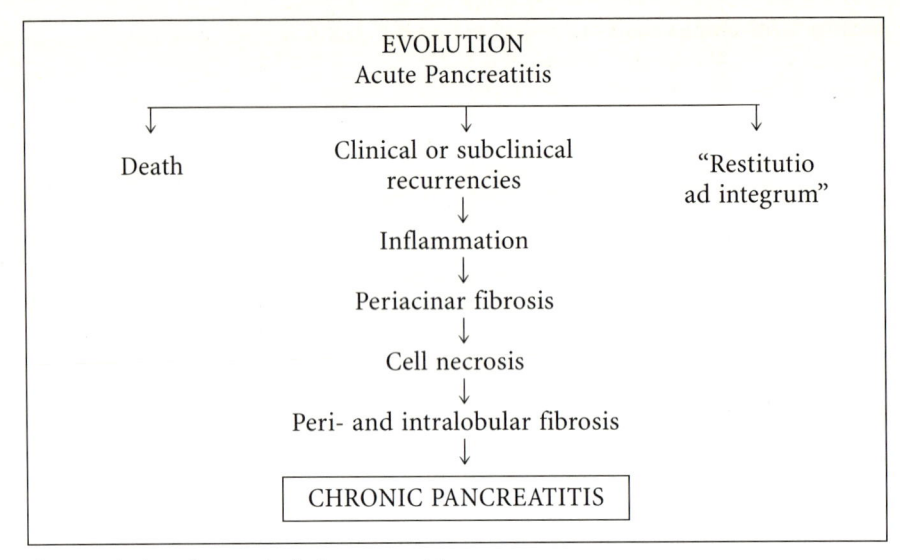

Fig. 2. Evolution of acute alcoholic pancreatitis

Acute alcoholic pancreatitis has to be considered a clinical entity apart from acute attacks complicating the evolution of chronic alcoholic pancreatitis. In fact just one bout of acute ingestion is sufficient to bring about an acute episode in unusual drinkers. Besides, these patients after recovery neither present signs of pancreatic damage at imaging studies nor functional abnormalities when submitted to secretory tests.

Histological evidence supports the concept that repeated outbursts of acute pancreatitis may result in chronic pancreatitis and may contribute to the acceleration of the disease [10].

Whether or not chronic pancreatitis is always a progressive disease has been questioned for a very long time. We have argued that, whenever the cause persists, chronic pancreatitis is always a progressive disease. However, the factors involved in this process are still controversial and enigmatic.

In 1977, a direct toxic-metabolic effect of ethanol on acinar cells was postulated [11]. The alcohol itself or one of its major metabolites, acetaldehyde, stimulated lipogenesis in acinar cells [12, 13]. Oxygen free radicals could also contribute to cell cytomembranes injury [14], and studies on this subject are now underway, one of them at our unit.

Recently, Cameron [15] concluded that oxidation of acetaldehyde releases free radicals which may be responsible for the peroxidation of cytomembranes, initiating the destructive process.

In alcoholic patients fulfilling the same characteristics in terms of sex, age, patterns of alcohol intake, undergoing surgery for other reasons than pancreatic disorders and with previous consent, we have studied on light and epon block thick sections the pathogenesis and progression of the pancreatic disease [16].

Concerning pathogenesis, in pancreatic biopsies we provided evidence for the first time that acinar cells are often injured very early, without clinical pancreatitis. The emphasis of this hypothesis is that acinar cells are injured first and secretory abnormalities then follow. Ductular abnormalities, stone formation and fibrosis are late sequelae to acinar injury.

Regarding progression, our findings have shown that the histopathology of more advanced stages is dominated by: (a) cellular degeneration followed by parenchymal atrophy and late diffuse fibrosis; (b) periacinar fibrosis may progress from the periphery to inner portions of the gland, isolating small groups of acini and setting off three forms of chronic pancreatitis: micronodular, macronodular and pancreatic atrophy.

Some important opposing views also exist (Pitchumoni and Bordalo 1996). Appealing hypotheses abound in the literature, and almost all of them agree that the pathogenesis and evolution of alcoholic pancreatitis is not well understood. Perhaps there is some truth in most of these hypotheses, and it is likely that pancreatitis is initiated and progresses by one or more of the mechanisms proposed so far (Pitchumoni and Bordalo 1996).

References

1. Noronha M, Batista A, Bordalo O (1984) Pancreatitis. concepts and classification. Gyr K, Singer M and Sarles H. Excerpta Medica, Amsterdam, New York, Oxford 61–65
2. Lerch MM and Adler G. Acute pancreatitis – recent developments and perspectivey. Urban und Schwarzenberg 64–69
3. Ranson JHC, Rifkind KM, Roses DF et al (1974) Prognostic signs and the role of operative management in acute pancreatitis. Surg Gynecol Obstet. 139: 69–81
4. Blainey SL, Imrie CW, O'Neill J et al (1984) Prognostic factors in acute pancreatitis. Gut 25: 1340–46
5. Larvin M, McMahon MJ (1989) APACHE II score for assessment and monitoring of acute pancreatitis. Lancet 2: 201–5
6. Domínguez-Muñoz JE, Carballo F, Garcia MJ et al (1991) Clinical usefulness of polymorphonuclear elastase in predicting the severity of acute pancreatitis: results of a multicenter study. Br J Surg 78: 1230–4
7. Viedma JA, Pérez-Mateo M, Domínguez-Muñoz JE et al (1992) Role of interleukin-6 in acute pancreatitis: comparison with C-reactive protein and phospholipase A. Gut 33: 1264–7
8. Gross V, Schölmerich J, Leser HG et al (1990) Granulocyte elastase in assessment of severity of acute pancreatitis: comparison with acute phase proteins C-reactive protein, α_1-antitrypsin, and protease inhibitor α_2-macroglobulin. Dig Dis Sci 35: 97–105
9. Domínguez-Muñoz JE, Malfertheiner P (1993) Management of acute pancreatitis. The Gastroenterologist 1: 248–256
10. Kloppel G, Maillet B (1991) Chronic pancreatitis. Evolution of the disease. Hepato-Gastroenterology 38: 408–412
11. Dreiling DA, Bordalo O (1977) A toxic-metabolic hypothesis of pathogenesis of alcoholic pancreatitis. Alcoholism Clin Exp Res 1: 293–299
12. Noronha M, Salgadinho A, Ferreira De Almeida MJ, Dreiling DA and Bordalo O (1981) Alcohol and the pancreas. I Clinical association and histopathology of minimal pancreatic inflammation. Am J Gastroenterol 76: 114–119
13. Noronha M, Bordalo O, Dreiling DA (1981) Alcohol and the pancreas. II Pancreatic morphology of advanced alcoholic pancreatitis. Am J Gastroenterol 76: 120–124
14. Guyan PM, Uden S, Braganza JM (1990) Heightened free radical activity in pancreatitis. Free Radical Biology & Medicine 8: 347–354
15. Cameron JL, Zuidema GD, Margolis S (1975) A pathogenesis for alcoholic pancreatitis. Surgery 77: 754–763
16. Noronha M, Dreiling DA, Bordalo MD (1983) Sequential changes from minimal pancreatic inflammation to advanced alcoholic pancreatitis. Z Gastroenterologie 21: 666–673

I
Imaging Procedures

Ultrasound in the Diagnosis and Grading of Acute Pancreatitis

R. Mahlke · C. Assmus · P. G. Lankisch

Introduction

Acute pancreatitis is usually diagnosed on the basis of characteristic symptoms and elevated serum amylase and lipase. With the help of supporting imaging procedures such as ultrasound (US), computed tomography (CT), and – in recent years – endoscopic ultrasound (EUS) and magnetic resonance (MR), severity of the disease, extent of complications, and etiology can be determined. Normally, only larger hospitals have CT, EUS, and MR, while US can be found even in small hospitals. Worldwide, abdominal US is the most frequently used initial imaging procedure for suspected acute pancreatitis.

The aim of this review is to evaluate the effectiveness of US in the diagnosis and grading of acute pancreatitis 10 years after Lees' review of the subject at the first meeting on Diagnostic Procedures on Pancreatic Disease [11].

Ultrasound in the Diagnosis of Acute Pancreatitis

Visualization of the Organ

As the most frequent complications of acute pancreatitis, meteorism and ileus may preclude or severely limit visualization of the pancreas. Many otherwise efficacious imaging techniques, such as scanning the pancreas in the erect position with large gastric fluid loads, examining the patient from the flank in the left- or right-sided position, or pressing away the air-filled small bowel loops, cannot be applied in severely ill patients [11]. Thus, expectedly, no study shows a high rate of visibility.

In a prospective study, Block et al. [4] found that the pancreas could not be visualized in 33% of patients with $\geq 50\%$ necrosis of the pancreas. In another prospective study, Schölmerich et al. [15] obtained full visualization of the pancreas in only 50% of the patients, and our own retrospective study demonstrated the gland in only 60% of cases. In contrast to others, in our study, non-visualization of the pancreas did not correlate with severity of morphological changes demonstrated on contrast-enhanced CT and scored according to Balthazar et al. (Table 1) [2, 3].

Table 1. Nonvisualization of the pancreas by initial ultrasound on admission to hospital in 120 consecutive patients with a first attack of acute pancreatitis compared to the results of contrast-enhanced computed tomography scored according to Balthazar et al. [2, 3]

CT score	n	Nonvisualization of the pancreas by ultrasound	
		n	%
0	16	5	31
1–2	32	14	44
3–4	53	20	38
>4	19	9	47
Total	120	48	40

The rate of nonvisualization did not significantly correlate with the severity of the disease (Mantel-Haenzel test [13]).

Sonographic Signs of Acute Pancreatitis

In the case of suspected acute pancreatitis, the ultrasound investigator especially examines the size and boundaries of the organ and parenchymal echogenicity, and combined with ultrasound-controlled palpation examines whether the gland causes pain.

Size of the Organ

In interstitial or clinically mild acute pancreatitis, localized or diffuse enlargement of the gland may or may not occur. The gland on admission, for example, appeared normal by ultrasound in the case of full visualization for 27 (38%) of 72 patients with acute pancreatitis of all severities (Fig. 1).

In interstitial acute pancreatitis, the boundaries of the organ may still be clearly determinable. Necrotizing or clinically severe acute pancreatitis necessarily entails enlargement of the pancreas, but it may be difficult to distinguish the organ boundaries due to the surrounding peri- and intrapancreatic accumulation of fluid.

Parenchymal Structure

Mild acute pancreatitis is characterized by a general reduction in parenchymal echogenicity, whereas in severe acute pancreatitis the parenchyma becomes heterogeneous with echo-poor and echo-free areas indicating necrosis and hemorrhages.

Pancreatic Duct Changes

In acute pancreatitis, the main pancreatic duct is usually not visible as it is compressed by pancreatic edema. An enlarged pancreatic duct may be a sign of an acute attack of chronic pancreatitis.

Painful Organ Palpation

In interstitial and clinically mild acute pancreatitis, the gland appears normal on ultrasound, but can be tested for pain by palpation with the index finger under ultrasound control, in which case acute pancreatitis would be indicated.

US score	CT score 0	CT score 1-2	CT score 3-4	CT score >4	Total
0	7	9	10	1	27
1	2	5	14	3	24
2	2	4	6	2	14
3	-	-	3	4	7
Total	11	18	33	10	72

Fig. 1. Comparison of the results of the initial ultrasound (*US*) and computed tomography (*CT*) performed within 72 h after admission to hospital in 72 consecutive patients with a first attack of acute pancreatitis and full visualization of the pancreas on US. For CT evaluation, the Balthazar score was used [2, 3]. US findings were scored as *0* (normal pancreas), *1* (localized enlargement of the organ or blurred boundary), *2* (diffuse organ enlargement), and *3* (2 plus pancreatic necrosis, pleural effusion, or ascites). Statistical analyses show that the gold standard, CT, demonstrated a significantly higher rate of severity of pancreatitis than the US (Bowker's test of symmetry [5], $p = 0.006$). In only 22 (31%) cases, both imaging procedures showed the same rate of severity of the disease. In 39 (54%) patients, the CT score was higher than the US score, i.e., US had underestimated the disease, and in the remaining 11 (15%) patients, US had overestimated the severity of morphological abnormalities

Summary of Sonographic Signs

In summary, in *interstitial acute pancreatitis*, the gland is usually fully visible, and the disease is characterized sonographically by an enlarged gland and reduced echogenicity. Boundaries of the organ are still determinable. In *necrotizing acute pancreatitis*, visualization is only partially, if at all, possible. The gland is enlarged, its boundaries indeterminable, and the inflammatory process extending beyond the confines of the gland causes increased echogenicity and heterogeneity of the surrounding retroperitoneal fat (Table 2) [11].

Sonographic Detection of Complications

Only CT can differentiate between pancreatic edema and necrosis or hemorrhages. So-called streets of necroses, which are echo-poor or constitute complex structures, frequently lead into pararenal space, more often on the left than right. Mesenterial streets are more difficult to demonstrate. Demonstrable even in small amounts are ascites and pleural effusions, the latter significantly correlating with CT-detected pancreatic damage [10]. US also readily diagnoses biliary obstruction, another complication of acute pancreatitis. Finally, US can diagnose pseudocysts, occurring in 14.3% of acute pancreatitis cases [9]; how-

Table 2. Sonographic signs of acute pancreatitis

Parameters	Interstitial pancreatitis	Necrotizing pancreatitis
Size	Normal/localized or diffuse enlargement	Always localized or diffuse enlargement
Boundaries	Determinable	Not determinable
Echogenicity	Reduced	Heterogenous
Peripancreatic area	Not involved	Involved

ever, CT shows more effectively the exact number and distribution of pseudocysts in the gland [11].

Nevertheless, even contrast-enhanced CT cannot reveal pancreatic necrosis or pseudocyst infections. A US- or CT-guided fine-needle aspiration of necrotic areas or pseudocysts is needed [7].

Ultrasound in Differential Diagnosis of Acute Pancreatitis

A number of abdominal and extra-abdominal diseases may mimic acute pancreatitis. US examinations have the advantage of being able to confirm or exclude such diseases by detecting their characteristic sonographical signs (Table 3).

Table 3. Ultrasound (US) findings in abdominal diseases with signs and symptoms mimicking acute pancreatitis

Disease	US findings
Peptic ulcer	Abnormal thickening of gastric or duodenal wall
Perforation of stomach, small or large intestine	Free air
Ileus (obstructive or paralytic)	Fluid-filled bowel loops, pendular peristalsis
Mesenterial arterial occlusion	Circular and longitudinal thickening of bowel loops
Acute cholecystitis	Stones and/or sludge in the gallbladder, gallbladder causing pain upon palpation, thickening of gallbladder wall
Biliary colic	Stones in the gallbladder and/or obstruction of the common bile duct
Ureter stone	Enlarged renal pelvis
Basal pleuritis	Pleural effusion or pulmonary infiltration
Aortic aneurysm	Dissecting membrane or aneurysmatic dilatation of the aorta

Ultrasonographic Detection of Etiology of Acute Pancreatitis

US investigation is ideal for diagnosing gallbladder stones. Stones in the common bile duct, in addition to cholelithiasis, justify a diagnosis of acute pancreatitis of biliary origin. However, most clinicians will assume biliary etiology if only gallbladder stones are found without common bile duct stones or signs of common bile duct obstruction. By comparison, US as well as CT were less accurate than endoscopic retrograde cholangiopancreatography (ERCP) in detecting gallbladder stones, common bile duct stones, and intrahepatic and/or extrahepatic dilatation of the biliary tree in a prospective study [14].

Alcohol-induced acute pancreatitis has no sonographical characteristics, but a fatty liver on US supports the assumption of alcoholism as the underlying etiology. In traumatic pancreatitis, US may show a mass or a cyst close to the point of ductal obstruction or stenosis shown on ERCP. In combination, both procedures provide a precise basis on which to plan effective, primarily surgical therapy [18].

In an acute attack of chronic pancreatitis, the presence of small focal areas of reduced echogenicity often associated with contiguous fluid accumulation indicates chronicity of the disease [11].

Ultrasound Assessment of the Severity of Acute Pancreatitis

In the acute stage of the disease, US is unable, for various reasons, to define the severity of the damage to the gland [11, 16]. First, the visibility of the organ in severe acute pancreatitis is poor [4]. Second, US cannot discriminate necrotic from nonnecrotic areas, with pancreatic necrosis of up to 25% of the gland being sonographically inapparent even in animal experiments [12], and it poorly demonstrates lesions in the anterior pararenal space and especially near the transverse mesocolon [8]. CT is better suited for detecting the extrapancreatic spread of acute pancreatitis in the lesser sac. Third, it is difficult to estimate the parapancreatic involvement of the disease on US.

All these disadvantages are overcome by contrast-enhanced CT, which is not inhibited by meteorism, can well define necrotic severity, and shows the parapancreatic state of the disease in detail. Because CT is not very widely available in hospitals, US remains a good viable alternative considering that the operator is highly experienced.

In this context, it should be stressed that acute pancreatitis is a rather rare disease. In a first epidemiological study in Germany, acute pancreatitis was found in the area of Lüneburg in $15.6/10^5$ inhabitants, i.e., in our Department of Internal Medicine with about 5000 admissions per year, we diagnosed acute pancreatitis in 15–20 patients per year [1]. Of these, 16% had necrosis on CT. This means that only a few doctors in our department have the opportunity to gain optimal experience in US investigation of severe acute pancreatitis. They often are not available when a patient with acute pancreatitis presents, for experience shows that these patients arrive most frequently outside working hours or on weekends.

It is probably due to the lack of experience with severe acute pancreatitis that there is no generally accepted US grading score as there is for CT [2, 3]. In a retrospective comparison between CT and US results, we found that CT, the gold standard, had a significantly higher rate for demonstrating pancreatic severity than the US (Fig. 1). In only 22 (31%) patients, both imaging procedures attained the same demonstration rate. In 39 (54%) patients, the CT score was higher than the US score, i.e., the US had underestimated the disease, and in the remaining 11 (15%) patients, the US had overestimated the severity of morphological abnormalities (Fig. 1).

Endoscopic Ultrasound

The efficacy of endoscopic ultrasound (EUS) in acute pancreatitis in comparison with established imaging procedures is not fully evaluated. Even recent reviews on imaging procedures in acute pancreatitis fail to mention this US technique [16]. Sugiyama et al. [17] prospectively compared the results of conventional US, EUS, and contrast-enhanced CT in 23 patients with acute pancreatitis. Conventional US depicted the pancreas in only 61% of the cases, compared to 100% for EUS. EUS was more sensitive than conventional US and CT in detecting common bile duct stones (100% vs. 43% and 57%, respectively). EUS was also more highly sensitive than CT in depicting inflammatory peripancreatic spread (Table 4). Further comparative studies would be of interest.

Due to the limited penetration depth of the US, peripancreatic complications are not always demonstrable in full. However, EUS does not require a contrast medium, the potential hazards of which are under discussion [6] and which may not be used in patients with severe renal insufficiency.

Table 4. Visualization of pancreas and bile duct by imaging techniques in 23 patients with acute pancreatitis (from [17])

Visualization	Endoscopic sonography	Conventional sonography	CT
Pancreas			
None	0	9	0
Partial	0	10	0
Total	23	4	23
Main pancreatic duct	18	6	8
Extrahepatic bile dict			
None	0	9	0
Partial	0	10	5
Total	23	4	18
Common bile duct stones			
($n = 7$)	7	3	4

Conclusions

With regard to advantages and disadvantages of US investigations in diagnosing and grading acute pancreatitis, little has changed during the past 10 years [11]. Costs of US examinations remain low, and there are no transport problems since it is a bedside procedure available worldwide in most hospitals. Full visualization enables diagnosis of acute pancreatitis in the majority of cases according to characteristic sonographic findings. In the case of mild acute pancreatitis, US investigation suffices even for further follow-up examinations, whereas severe acute pancreatitis with its localized complications advisedly requires contrast-enhanced CT.

Disadvantages of US in acute pancreatitis are the nonvisualization of the gland in up to 50 % of patients, primarily in severe acute pancreatitis, and the difficulties in demonstrating intra- and extrapancreatic necroses. Experience is essential for the quality of US investigations, but difficult to obtain since severe acute pancreatitis is rare. EUS seems to overcome most of these disadvantages, but requires upper gastrointestinal endoscopy, which may be too risky for severely ill patients; in addition, it certainly requires an experienced investigator. Further studies of this US technique will be of great interest.

References

1. Assmus C, Petersen M, Gottesleben F, Dröge M, Lankisch PG (1996) Epidemiology of acute pancreatitis in a defined German population. Digestion 57: 217 (abstr)
2. Balthazar EJ, Ranson JHC, Naidich DP, Megibow AJ, Caccavale R, Cooper MM (1985) Acute pancreatitis: prognostic value of CT. Radiology 156: 767–772
3. Balthazar EJ, Robinson DL, Megibow AJ, Ranson JHC (1990) Acute pancreatitis: value of CT in establishing prognosis. Radiology 174: 331–336
4. Block S, Maier W, Clausen C, Büchler M, Malfertheiner P, Beger HG (1985) Diagnostik der nekrotisierenden Pankreatitis. Vergleich von Kontrastmittel-CT and Ultraschall in einer klinischen Studie. Dtsch Med Wochenschr 110: 826–832
5. Bowker AH (1948) A test for symmetry in contingency tables. J Am Statist Assoc 43: 572–574
6. Foitzik T, Bassi DG, Schmidt J, Lewandrowski KB, Fernandez-del Castillo C, Rattner DW, Warshaw AL (1994) Intravenous contrast medium accentuates the severity of acute necrotizing pancreatitis in the rat. Gastroenterology 106: 207–214
7. Gerzof SG, Banks PA, Robbins AH, Johnson WC, Spechler SJ, Wetzner SM, Snider JM, Langevin RE, Jay ME (1987) Early diagnosis of pancreatic infection by computed tomography-guided aspiration. Gastroenterology 93: 1315–1320
8. Jeffrey RB, Jr., Laing FC, Wing VW (1986) Extrapancreatic spread of acute pancreatitis: new observations with real-time US. Radiology 159: 707–711
9. Lankisch PG, Burchard-Reckert S, Petersen M, Lehnick D, Schirren CA, Köhler H, Stöckmann F, Peiper HJ, Creutzfeldt W (1996) Morbidity and mortality in 602 patients with acute pancreatitis seen between the years 1980–1994. Z Gastroenterol 34: 371–377
10. Lankisch PG, Dröge M, Becher R (1994) Pleural effusions: a new negative prognostic parameter for acute pancreatitis. Am J Gastroenterol 89: 1849–1851
11. Lees WR (1986) Ultrasound in acute pancreatitis: In: Malfertheiner P, Ditschuneit H (eds) Diagnostic procedures in pancreatic disease. Springer, Berlin-Heidelberg, pp 21–31
12. Maier W (1988) Experimentelle Untersuchungen zur echographischen Frühestmanifestation der inzipienten Pankreatitis und Pankreasnekrose. Fortschr Röntgenstr 149: 522–525
13. Mantel N (1963) Chi-square tests with one degree of freedom: extensions of the Mantel-Haenszel procedure. J Am Statist Assoc 58: 690–700

14. Schölmerich J, Gross, W, Farthmann EH (1989) Detection of biliary origin of acute pancreatitis. Comparison of laboratory tests, ultrasound, computed tomography, and ERCP. Dig Dis Sci 34: 830–833
15. Schölmerich J, Johannesson T, Brobmann G, Wimmer B, Thiedemann B, Pankreatitis – Diagnose, Ätiologieklärung und Prognoseabschätzung. Ultraschall 10: 290–294
16. Stoupis C, Becker C, Vock P, Uhl W, Büchler MW (1994) Imaging procedures in acute pancreatitis. Dig Surg 11: 209–213
17. Sugiyama M, Wada N, Atomi Y, Kuroda A, Muto T (1995) Diagnosis of acute pancreatitis: value of endoscopic sonography. Am J Roentgenol 165: 867–872
18. Vallon AG, Lees WR, Cotton PB (1979) Grey-scale ultrasonography and endoscopic pancreatography after pancreatic trauma. Br J Surg 66: 169–172

Computed Tomography in Acute Pancreatitis: Diagnosis, Staging, and Detection of Complications

P. C. Freeny

Introduction

Acute pancreatitis is characterized by a spectrum of inflammatory disease ranging from mild (interstitial or edematous pancreatitis) to severe (pancreatitis with associated parenchymal and/or peripancreatic fat necrosis, pancreatic abscess, pseudocyst, or other local or systemic complications). In a series of 897 patients with acute pancreatitis reported by Beger, 75% (679) had acute interstitial pancreatitis, 18% (157) had necrotizing pancreatitis, 5% (41) developed pseudocysts, and 2% (20) developed a pancreatic abscess [1]. As the severity of the inflammatory process increases, the associated morbidity and mortality also increase. In Beger's series, the mortality rate for patients with acute interstitial pancreatitis was only 0.4%, while it rose to 12% in patients with necrotizing pancreatitis and to 17% if a pancreatic abscess was present. Thus, staging and early detection of complications of acute pancreatitis are important for appropriate patient management [2, 3].

Dynamic contrast-enhanced computed tomography (CT) currently is the most accurate single imaging modality for diagnosis, staging the severity of the inflammatory process, and detecting complications of acute pancreatitis [4-7]. Most importantly, CT has been shown to have a sensitivity of 87% and an overall detection rate of over 90% for pancraetic gland necrosis [5, 8, 9].

Computed Tomography Techniques

Scan technique. The examination is performed using 5-mm collimated scans at 8-mm intervals for incremental CT and 5-7-mm collimation for helical CT. An oral contrast agent should be given if possible to opacify the gastrointestinal tract, permitting differentiation of pancreatic fluid collections from loops of bowel and facilitating detection of involvement of the gastrointestinal tract by the inflammatory process.

Intravenous Contrast. For incremental CT, a 150- to 180-ml bolus of a 60% iodinated contrast agent should be administered during the scanning sequence using a monophasic (2-3 ml/s) injection sequence and a 30-s scan delay. For helical CT, a bolus of 150 ml of a 60% contrast agent is injected at a rate of 3 ml/sec with a 60-s scan delay. Normal pancreatic parenchyma will show an increase in attenuation of 40–60 HU above baseline attenuation of normal non-enhanced parenchyma. In addition, the peripancreatic vascular structures will show intense contrast enhancement, allowing detection of vascular complications associated with acute pancreatitis. If acute or active hemorrhage is suspected, an initial non-contrast-enhanced scan should be obtained because IV contrast can mask or obscure the presence of blood which is seen as a collection of high attenuation material.

Contraindications to the use of intravenous contrast include a previous severe (anaphylactic) allergic reaction to iodinated contrast material and markedly diminished renal function not yet requiring dialysis (if the patient is on dialysis, then contrast is not contraindicated). In these two cases, a non-contrast-enhanced scan should be obtained and evaluated for its adequacy (i.e., does the scan provide sufficient information to manage the patient appropriately?). If the scan is considered inadequate, patients with contrast allergies are premedicated with 50 mg prednisone po every 6 h for four doses prior to the scan and 50 mg Benadryl (diphenhydramine hydrochloride) po 1–2 h prior to the scan, and a nonionic conrast agent is used. If the patient not to receive anything po (NPO), intramuscular injections of 40 mg methylprednisolone (Solu-Medrol Upjohn, Kalamazoo, MI) every 6 h for four doses prior to the scan, plus 25–50 mg Benadryl IM 30 min prior to the scan, can be utilized.

In the case of diminished renal function, the potential for contrast-induced nephropathy leading to dialysis must be weighed against the potential benefit of a contrast-enhanced CT. If contrast enhancement is believed to be necessary, the patient is hydrated with intravenous fluid for 3–6 h prior to and following the scan and is given 25–50 g mannitol immediately after the contrast bolus. The volume of contrast is reduced to 90–100 ml and a nonionic agent is used.

Indications for Computed Tomography for Acute Pancreatitis

CT has two major roles in evaluation of patients with known or suspected acute pancreatitis: (1) initial staging of the severity of the inflammatory process; and (2) early detection of complications, particularly the identification and quantification of parenchymal and peripancreatic necrosis. In patients in whom the clinical diagnosis of acute pancreatitis is equivocal, CT also can be used for diagnosis.

Computed Tomography Staging of the Severity of Acute Pancreatitis

The ability to stage accurately the severity of acute pancreatitis may have important prognostic and treatment implications [2, 5, 10–13]. Several studies have shown that initial clinical evaluation may be able to identify only between 34% and 39% of patients with severe acute pancreatitis or patients who are likely to have high morbidity [14–17]. However, recent studies have shown that CT performed early in the course of acute pancreatitis can better identify those patients with severe pancreatitis [5, 12, 18]. This is because clinical criteria alone measure only the physiologic or systemic response of the patient, while CT can depict both the existing extent of damage to the pancreas, particularly the presence of gland necrosis, as well as identify other complications prior to their clinical manifestations that subsequently will likely result in major sequelae, such as extensive peripancreatic fluid collections, abscess formation, and vascular, biliary, or gastrointestinal tract involvement [5].

The morphologic severity of acute pancreatitis can be defined precisely using the CT severity index (CTSI) developed by Balthazar and coworkers [5].

First, the severity of the acute inflammatory process is categorized into stage A through E, corresponding to scores of 0–4, respectively.

Stage A: Normal Pancreas (Score 0). Patients with acute edematous or interstitial pancreatitis may have a normal pancreatic CT in 20%–25% of cases [19]. This is because the inflammatory process is so mild that no peri or intrapancreatic fluid collections form and no changes occur in the peripancreatic soft tissues. The gland may be slightly enlarged, but without a baseline scan performed prior to the onset of the acute attack, this change may be too subtle to detect.

Stage B: Intrinsic Pancreatic Changes (Score 1). Stage B acute pancreatitis represents a spectrum of changes including focal or diffuse gland enlargement, mild heterogeneity of the gland parenchyma, and small intrapancreatic fluid collections caused by rupture of a small lateral sidebranch duct or a small zone (less than 3 cm) of parenchymal necrosis and ductal rupture.

Stage C: Intrinsic and Extrinsic Inflammatory Changes (Score 2). Stage C acute pancreatitis is manifested by intrinsic gland abnormalities as described for stage B, but also includes mild inflammatory changes of the peripancreatic soft tissues (Fig. 1).

Stage D: Extrinsic Inflammatory Changes (Score 3): Patients with Stage D acute pancreatitis manifest more prominent peripancreatic inflammatory changes but not more than one pancreatic fluid collection (Fig. 2).

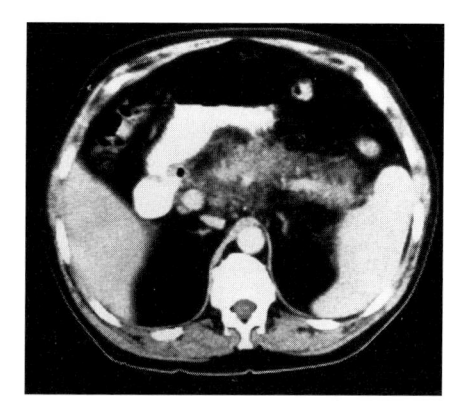

Fig. 1. Grade C acute pancreatitis, computed tomography (CT) severity index 2. Contrast-enhanced CT shows heterogeneous pancreatic parenchyma and mild peripancreatic soft tissue inflammatory changes

Fig. 2. Grade D acute pancreatitis, computed tomography (CT) severity index 3. Contrast-enhanced CT shows a single fluid collection anterior to the pancreas (*arrow*) and peripancreatic soft tissue inflammatory changes around the pancreatic tail

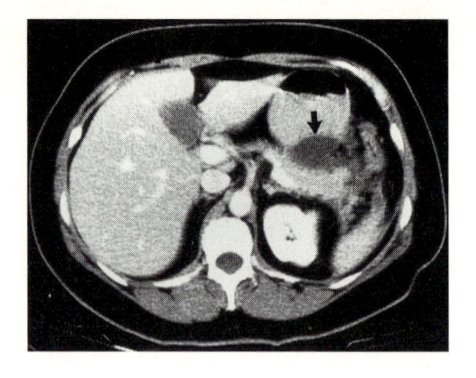

Stage E: Multiple or Extensive Extrapancreatic Fluid Collections or Abscess (Score 4): This is the most severe CT stage of acute pancreatitis and is manifested by marked intrapancreatic (fluid collections, necrosis) and peripancreatic (fluid collections, extraglandular fat necrosis), inflammatory changes, or frank pancreatic abscess formation (Fig. 3). These patients have a high morbidity owing to systemic complications (respiratory and renal failure, cardiovascular collapse) and a high mortality. Thus serial CT scans are important for following the progression of the disease and for detecting additional complications.

Second, the presence and extent or the absence of gland necrosis are assessed. If necrosis is present, the extent is estimated as less than one third, one half, or greater than one half on the basis of the area of gland parenchyma involved as demonstrated on axial scans. A score of 0 is given if no necrosis is present, and scores of 2, 4, and 6 for less than one third, up to one half, and greater than ohne half, respectively.

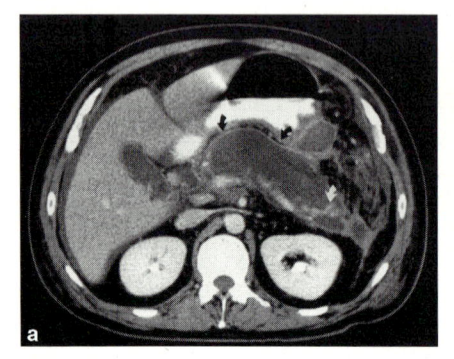

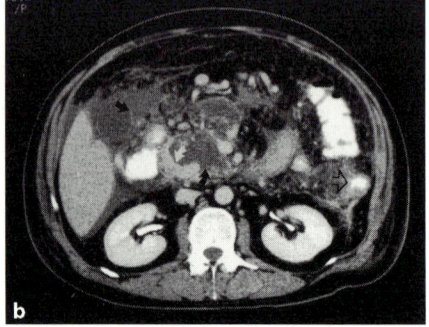

Fig. 3a, b. Grade E acute pancreatitis with subtotal necrosis, computed tomography (CT) severity index 10. CT scans show multiple fluid collections and peripancreatic fat necrosis around the pancreas (*black arrows*), pancreatic ascites (free fluid around the liver), and subtotal gland necrosis. Only small segments of the pancreas show normal contrast enhancement (*white arrows*). Inflammatory process also extends to involve the descending colon (*open arrow*)

Fig. 4. Grade D acute pancreatitis with subtotal pancreatic necrosis, computed tomography (CT) severity index 9. Contrast-enhanced CT shows no enhancement of the body and tail of the pancreas (*cursor 1*). Only a small fragment of parenchyma in the tail shows enhancement (*arrow*). Other levels (not displayed) showed a small residual are of parenchymal enhancement in the head

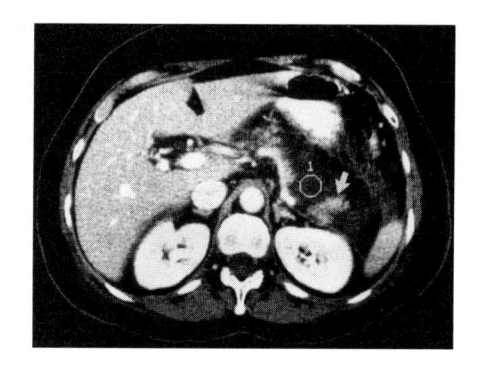

Necrosis can be detected by CT as a focal or diffuse area of diminished pancreatic parenchymal contrast enhancement (Fig. 4) [7, 9, 20, 21]. The accuracy of CT detection of parenchymal necrosis was investigated by Beger and colleagues in a large series of patients who underwent both CT and surgery [21]. The overall accuracy for CT was 87%. The false negative rate was 21% in patients with minor necrosis, but in cases of major or extended necrosis (>50%), the false negative rate was only 11%. There were no false positive CT scans, giving a specificity of 100%. Bradley and coworkers subsequently confirmed these results and indicated that CT detection of gland necrosis had important prognostic implications [22]. In Balthazar's series, patients who had a CT severity index of 0-1 had no mortality or morbidity, while those with an index of 2 had a 4% morbidity, and those with an index of 7-10 had a 17% mortality and a 92% morbidity [4] (Fig. 5).

In a recent study at the University of Washington (K.C. Carpenter et al., unpublished results, 1995), we found no difference in the total number of complications in patients with a moderate CT severity index [4-6] versus those with a severe CT severity index [7-10]. However, if patients with no prior episode of

Fig. 5. Computed tomography (CT) severity index. (Modified from Balthazar et al. 1990)

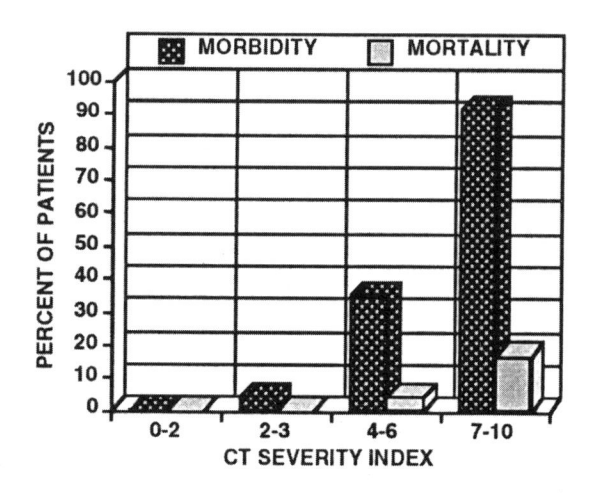

acute pancreatitis are excluded, then there was statistical difference in the number of complications and the CT severity index. Thus we postulate that a prior episode of acute pancreatitis may leave residual morphologic changes (e.g., previous necrosis may result in atrophy of the involved portion of the gland) that will cause overestimation of the CT severity index. Thus caution must be exercised when interpreting and grading CT scans in patients with a prior episode of acute pancreatitis.

The presence of necrosis as an isolated finding also correlated with subsequent patient morbidity and mortality [5]. Patients with no necrosis had no mortaliy and only a 6% morbidity, while those with 50% necrosis had a 25% mortality and a 75% morbidity, and those with greater than 50% necrosis had an 11% mortality and a 100% morbidity. These figures are similar to those from Beger's series [1].

It should be noted that most patients with acute pancreatitis who develop necrotizing pancreatitis do so within the first 24 h and virtually all within the first 72 h following the onset of clinical symptoms (Büchler, personal communication). Because the CT findings of necrosis may be equivocal within the first 24-48 h, the initial CT scan obtained in patients with clinically severe acute pancreatitis should be postponed until 72 h unless the patient is critically ill and in need of emergent surgery.

The presence or absence of secondary infection of necrotic pancreatic tissue also has a significant effect on patient morbidity and mortality. In Beger's series of 114 patients with pancreatic necrosis, intestinal microorganisms were cultured from the necrotic tissue in 39.4% of cases [23]. Patients with less than 50% gland necrosis showed an increase in mortality from 12.9% to 38.9% if the necrotic tissue was infected, and patients with subtotal necrosis (>50%), showed an increase in mortality from 14.3% to 66.7% in the presence of infection.

In about one-half of patients with clinically suspectes sepsis (fever, leukocytosis), no infection will be present. Thus, because CT cannot determine if necrotic tissue is infected or sterile, patients with necrosis who manifest clinical signs of sepsis should undergo fine-needle aspiration of the necrotic areas under CT or ultrasound guidance to determine the presence of bacterial con-

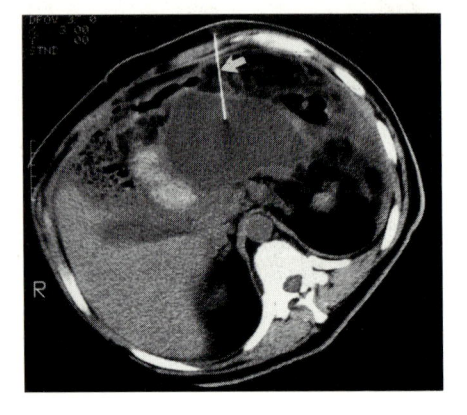

Fig. 6. Infected pancreatic necrosis. Computed tomography (CT) scan shows 20-gauge needle (*arrow*) directed into area of pancreatic necrosis. Cultures showed a polymicrobial infection

tamination (Fig. 6) [24, 25]. In the patients, a gram-positive stain or culture indicate the need for surgical or percutaneous intervention.

Computed Tomography Detection of Complications of Acute Pancreatitis

Many of the complications of acute pancreatitis can be detected by CT. One of the most important is the presence of gland necrosis as discussed above. Others include pancreatic fluid collections, pancreatic abscess, and involvement of the vascular system, biliary and gastrointestinal tract and the contiguous solid organs (liver, spleen, kidney). Early recognition of these complications can be expected to result in reduction of morbidity and mortality by leading to early and appropriate surgical, radiologic, or endoscopic treatment.

Fluid Collections. Fluid collections develop in or around the pancreas in as many as 50% or more of patients with acute pancreatitis [26, 27]. In many cases, the collections resolve spontaneously and never produce clinical symptoms (Fig. 7). In other patients, however, the collections can persist, enlarge, become secondarily infected, or erode into contiguous structures. These persistent or enlarging collections and their secondary complications can be detected by CT and a decision regarding surgical, endoscopic, or percutaneous drainage can be made.

Large peripancreatic fluid collections often can be associated with coexisting peripancreatic fat necrosis (see Fig. 3). It is usually not possible to make this differentiation by CT. However, if the peripancreatic process has low CT attenuation numbers (< 15 HU), it is most likely a simple peripancreatic fluid collection, while higher numbers (> 25 HU) are highly indicative of coexisting fat necrosis. The presence or absence of secondary infection within these peripancreatic collections also cannot be determined accurately on the basis of CT mor-

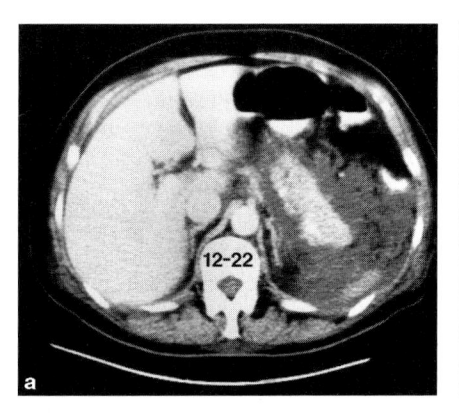

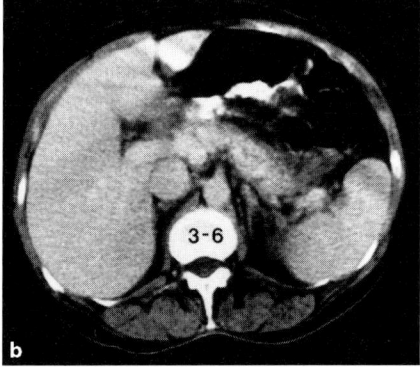

Fig. 7a, b. Acute pancreatic fluid collection: spontaneous resolution. a Computed tomography (CT) scan on 22 December shows large fluid collection surrounding the pancreatic tail. b Patient had slow, but progressive clinical improvement. Follow-up CT on 6 March shows complete resolution of the fluid collection

phology. The presence of gas within a collection may be caused by gasforming bacteria, but also can be caused by a gastrointestinal fistula in the absence of infection [28]. The presence of infection within a fluid collection can be confirmed with CT-guided fine-needle aspiration. If percutaneous drainage is to be performed, CT always should be obtained to define the precise anatomic relationship of the collection to surrounding structures so that catheter can be placed safely in the appropriate location [29].

Percutaneous Catheter Drainage. Infected fluid collections can be treated effectively by percutaneous catheter drainage (PCD) [3, 29, 30]. The initial fine-needle aspiration should be used to determine the presence of infection and the quality of the fluid (i.e., sufficiently liquid to be drained via catheter).

CT should be obtained prior to PCD to define precisely the location, size, and number of collections, their relationship to surrounding structures, and to identify vascular involvement, such as pseudoaneurysm or venous obstruction with large varices, which could result in major complications following PCD.

Patients with pancreatic fluid collections, particularly those with chronic pancreatitis, should have an endoscopic retrograde cholangiopancreatography (ERCP) prior to nonemergent PCD to determine whether a pancreatic duct fistula is present and to assess the patency of the main duct. If the main pancreatic duct between a communicating fluid collection and the papilla is obstructed by a calculus or stricture, PCD is likely to result in a pancreatic-cutaneous fistula and should be performed only for temporary palliation of sepsis if the patient is a prohibitive operative risk.

In a collected series of 207 patients with pancreatic fluid collections, 57% of the were infected. Overall success for PAD was 82%, with a range of 67%–93%. Catheter drainage times ranged from 7 to 210 days, with a mean of 33 days (one patient not included in the range or mean calculations had catheters in place for 2.5 years). In one series, prolonged drainage time reflected the presence of gastrointestinal or pancreatic duct fistulae. In the patients with isolated collections, drainage time averaged 29 days, while it was prolonged to 96–104 days in patients with pancreatic or gastrointestinal fistulae, respectively [29]. The drainage times in the cases reported by van Sonnenberg were less: mean 19.6 days (range 3–38 days in 75 patients; 72 and 102 days in two patients); mean 28.3 days in patients with a pancreatic duct fistula [30]. There was only a slight difference in drainage times between patients with infected (16.7 days) and noninfected (21.2 days) collections. Six patients (7.8%) required surgery for persistent drainage. In both series, frequent contrast studies and catheter manipulations and changes were necessary to maintain adequate drainage.

It has been suggested by some authors that transgastric drainage may prevent recurrence of fluid collections by allowing drainage to occur through the catheter tract from the collection to the stomach following catheter withdrawal [31, 32]. However, results and recurrence rates in patients treated with transgastric versus transperitoneal drainage were not significantly different in an analysis of several series [29–32]. It has been shown with endoscopy that even a surgically created cystgastrostomy often closes shortly after operation. Thus, the communication created between a fluid collection and the stomach using a catheter only 8–12 F in diameter would be unlikely to remain patent for any length of time following catheter removal.

The overall complication rate following PCD of acute fluid collections or pseudocysts is about 18%. However, major complications occur in only 8.6% (18 patients). This compares favorably with surgical drainage where operative mortality rates of 5% to 18% have been reported. In the collected series of 207 patients, no mortality occurred as a result of the PCD, although 11 patients died following catheter placement. These deaths all occurred in critically ill patients with multi-system failure and sepsis who were deemed prohibitive operative risks and PCD was attempted only as a last resort.

Endoscopic placement of pancreatic duct stents recently has been used to decompress fluid collections which communicate with the pancreatic duct [33]. The stent is placed via the major a minor papilla into the main pancreatic duct and either directly into the fluid collection through the rent in the duct, or across the rent, bidging the ductal defect and facilitating duct healing. The pancreatic duct stent also can be used in concert with PCD to decrease catheter drainage times when ductal disruption is present.

Vascular Complications. Involvement of the peripancreatic arteries and veins by the inflammatory process associated with acute pancreatitis is common and can be detected accurately by CT. Complications include erosion of intrapancreatic or peripancreatic arteries with acute hemorrhage, formation of arterial pseudoaneurysms, and thrombosis of branches of the portal venous system with formation of varices or acute mesenteric infarction (see Fig. 6) [28–31].

In many cases, acute pancreatic hemorrhage is a catastrophic event heralded by pain and shock. In these patients, emergency angiography and transcatheter embolotherapy or surgery are required and CT has little to offer and may delay diagnosis and treatment.

Arterial pseudoaneurysms can develop within the pancreatic parenchyma, adjacent to the gland, or within a pseudocyst. They can be diagnosed by angiography or CT by demonstrating a contrast-enhancing mass. They can be treated treated surgically, but transcatheter embolotherapy is efficacious and can be performed at the time of diagnostic angiography [34–39].

Fig. 8. Arterial pseudoaneurysm. Patient had a previous of severe acute pancreatitis. Continued pain prompted a contrast-enhanced computed tomography (CT) scan which shows an enhancing arterial pseudoaneurysm (*A*) adjacent to the tail of the pancreas

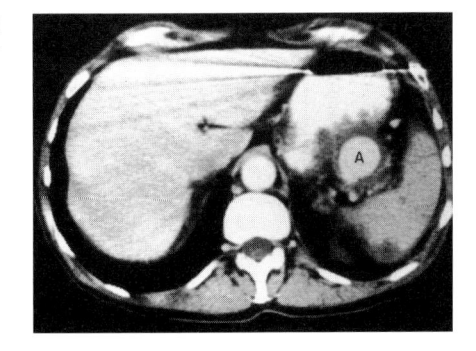

Biliary Tract Involvement. CT is quite accurate in detecting involvement or associated abnormalities of the biliary tract. The most common biliary tract abnormality associated with acute pancreatitis is choledocholithiasis. Biliary tract involvement by the inflammatory process associated with acute pancreatitis can be manifested by transient obstruction of the intrapancreatic segment of the common bile duct owing to periductal inflammation or to compression by an adjacent pseudocyst or fluid collection, or chronic obstruction owing to a ductal stricture caused by the surrounding inflammatory process. Pancreatic pseudocysts also can involve the common bile duct directly or they can invade into the liver resulting in an intrahepatic biliary fistula [40].

Biliary obstruction can be treated with surgical bypass if it is caused by a ductal stricture, or by surgical or percutaneous drainage of an adjacent pseudocyst if it is caused by extrinsic pressure. Patients who are poor operative risks, or who are critically ill with cholangitis, can be temporarily or permanently treated with percutaneous or endoscopic biliary decompression [34].

Gastrointestinal Tract Involvement. While both CT and contrast studies can detect abnormalities of the gastrointestinal tract caused by acute pancreatitis, CT provides important information concerning the extent of the inflammatory process extrinsic to or surrounding the involved segment of the gastrointestinal tract [41–44]. The etiology of the involvement usually can be elucidated (e.g., fluid collection, pseudocyst, or direct extension of the inflammatory process) and the appropriate surgical or interventional treatment can be planned.

Solid Organ Involvement. The inflammatory process of acute pancreatitis can extend to involve the contiguous solid organs, particularly the spleen, left kidney, and the liver [34, 45–47].

Recommendations for Use of Computed Tomography in Acute Pancreatitis

The following guidelines for the use of CT in patients with acute pancreatitis are suggested:

1. Initial CT scan
   a) Patients with clinically severe acute pancreatitis at the time of initial evaluation (based on Ranson criteria or APACHE II score) who do not manifest rapid clinical improvement within 72 h of conservative medical treatment;
   b) Patients who demonstrate clinical improvement during initial medical therapy but then manifest an acute change in clinical status indicating a developing complication (e.g., fever, pain, inability to tolerate oral intake, hypotension, falling hematocrit).
2. Follow-up CT scan
   a) A follow-up scan subsequent to an initial CT which shows only Grade A–C pancreatitis without parenchymal necrosis (CT severity index score

of 0–2) is recommended only if there is a change in the patient's clinical status which suggests a developing complication;

b) A follow-up scan is recommended at 7–10 days if the initial scan shows grade D–E pancreatitis with or without parenchymal necrosis (CT severity index score of 3–10). Resolution of the CT manifestations of pancreatic and peripancreatic inflammation virtually always lags behind the improving clinical status of the patient. Thus, if the patient shows an improving clinical status, additional follow-up scans during hospitalization are recommended only if the patient's clinical status deteriorates or fails to show continued improvement. However, because some important complications can develop without becoming clinically evident, such as evolution of a fluid collection into a pseudocyst or development of an arterial pseudoaneurysm, a scan should be obtained at the time of hospital discharge to confirm reasonable resolution of initial grade D or E (CT severity index of 3–10) pancreatitis.

References

1. Beger H (1991) Surgery in acute pancreatitis. Hepatogastroenterology 38: 92–96
2. London N, Leese T, Lavelle J, et al (1991) Rapid-bolus contrast-enhanced dynamic computed tomography in acute pancreatitis: a prospective study. Br J Surg 78: 1452–1456
3. Balthazar E, Freeny P, vanSonnenberg E (1994) Imaging and intervention in acute pancreatitis. Radiology 193: 297–306
4. Freeny P (1993) Incremental dynamic bolus computed tomography of acute pancreatitis-state-of-the-art. Internatl J Pancreatol 13: 147–158
5. Balthazar E, Robinson D, Megibow A, et al (1990) Acute pancreatitis: value of CT in establishing prognosis. Radiology 174: 331–336
6. Freeny P (1991) Angio-CT: diagnosis and detection of complications of acute pancreatitis. Hepatogastroenterol 38: 109–115
7. Larvin M, Chalmers A, McMahon M (1990) Dynamic contrast enhanced computed tomography: a precise technique for identifying and localising pancreatic necrosis. Br Med J 300: 1425–1428
8. Block S, Maier W, Bittner R, et al (1986) Identification of pancreas necrosis in severe acute pancreatitis: imaging procedures versus clinical staging. Gut 27: 1035–1042
9. Kivisaari L, Somer K, Standertskjold-Nordenstam C-G, et al (1983) Early detection of acute fulminant pancreatitis by contrast-enhanced computed tomography. Scand J Gastroenterol 18: 39–41
10. Balthazar E (1989) CT diagnosis and staging of acute pancreatitis. Radiologic Clinics of North Am 27: 19–37
11. Balthazar E, Ranson J, Naidich D, et al (1985) Acute pancreatitis: prognostic value of CT. Radiology 156: 767–772
12. Beger H, Maier W, Block S, et al (1986) How do imaging methods influence the surgical strategy in acute pancreatitis? In: Malfertheiner P, Ditchuneit H, ed. Diagnostic Procedures in Pancreatic Disease. Berlin: Springer-Verlag, 54–60
13. Beger H, Büchler M (1986) Outcome of necrotizing pancreatitis in relation to morphological parameters. In: Malfertheiner P, Ditchuneit H, ed. Diagnostic Procedures in Pancreatic Disease. Berlin: Springer-Verlag, 130–132
14. MacMahon M, Playforth M, Pickford I (1980) A comparative study of methods for the prediction of the severity of attacks of acute pancreatitis. Br J Surg 67: 22–25
15. Corfield A, Williamson R, McMahon M, et al (1985) Prediction of severity in acute pancreatitis: prospective comparison of three prognostic indices. Lancet 2: 403–406
16. Agarwal N, Pitchumoni C (1991) Assessment of severity in acute pancreatitis. Am J Gastroenterology 86: 1385–1391
17. Wilson C, Heath D, Imrie C (1990) Prediction of outcome in acute pancreatitis: a comparative study of APACHE II, clinical assessment and multiple factor scoring systems. Br J Surg 77: 1260–1264

18. Büchler M (1991) Objectification of the severity of acute pancreatitis. Hepatogastroenterology 38: 101–108
19. Hill M, Barkin J, Isikoff M, et al (1982) Acute pancreatitis: clinical vs. CT findings AJR 139: 263–269
20. Johnson C, Stephens D, Sarr M (1991) CT of acute pancreatitis: correlation between lack of contrast enhancement and pancreatic necrosis. AJR 156: 93–95
21. Maier W (1987) Early objective diagnosis and staging of acute pancreatitis by contrast enhanced CT. In: Beger H, Büchler M, ed. Acute Pancreatitis. Berlin: Springer-Verlag 132–140
22. Bradley E III, Murphy F, Ferguson C (1989) Prediction of pancreatic necrosis by dynamic pancreatography. Ann Surg 210: 495–504
23. Beger H, Bittner R, Block S, et al (1986) Bacterial contamination of pancreatic necrosis. A prospective study. Gastroenterology 91: 433–438
24. Banks P (1991) Infected necrosis: morbidity and therapeutic consequences. Hepatogastroenterology 38: 116–119
25. Banks P, Gerzof S (1987) Indications and results of fine needle aspiration of pancreatic exudate. In: Beger H, Büchler M, ed. Acute Pancreatitis. Berlin: Springer-Verlag 171–174
26. Kourtesis G, Wilson S, Williams R (1990) The clinical significance of fluid collections in acute pancreatitis. Am Surgeon 56: 769–799
27. Yeo C, Bastidas J, Lynch-Nyhan A, et al (1990) The natural history of pancreatic pseudocysts documented by computed tomography. Surg Gynec Obstet 170: 411–417
28. Mendez G, Isikoff M (1979) Significance of intrapancreatic gas, demonstrated by CT: a review of nine cases. AJR 132: 59–62
29. Freeny P, Lewis G, Traverso L et al (1988) Infected pancreatic fluid collections: percutaneous catheter drainage. Radiology 167: 435–441
30. vanSonnenberg E, Wittich G, Casola G, et al (1989) Percutaneous drainage of infected and noninfected pancreatic pseudocysts: experience in 101 cases. Radiology 170: 757–761
31. Grosso M, Gandini G, Cassinis M, et al (1989) Percutaneous treatment (including pseudocystogastrostomy) of 74 pancreatic pseudocysts. Radiology 173: 493–497
32. Matzinger F, Ho C-S, Yee A, et al (1988) Pancreatic pseudocysts drained through a percutaneous transgastric approach: further experience. Radiology 167: 431–434
33. Kozarek R, Ball T, Patterson D, et al (1991) Endoscopic transpapillary therapy for disrupted pancreatic duct and peripancreatic fluid collections. Gastroenterology 1362–1370
34. Freeny P, Lawson T (1982) Radiology of the Pancreas. New York: Springer-Verlag
35. Freeny P (1984) Computed tomography of the pancreas. Clinics in Gastroenterology 13: 791–818
36. Vujic I, Seymour E, Meridith H (1980) Vascular complications associated with sonographically demonstrated cystic epigastric lesions: an important indication for angiography. Cardiovasc Intervent Radiol 3: 75–79
37. Vujic I, Anderson B, Stanley J, et al (1984) Pancreatic and peripancreatic vessels: embolization for control of bleeding in pancreatitis. Radiology 150: 51–55
38. Vujic I (1989) Vascular complications of pancreatitis. Radiologic Clinics of North Am 27: 81–91
39. Waltman A, Luers P, Athanasoulis C, et al (1986) Massive arterial hemorrhage in patients with pancreatitis. Complementary roles of surgery and transcatheter occlusive techniques. Arch Surg 121: 439–443
40. Rohrmann C, Baron R (1989) Biliary complications of pancreatitis. Radiologic Clinics of North Am 27: 93–104
41. Lindahl F, Vejlsted H, Backer O (1972) Lesions of the colon following pancreatitis. Scand J Gastroenterol 7: 375–378
42. Meyers M, Evans J (1973) Effects of pancreatitis on the small bowel and colon. AJR 119: 151–165
43. Safrit H, Rice R (1989) Gastrointestinal complications of pancreatitis. Radiologic Clinics of North Am 27: 73–79
44. Thompson W, Kelvin F, Rice R (1977) Inflammation and necrosis of the transverse colon secondary to pancreatitis. AJR 128: 943–948
45. Farman J, Dallemand S, Schneider M, et al (1977) Pancreatic pseudocysts involving the spleen. Gastrointest Radiol 1: 339–343
46. Lilienfeld R, Lande A (1976) Pancreatic pseudocysts presenting as thick walled renal and perinephric cysts. J Urol 115: 123–125
47. Fishman E, Soyer P, Bliss D, et al (1995) Splenic involvement in pancreatitis: spectrum of CT findings. AJR 164: 631–635

Diagnosis of Infected Pancreatic Necrosis

C. Bassi · M. Falconi · A. Bonora · N. Sartori · E. Caldiron
R. Salvia · R. Girelli · P. Pederzoli

Introduction

No more than a decade ago, the whole issue of the clinical significance, diagnosis, therapy and prevention of infected pancreatic necrosis was only barely perceived by pancreatologists. It was only as recently as 1986 and 1987 that two elegant prospective studies were published by Beger et al. [1] and Gerzof et al. [2], respectively, which were to become the cornerstones of the scientific frame of reference serving as a basis for our concrete understanding of the actual impact of infected necrosis on the natural history of acute pancreatitis and of how an early, reliable diagnosis could be achieved with certainty.

The same period has witnessed both the most modern contributions towards the surgical treatment of the condition [3-5] and, in the last few years, a tendency to devote attention more specifically to the prevention of such infections [6-13].

Infection is a complication which develops in 5%-10% of all cases of acute pancreatitis. In actual fact, infection is possible only if the substrate consists of necrosis as a non-viable area of pancreatic parenchyma [14]. If, then we consider only cases of necrotic pancreatitis, the incidence of infection rises to 30%-70% of the cases reported in the literature and proves more frequent, the more extensive the area of pancreatic necrosis is [6, 15]. From the point of view of clinical timing, the complication tends to manifest itself mainly after the second week of acute pancreatitis (Fig. 1). Last but not least, infected necrosis and pancreatic abscesses are now the main causes of mortality in patients with acute pancreatitis [6]. Thus the earliest possible detection of onset of infection is a vital factor for the prompt implementation of therapy to save the patient's life.

In this chapter, we shall attempt to identify and discuss those clinical aspects as well as the biochemical and radiological evidence suggesting the possible occurrence of the septic complication in the clinical couse of acute pancreatitis.

"Natural" and "Unnatural" Clinical Course of Necrotic Pancreatitis

Few diseases in medical practice have such a bizarre and unpredictable course as acute pancreatitis. Though the present prognostic staing is fairly reliable [16-18], in practice it is very difficult to codify and predict patterns of clinical trends in individual cases.

Fig. 1. Frequency of positive cultures versus time in surgically treated patients ($n = 45$) [1]

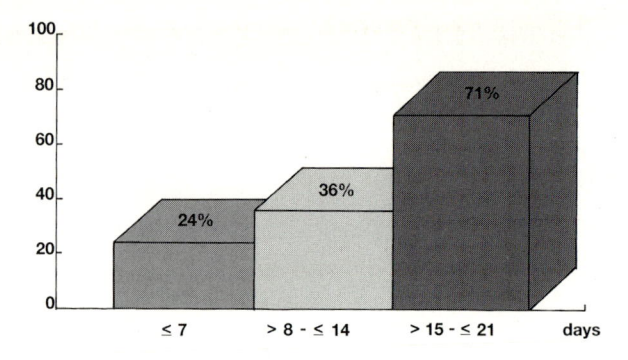

Since, however, some kind of "didactic" schematic representation is necessary, we might attempt to distinguish between three types of clinical course: the first of these, the most "natural and desirable", is dominated by abdominal pain and by more or less severe signs of toxicity related to the release of vasoactive substances and enzymes into the bloodstream which damage target organs and apparati (lungs, kidneys, heart, circulatory and nervous systems). Fortunately, in most cases, there is more or less major impairment of these targets, which is

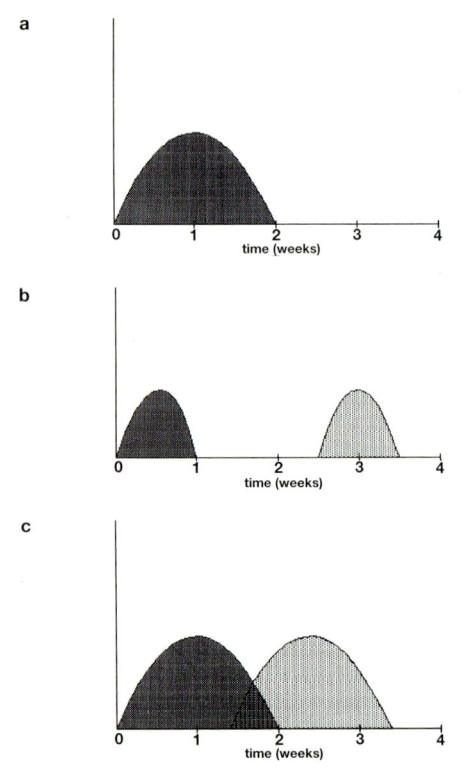

Fig. 2a–c. Clinical patterns of acute pancreatitis *Dark shading,* toxic phase; *light shading,* septic phase. **a** Acute pancreatitis without infection. **b** Pancreatic abscess. **c** Infected necrosis

generally readily amenable to medical treatment, as a result of undoubted improvements in intensive care. More rarely, despite the necessary abundant rehydration, severe failure of one or more organs can occur and even fulminating or irreversible situations of multiorgan failure.

In the past, prior to the advent of the above-mentioned improvements in intensive care and resuscitation therapy, these were the main causes of pancreatitis-associated mortality. Most patients now survive this phase, thus increasing the risk of later sepsis, which would explain the present greater number of infections and deaths associated with them.

This "monophasic" trend (Fig. 2A) is almost always characterised both by the occurrence of fever (not, however, with a septic trend nor, generally speaking, above 38 °C) and neutrophil leukocytosis. In actual fact, however, initially the pancreatic necrosis and peripancreatic fluid collections, when present, are sterile. The fever and leukocytosis are of toxic origin or may be an expression, as may be the case later, of non-pancreatic infection foci (e.g. pleura, pulmonary parenchyma, urinary tract). In the latter eventuality, these septic foci must be promptly recognised and treated so as to avoid bacteriaemia capable of colonising the pancreas [6, 19, 20].

The timing of these phenomena may vary, depending upon the clinical severity, from a few days to approximately 2 weeks after the acute pancreatitis attack.

The second type of clinical expression is characterised by a trend which can be defined as "biphasic" (Fig. 2B) in that, after completion of the phase outlined above, we witness a variable period (from a few weeks to 1–2 months) of relative or even absolute well-being: the patient regains performance capability, is able to cope independently and is regular in his or her eating habits up to the onset of marked signs of sepsis (bouts of fever > 38 °C), abdominal pain with or without disorders attributable to a "mass" and, albeit not necessarily, leukocytosis with an increase in erythrocyte sedimentation rate and in the other common blood-chemistry indices of acute inflammation.

Generally speaking, this clinical trend is relatively rare and corresponds to the occurrence of a pancreatic abscess, which is a severe clinical condition requiring immediate drainage, but which, compared to infected necrosis, carries a significantly lower mortality rate, if treated promptly [4, 14].

The third and last clinical pattern is the most frequent and the one most difficult to interpret, being characterised by an "overlapping biphasic" trend (Fig. 2C). In practice, after an initial "toxic" phase, the latter blends with clinical elements which are an expression of concomitant sepsis and whose differentiation is not always a foregone conclusion. It is at this point, generally between the second and third week after onset of the symptoms, that the clinician encounters the greatest difficulty, when called upon to interpret fever, hypotension and various organ impairments which could be explained in both toxic and septic terms. The frequent presence of the above-mentioned extrapancreatic infection foci certainly does not facilitate the task of making a differential diagnosis. It is in this phase that the biochemical and radiological evidence takes on primary importance and, as we shall see later, analysis of cultures of necrotic material obtained by aspiration is almost always mandatory.

This third clinical pattern outlined here above is typical of cases of infected necrosis [6, 14].

Biochemical Evidence

Table 1 lists the clinical and laboratory elements which have been suggested as being useful for the identification of patients suffering from sepsis of pancreatic origin. However, only 25% of infected cases exhibit three positive indicators [21].

In our experience [15], univariate statistical comparison of Ranson scores (RS) and C-reactive protein (CRP) values have proved significant with regard to the risk of onset of sepsis. The RS in patients with infected necrosis is 3.9 (range, 2–6) compared to 3.2 (range, 2–4) in the sterile cases. The mean CRP value in patients not presenting septic complications was 82 mg/l (at onset of acute pancreatitis) as against 130 mg/l in cases later presenting the complication. Multivariate analysis, however, showed that the predominant risk factor is the extent of the necrosis as determined by computed tomography (CT) with intravenous injection of contrast medium. The amount of pancreatic necrosis correlates significantly with the development of infection of the necrosis with a coefficient of risk of 5.32. In practice, then, the simple, gross distinction based on the necrotic process extending to 30%, 50% or more than 50% of the glandular volume is a basic reference element when it comes to estimating "risk of infection". For this reason, all patients suffering from necrotizing pancreatitis should also be typed for radiological extent of necrosis, particularly when included in controlled clinical trials the purpose of which is to assess drugs and/or diagnostic or therapeutic procedures suitable for the identification, prevention and treatment of infected necrosis and pancreatic abscesses

Radiological Evidence

As described above, CT is today the gold standard for the diagnosis of pancreatic necrosis [6]. Unfortunately, however, despite the very impressive resolution capability of modern CT equipment, it does not yet possess the ability to detect micro-organisms. In other words, CT is capable of informing us as to the pres-

Table 1. Clinical and laboratory data suggesting the presence of infected pancreatic necrosis or pancreatic abscess

Parameter	Value
Fever	$> 38\,°C$
Haematocrit	$< 35\%$
Base excess	< 4 mmol/l
PaO	< 60 mmHg
PaCO$_2$	< 30 mmHg
Serum albumin	< 3 g/dl
Platelet count	$> 450\,000/mm^2$

Diagnosis of Infected Pancreatic Necrosis

Fig. 3. Typical "soap bubble" suggesting the presence of a pancreatic abscess. The patient presented with signs of sepsis. In thic case, faced with clinical and radiological evidence of sepsis, we proceeded to treated the condition immediately without resorting to fine-needle aspiration (FNA) of the lesion

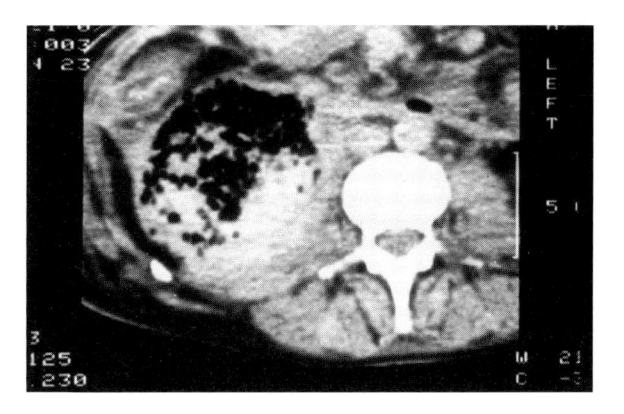

ence of necrosis, its intrapancreatic and retroperitoneal extension and the topography of collections of pancreatic origin, but it is incapable of revealing with absolute certainty the presence of superinfection of such lesions.

The identification of so-called "soap bubbles" (Fig. 3) as radiological evidence of the presence of anaerobic micro-organisms is a fairly rare event (18 % in our experience and occurring late when the necrosis has left space, after its colliquation, for a pancreatic abscess in the strict sense of the term). Moreover, the presence of gas may derive either from spontaneous fistulisation of the peripancreatic fluid collections into the digestive tract or from spontaneous production of gas in the context of a voluminous necrosis which is itself sterile [6].

Fine-Needle Aspiration

In view of the poor reliability of both clinical findings and laboratory and radiological data in the differential diagnosis of septic versus sterile necrosis, ultrasound (US)- or CT-guided puncture of the necrotic collections and subsequent culture examinations of the material obtained has progressively gained widespread popularity (Fig. 4). This is due not only to the diagnostic reliability of the procedure (when performed by an expert and with only a few, precise manoeuvres) but also to its relatively limited invasiveness, its simplicity and safety [2, 6, 11, 15].

The risk of infecting collections which are in themselves sterile is purely theoretical, in that the needle is not left in place except for the few seconds necessary for obtaining a few drops or microscopic fragments of necrotic material.

We generally use 19- to 21-gauge needles under CT guidance (more precise in its "tracking" mechanisms), except in the case of very voluminous collections, where US can also easily be used and is less expensive and more manageable.

The amount of material to be aspirated is minimal and the aspiration can be performed from any site in the lesion, inasmuch as the infection in severe acute pancreatitis is a widespread contamination with a widespread distribution. The

Fig. 4. Computed tomography (CT)-guided fine-needle aspiration (FNA) of voluminous post-pancreatitis collection. In this specific case, we proceeded to perform a partial drainage of the collection, as can be seen in the *bottom image*, since the lesion caused compression symptoms and pain due to abdominal distension

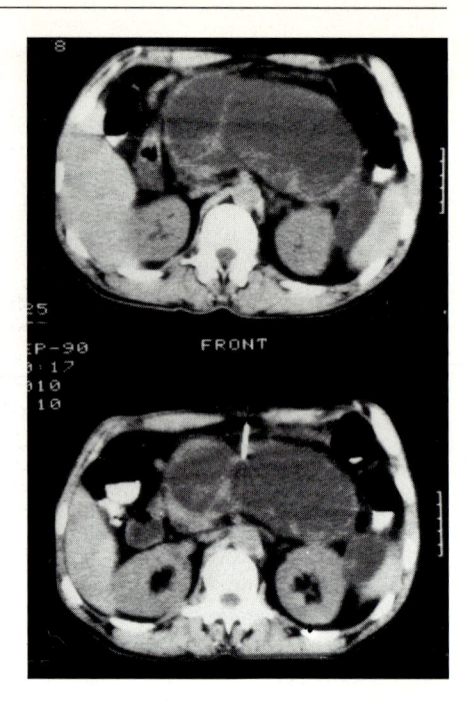

correspondence between fine-needle aspiration (FNA) and intra-operative isolates is constant.

The risk of false positivity must be considered either due to skin contamination (*Staphylococcus epidermidis*) or to aspiration of large bowel contents (*Escherichia coli*). The latter type of false positive can easily be avoided by an expert reader of radiological images and, particularly, by using CT-guided "tracking".

It should not come either as a surprise or as a matter of concern if some patients complain of spontaneous abdominal tenderness accentuated by palpation for a few hours after the examination: a slight leakage due to fissurisation of peripancreatic inflammatory collections due to the exploratory puncture is to be expected, but is resolved rapidly thanks to the well-known reabsorption capability of the retro-intraperitoneal serous membrane. The fact that FNA is a safe procedure is further demonstrated if we consider that the cyto-histological aspiration of expansive pancreatic lesions (in addition to necrosis and pancreatic infections) has now become an integral part of the routine diagnostic staging of such lesions.

Fine-Needle Aspiration: Always? When? How often?

In clinical practice, then, should all patients suffering from pancreatic necrosis be submitted to FNA of the pancreatic necrotic tissue? The answer is no. In practice, we perform FNA whenever a patient with proven necrotizing pancreatitis presents a clinical course characterised by the onset of fever $> 38\,°C$, particularly if not due to other infection foci. The number of white blood cells is of only relative importance, since, as is well known, it is influenced by the type of micro-organisms responsible for the infection, just as there is also considerable variability of the other clinical and laboratory elements bearing witness to a septic – toxic state reported in the table.

Returning for a moment to the previous description of the clinical phases which generally characterise the course of acute pancreatitis, it is obvious that the period when as a rule FNA most needs to be performed is precisely the period straddling the toxic and septic phases of the disease (weeks 2–3 after onset), when the disease presents the pattern defined above as "overlapping biphasic".

However, in view of the safety and accuracy of FNA, the problem is not so much if and when to perform it in the presence of suspected necrosis, but whether it should always be performed even when clinical evidence of sepsis is available.

An example is the situation in Fig. 3 which refers to a patient transferred to our department 1 month after the onset of the disease with a clinical picture of septic shock. Faced with the CT scan in association with the clinical picture, we did not waste time with other diagnostic procedures, but immediately performed the drainage of the abscess, obtaining the microbiological analysis intraoperatively.

Finally, we should stress the importance of repeating FNA in the course of pancreatitis whenever the clinical evidence suggests the need for it. In the controlled trial conducted by the Boston team [2], repetition of FNA in 17 patients out of 87 led to positive results (eight of 17) in a percentage of patients comparable to those undergoing the investigation only once (36 of 70).

In the light of what we have said, only 10 years after the first reports on the clinical and prognostic significance of infected pancreatic necrosis, we can now claim that modern diagnostic techniques, thanks mainly to FNA, have achieved an acceptable degree of reliability and safety.

What has still to be clarified in the immediate future is the clinical significance of patients who are contaminated, but not infected; we refer here to those cases in which, though sepsis is not present, FNA yields positive findings. This generally happens in early phases of the disease, almost as if to show that contamination is an early phenomenon followed later, and not necessarily always, by its clinical expression, namely infected necrosis and pancreatic abscess.

References

1. Beger HG, Bittner R, Block S, Büchler M (1986) Bacterial contamination of pancreatic necrosis. Gastroenterology 91: 433–438
2. Gerzof SG, Banks PA, Robbins AH, Johnson WC, Spechler SJ, Wetzner SM, Snicer JM, Langevin RE, Jay ME (1987) Early diagnosis of pancreatic infection by computed tomography-guided aspiration. Gastroenterology 93: 1315–1320
3. Beger HG, Büchler M, Bittner R, Block S, Nevalainen T, Roscher R (1988) Necrosectomy and postoperative local lavage in necrotizing pancreatitis. Br J Surg 75: 207–212
4. Bassi C, Vesentini S, Nifosì F, Girelli R, Falconi M, Elio A, Pederzoli P (1990) Pancreatic abscess and other pus harboring collections related to pancreatitis: a review of 108 cases. World J Surg 14: 505–512
5. Pederzoli P, Bassi C, Vesentini S, Girelli R, Cavallini G, Falconi M et al (1990) Retroperitoneal and peritoneal drainage and lavage in the treatment of severe necrotizing pancreatitis. Surg Gynecol Obstet 170: 197–203
6. Bassi C (1994) Infected pancreatic necrosis. Int J Pancreatol 16: 1–10
7. Bradley, EL (1989) Antibiotics in acute pancreatitis. Am J Surg 158: 472–478
8. Uhl W, Schrag HJ, Wheatley AM, Büchler MW (1995) The role of infection in acute pancreatitis. Dig Surg 11: 214–219
9. Büchler M, Malfertheiner P, Friess H, Isenmann R, Vanel E, Grimm H, Schlegel P, Friess T, Beger HG (1992) Human pancreatic tissue concentration of bactericidal antibiotics. Gastroenterology 103: 1902–1908
10. Bassi C, Pederzoli P, Vesentini S, Falconi M, et al (1994) Behavior of antibiotics in human necrotizing pancreatitis. Antimicrob Ag Chemother 38: 830–836
11. Pederzoli P, Bassi C, Vesentini S, Campedelli A (1993) A randomized multicenter clinical trial of antibiotic prophylaxis of septic complications in acute necrotizing pancreatitis. Surg Gynecol Obstet 176: 480–483
12. Sainio V, Kemppainen E, Puolakkainen P, Taavilsainen M, Kivisaari L, Valtonen V, Haapiainen R, Schröder T, Kivilaakso E (1995) Early antibiotic treatment in acute necrotising pancreatitis. Lancet 346: 633–667
13. Luiten EJT, Hop WCJ, Lanje JF, Bruining HA (1995) Controlled clinical trial of selective decontamination for the treatment of severe acute pancreatitis. Ann Surg 222: 57–65
14. Bradley EL (1993) A clinically based classification system for acute pancreatitis. Arch Surg 128: 586–590
15. Vesentini S, Bassi C, Talamini G, Cavallini G, Campedelli A, Pederzoli P (1993) Prospective comparison of C-reactive protein level, Ranson score and contrast-enhanced computed tomography in the prediction of septic complications of acute pancreatitis. Br J Surg 80: 755–757
16. Malangoni MA, Richardson JD, Shallcross JC, Seiler JG, Polk HC (1986) Factors contributing to fatal outcome after treatment of pancreatic abscess. Ann Surg 203: 605–613
17. Karimgani I, Porter KA, Langevin ER, Banks PA (1992) Prognostic factors in sterile pancreatic necrosis. Gastroenterology 103: 1636–1640
18. Banks PA (1994) Acute pancreatitis: conservative management. Dig Surg 11: 220–225
19. Widdison AL, Karanjia ND (1993) Pancreatic infection complicating acute pancreatitis. Br J Surg 80: 148–154
20. Widdison AL, Karanjia ND, Reber HA (1990) Routes of spread of bacteria to the pancreas in acute necrotizing pancreatitis. Pancreas 5: A736
21. Block S, Büchler M, Beger HG (1987) Sepsis indicators in acute pancreatitis. Pancreas 2: 499–505

Endoscopic Retrograde Cholangiopancreatography in Acute Pancreatitis: Indications and Limitations

P. G. Wilson · J. D. Evans · J. P. Neoptolemos

Introduction

With the developoment of endoscopic techniques for the instrumentation of the biliary tree there has been an explosion in the potential for diagnostic and therapeutic procedures that can be performed. Over the last ten years the indications for intervention using endoscopic retrograde cholangiopancreatography (ERCP) in acute pancreatitis have become gradually more clearly defined in the areas of both diagnosis and treatment. It is recognised, however, that this procedure is not without some degree of risk to the patient with acute pancreatitis and therefore should only be performed by experienced operators in those subjects who are most likely to benefit from endoscopic therapeutic intervention.

Background

It was Eugeine Opie who first recognised the association between acute pancreatitis and gallstones [1] in 1901 when he described a patient who had died of an attack of necrotising pancreatitis and was found to have a gallstone impacted at the ampulla of Vater at necropsy. Opie assumed that there was bile reflux into the pancreas [2] as a result of the impacted stone and this had led to the overwhelming inflammatory reaction he had observed. However postmortem studies over the years [3–5] have demonstrated that the situation described by Opie was uncommon in acute pancreatitis. It was proposed in 1974 that it was infact the gallstone passage through the ampulla of Vater that led to the majority of attacks of acute biliary pancreatitis [6]. At this stage it was unknown whether temporary stone impaction was important or if it was just the passage of a stone that was sufficient to precipitate an attack.

Following this initial investigation and subsequent confirmatory studies [7, 8], it became clear that the larger the number of gallstones that were passed, generally the more severe the attack of pancreatitis. This observation along with Opie's original theory promoted the idea that biliary decompression and stone extraction may be of some benefit in those with acute biliary pancreatitis. Intense discussion took place in the 1970s and 1980s about the need for urgent surgical intervention in these patients. With the publication of prospective randomised studies [9, 10], the picture became clearer. The first study done by Stone [9] was unable to demonstrate a difference between urgent or delayed surgery but there were no predictive criteria of severity applied to the patients. The second study by Kelly [10], however, showed that those with a predicted severe attack of acute pancreatitis did worse with urgent surgery both from the point of view of mortality and morbidity. Thus urgent surgical intervention was abandoned and patients were managed conservatively in the acute phase of the attack.

The first description of endoscopic intervention in 1978 for acute biliary pancreatitis [11] was not well received in view of the recognised complications of ERCP, the most feared of which was acute pancreatitis itself. The first prospectively stratified randomised study of endoscopic sphincterotomy (ES) for acute gallstone pancreatitis reported in 1988 however showed an improved outcome in those with a predicted severe attack of acute pancreatitis [12], thus leading to ERCP gaining acceptance as a tool for management of acute pancreatitis in the acute phase.

Endoscopic Retrograde Cholangiopancreatography and Diagnosis

Detection of Aetiological Factors

The commonest cause of acute pancreatitis in the Western world is gallstones or biliary sludge [13]. If recurrent attacks of acute gallstone pancreatitis are to be prevented then the diagnosis needs to be confirmed and treatment (usually surgical) instituted. Abdominal ultrasound scanning (USS) has a detection rate of greater than 95% for uncomplicated cholelithiasis, but is much lower in acute pancreatitis [14, 15] due to the associated ileus and loops of gas-filled bowel obscuring the view for the ultrasonographer. In addition to this, there is a tendency for smaller gallstones to bring about attacks of acute pancreatitis [16, 17], which means that up to 30% of gallstones leading to acute pancreatitis will be missed [14]. The sensitivity of detection can be increased by a further 10%–20% by measuring the aspartate aminotransferase (AST) or the alanine aminotransferase (ALT). If the AST or ALT are greater than 60 IU/l then an attack of acute pancreatitis is more likely to be due to gallstones (sensitivity, 75%; specificity, 74%) [18].

By far the best way of detecting gallstones in acute pancreatitis is by ERCP [19]. The sensitivity is in excess of 95%, but there is an associated morbidity and mortality [20] and the procedure should not be performed in the acute phase of an attack unless therapeutic intervention is intended.

Because ERCP is not without risk it is important to mention ways in which alcoholic acute pancreatitis may be distinguished from other causes and thus negate the need for expensive, time consuming and sometimes dangerous investigation. It had been suggested by Gumaste et al. that the serum lipase to amylase ratio may distinguish alcoholic from non-alcoholic causes of acute pancreatitis but unfortunately this initial promising study [21] has not been borne out by subsequent investigators [22–24]. A potentially more useful biochemical discriminant is the level of carbohydrate deficient transferrin (CDT). A study performed by Jaakkola et al. in 1995 [24] looked at 86 consecutive patients admitted to hospital with acute pancreatitis. CDT levels were found to correlate significantly with the reported 2-month and 7-day ethanol consumption and was more specific than erythrocyte mean cell volume and the gamma glutamyl transferase. A CDT level of over 17 U/l was found only in those patients with acute alcoholic pancreatitis and the sensitivity of CDT to detect a weekly ethanol consumption of over 560 g was 75 %. This clearly needs to be confirmed by further studies but nonetheless looks very hopeful.

There are many other causes of acute pancreatitis that could be potentially detected by ERCP though the proportion in terms of the overall causes of acute pancreatitis is small. In western countries other endoscopically detectable causes of acute pancreatitis include malignancy [25], pancreas divisum [26, 27] and other anatomical abnormalities such as a bifid pancreatic duct or choledochal cyst [28] and, with the use of biliary manomatory, sphincter of Oddi dysfunction [29, 30]. In Third World countries in addition to these causes, parasites such as ascariasis [31] and clonorchiasis [32] constitute a significant proportion of aetiological agents and can account for upto a quarter of all cases [31].

Pancreatic Duct Integrity

Studies have shown that in clinically mild acute pancreatitis and in servere pancreatitis with less than 50 % necrosis the integrity of the main pancreatic duct (MPD) is maintained though there may some irregularity of the MPD [33, 34]. The MPD becomes disrupted only in those patients with severe pancreatitis and extensive pancreatic necrosis. The disruption may occur at a single site or in particularly severe cases at multiple sites [33, 35]. Disruption of the MPD in the pancreatic head is associated with almost entire parenchymal necrosis whereas if the MPD becomes disrupted in the tail of the gland there seems to be left sided necrosis only [33]. The aetiology does not determine the pattern of MPD damage and disruption [33, 35] which is related more closely to the severity of the disease. How useful an ERP is in this situation is unclear, but in patients with a disrupted MPD studies have suggested that surgical intervention is required [33, 36] and it may therefore be useful in decision making. The site of MPD disruption may refine the surgical technique by determining the extent of debridement in order to ensure that this area of tissue is removed. More studies are obviously required in an attempt to clarify the role of ERCP in this situation.

Preoperative Assessment

For determining the anatomy prior to surgery ERCP is not only useful but in certain situations may be essential. Anatomical communications between the pancreatic duct and pseudocysts (which can occur in up to 50 % of cases [37]) may be detectable and the ERCP will therefore demonstrate those who are going to be inadequately managed by drainage of the cyst alone. Preoperative ERCP in this situation also allows for the insertion of a pancreatic stent should one be required.

Patients who have suffered an attack of acute gallstone pancreatitis should undergo a cholecystectomy on the same admission as there is a 30%–40% risk of a further attack [8, 38]. In many centres until a few years ago the majority of patients in whom a laparoscopic cholecystectomy was to be performed would have had a preoperative ERCP to ensure that the bile duct was clear of stones. However this meant that a large number of patients were having an unnecessary procedure and it did not negate the need for intraoperative biliary imaging as gallstones could still migrate into the main bile duct (MBD) between the time of ERCP and surgery.

A more efficient method of coping with the possibility of MBD stones is to select those with a high probability of MBD stones for preoperative ERCP. This can be done on the basis of clinical, biochemical and ultrasound findings [39, 40]. Patients with a high probability of MBD stones are those with cholangitis, obstructive jaundice, persistent hyperamylasaemia or MBD stones on USS. The rate of unnecessary preoperative ERCPs can be reduced to less than 10% by careful selection of the patients [40]. If intraoperative imaging demonstrates the presence of MBD stones then they can be removed at the time of surgery or by means of postoperative ERCP and ES prior to the patients discharge form hospital. The particular technique chosen depends on local expertise but at the present time the latter procedure seems to be the most popular.

Therapeutic Endoscopic Retrograde Cholangiopancreatography

One of the great advantages of ERCP is that it offers the opportunity not only to determine the cause of an attack of pancreatitis but also to undertake therapeutic manoeuvres should they be indicated. There has over the last ten years or so been an increasing body of evidence supporting the rationale for endoscopic intervention and biliary decompression in patients with gallstone acute pancreatitis. It has been shown that the passage of an MBD stone can cause the biliopancreatic duct to behave as a common channel [41, 42] presumably by causing a functional stenosis of the ampulla of Vater. One study [41] examined 21 patients who had undergone open cholecystectomy, common bile duct exploration and insertion of a T tube. The patients were divided into three groups, namely, those with gallstones alone, those with gallstones and MBD stones and those with gallstone acute pancreatitis. The T-tube fluid from those with acute pancreatitis had an elevated resting and elevated stimulated amylase activity. In addition to this interesting finding there was a high level of inactive trypsinogen and no activated duodenal brush border trypsin in those with recent attacks of acute biliary pancreatitis. This tells us that in these patients there had been direct reflux of pancreatic juice along a common channel as opposed to the regurgitation of pancreatic juice from the duodenum. There was no brush border trypsin and negligible amounts of trypsinogen in the other two groups.

Of course this does not directly indicate that reflux of bile up the pancreatic duct is the cause of biliary pancreatitis but it demonstrates very nicely that a common channel situation can arise and that duodenal contents do not reflux into the biliary tree in significant amounts in this group of patients. It is possible however that the pressure in the biliary tree can sometimes exceed that in the pancreatic duct (for example, when there is contraction of the gallbladder) and thus bile may reflux into the pancreatic duct which can lead to in situ activation of trypsinogen [43].

Further evidence that decompression of the biliary tree may be of benefit in acute gallstone pancreatitis comes from Steer's group which showed that decompression of the biliary tree in the opossum model of acute pancreatitis was associated with a more favourable outcome [44]. They induced haemorrhagic acute pancreatitis in the opossum using a balloon catheter to obstruct the MPD and demonstrated that by letting the ballon down and relieving the MPD obstruction that the progression of the pancreatitis was arrested. Hirano and Manabe have shown that the outcome in pancreatitis induced in rats is more severe if the MPD is repeatedly obstructed [45], giving support to the observation that the more gallstones a patient passes the more severe an attack of pancreatitis they will suffer.

Acute Attack

The experimental and observational work described above lends support to the theoretical reasons why ERCP and MBD clearance and decompression should be undertaken in acute gallstone induced pancreatitis. To date, there have been four randomised trials into the effects of urgent ERCP and ES in acute gallstone induced pancreatitis. The first of these was done in 1988 in Leicester [12]. This trial reported on 121 patients who were prospectively stratified for severity according to modified Glasgow criteria and *then* randomised to undergo ERCP (and ES if stones were present in the bile duct) within 72 h or conservative treatment only (ERCP prohibited for at least 5 days). The outcome was the same in those patients with predicted mild attacks (morbidity, 12 %; mortality, 0 %), but was significantly improved when urgent ES was performed in those with a predicted severe attack (morbidity, 24 % vs. 61 %; mortality, 1.7 % vs. 18 %; $p < 0.0001$). A total of 63 % of patients in the severe group who underwent ERCP had ES for confirmed MBD stones. It has been suggested that the benefits observed were due to relief of concomitant cholangitis but if those patients are excluded from the analysis there is still a pronounced benefit in severe cases. Furthermore median hospital stay was reduced from 17 days in the conservatively managed group to 9.5 days in the urgent ERCP and ES group.

The second trial from Katowice in Poland [46, 47] looked at 250 patients undergoing ERCP within 24 h of admission, though the patients were mainly tertiary referrals and the mean time of delay was 3.5 days between the onset of symptoms and endoscopic intervention. All patients with ampullary appearances suggestive of an impacted stone had ES performed ($n = 62$) and the remaining 188 patients were randomised to undergo ES or conventional treatment (no prospective stratification for severity was done). Patients significantly benefited from ES (morbidity, 14 % vs. 34 %; mortality, 1 % vs. 11 %) even though there was a delay from onset of symptoms to the time of ES.

In the third trial from Hong Kong [48], 195 patients were randomised to ERCP with or without ES within 24 h of admission. The only benefit demonstrated by this study was a reduction in biliary sepsis in those undergoing urgent ERCP and ES (0% vs. 12%). However their severity assessment was derived from the blood glucose and urea measurements which was based on previous work done by this group [49]. It has been subsequently shown that this method of assessment is inadequate when compared to the Ranson and Glasgow methods of scoring [50]. In fact, patients were not stratified prior to randomisation and when it came to the ERCP only 127 patients actually had gallstones, the remainder having other diagnoses. If this group of non-gallstone patients are excluded from analysis then the results are similar to those of the Leicester group.

The fourth study performed in Germany was a multicentre study [51]. Patients were randomised to ERCP and ES within 72 h of admission or to conventional treatment. Jaundiced patients all underwent urgent ERCP and ES and were thus excluded form the study, which is important as those with a bilirubin of greater than 40 μmol/l are those most likely to have MBD stones and thus have the greatest benefit from endoscopic intervention. The patients were not prospectively stratified for severity (which was determined retrospectively) and there were some patients in each group in whom the predicted severity was "undefined". Equal numbers of patients in each group ($n = 11$) developed cholangitis, which suggests that the quality of ES and biliary drainage, at least in some of the centres, was inadequate. These shortcomings in study design may explain why there was no demonstrable benefit.

Endoscopic Stent Placement

Stent placement into the biliary tree has for many years been a standard treatment for certain types of stricture and also for the decompression of the biliary tree when sepsis is a problem. Only more recently has the concept of pancreatic duct stenting become popular. The requirement for this in the setting of acute pancreatitis is fairly limited but nonetheless there are some applications. There is still much debate about whether pancreas divisum can give rise to acute pancreatitis but recently there is an increasing body of evidence suggesting it can be a cause [26, 27, 52]. The most convincing evidence comes from a recent prospective randomised controlled trial [27]. This showed that in those with an endoscopic endoprosthesis placed across the minor papilla subsequently had significantly less attendance with episodes of pain to the emergency room than controls ($p < 0.05$). In addition, there were significantly less documented episodes of acute pancreatitis in the stented group ($p < 0.05$), suggesting that this is a useful treatment for this small group of patients.

Patients with pseudocysts as a result of acute pancreatitis often present something of a management problem. There is increasing interest in treating the complications of acute pancreatitis endoscopically [53–56], either instead of or as an adjunct to surgery. It has been shown by Barthet et al. [56] that in some patients insertion of a stent into the pancreatic duct may be sufficient to bring about resolution of the pseudocyst and obviate the requirement for surgery. Clearly, the pseudocyst needs to be communicating with the pancreatic duct for this to be effective and more studies are required to determine with greater accuracy which patients are going to benefit from endoscopic stenting alone.

There is also anecdotal evidence in the literature that stenting across a disrupted MPD may promote the resolution of pancreatic ascites and pleural effusion [55]. Again, this needs further evaluation, but is an exciting development in the area of endoscopic management of these patients.

Endoscopic Sphincterotomy with Gallbladder In Situ

There are going to be a small number of patients, predominantly the elderly who, due to co-morbidity, will be unfit for either open or laparoscopic cholecystectomy. However these patients are still at considerable risk of a further attack of pancreatitis and because of their other medical problems will not cope as well as those younger and fitter patients. Clearly, these patients need something done to try and prevent further attacks. ERCP with ES in this group of patients has been shown to be very succesful [57]. In fact, if there is a further attack of pancreatitis it usually means that the sphincterotomy has stenosed and this can be enlarged by repeat ES. However, these patients are at risk of gallbladder-related complications of up to 20 %, and there is a mortality rate associated with this [58]. For that reason, all patients should have a cholecystectomy performed if at all possible.

Conclusions

The role of endoscopic intervention in the setting of acute pancreatitis is now becoming more clearly defined. Indeed there is now a large experience with 20 worldwide trials for ERCP and ES in acute biliary pancreatitis. Urgent ERCP and ES is now gaining acceptance and is of particular benefit in those with concomitant cholangitis. It is inappropriate based on current levels of knowledge to subject those with a predicted mild attack to ERCP and ES but those with a severe attack of gallstone-induced pancreatitis should have an ERCP if local expertise is available. The Leicester, Hong Kong and Katowice studies showed a reduction in both local and systemic complications in those severe patients who underwent ERCP and ES.

The role of therapeutic ERCP is still predominantly limited to those who have acute pancreatitis induced by gallstones but evidence is growing for those with sphincter of Oddi dysfunction or anatomical abnormalities causing recurrent acute pancreatitis. There is also the exciting prospect that a certain subgroup of patients with complications of acute pancreatitis may benefit from therapeutic endoscopic intervention, but this needs further clarification through clinical trials. It should be remembered, however, that ERCP may exacerbate an attack of pancreatitis and thus should only be performed in the acute phase of an attack if there is indication and intent to undertake therapeutic intervention.

Patients who have recurrent attacks of acute pancreatitis though there is no ultrasound evidence of gallstones should have an ERCP to rule out microlithiasis once the acute attack has subsided. In addition, ERCP will give information about other causes, such as pancreas divisum, small pancreatic tumours, choledochocele and sphincter of Oddi dysfunction.

ERCP now is getting a much more clearly defined role prior to laparoscopic surgery and should be performed in those patients who have a high probability of MBD stones. ERCP may be required postoperatively to extract stones from the MDB that have been discovered by intraoperative imaging. In addition, ERCP and ES is indicated in those with gallstone-induced pancreatitis who are not fit enough to have a cholecystectomy, but there are limitations to this procedure, and the gallbladder should be removed if possible.

References

1. Opie EL (1901) The relation of cholelithiasis to disease of the pancreas and to fat necrosis. American Journal of the Medical Sciences 121: 27–43
2. Opie EL (1901) The etiology of acute haemorrhagic pancreatitis. Bulletin of the Johns Hopkins Hospital 121: 182–8
3. Bell ET (1958) Pancreatitis: a study of 179 fatal cases. Surgery 43: 527–37
4. Shader AE, Paxton JR (1966) Fatal Pancreatitis. American Journal of Surgery 111: 369–73
5. Storck G, Pettersson G, Edlund Y (1976) A study of autopsies upon 116 patients with acute pancreatitis. Surgery Gynecology and Obstetrics 143: 241–5
6. Acosta JL, Ledesma CL (1974) Gallstone migration as a cause for acute pancreatitis. New England Journal of Medicine 190: 484–7
7. Kelly TR (1976) Gallstone pancreatitis: pathophysiology. Surgery 80: 88–92
8. Kelly TR (1980) Gallstone pancreatitis: The timing of surgery. Surgery 88: 345–9
9. Stone HH, Fabian TC, Dunlop WE (1981) Gallstone pancreatitis: biliary tract pathology in relation to time of operation. Annals of Surgery 194: 305–10
10. Kelly TR, Wagner DS (1988) Gallstone pancreatitis: a prospective randomised trial of timing of surgery. Surgery 104: 600–5
11. Classen M, Ossenberg W, Wurbs D, Dammermann R, Hagenmuller F (1978) Pancreatitis – an indication for endoscopic papillotomy? Endoscopy 10: 223 (Abstract)
12. Neoptolemos JP, London NJ, James D, Carr-Locke DL, Bailey IA, Fossard DP (1988) Controlled trial of urgent endoscopic retrograde cholangiopancreatography and endoscopic sphincterotomy versus conservative treatment for acute pancreatitis due to gallstones. Lancet ii: 979–83
13. Corfield AP, Cooper MJ, Williamson RCN (1985) Acute pancreatitis: a lethal disease of increasing incidence. Gut 26: 724–9
14. Neoptolemos JP, Hall A, Finlay DF, Berry JM, Carr-Locke DL, Fossard DP (1984) The urgent diagnosis of gallstones in acute pancreatitis: a prospective study of the methods. British Journal of Surgery 71: 230–47
15. Wang SS, Lin XZ, Tsai YT, Lee S, Pan HB, Chou YH, Su CH, Lee C, Shiesn SC, Lin CY, et al (1988) Clinical significance of ultrasonography, computed tomography, and biochemical tests in the rapid diagnosis of gallstone-related pancreatitis: a prospective study. Pancreas 3: 153–8
16. Houssin D, Castain GD, Lemoine J, Bismuth H (1983) Microlithiasis of the gallbladder. Surgery, Gynecology and Obstetrics 157: 20–40
17. Farinon AM, Sianesi M and Zannella E (1987) Physiopathological role of microlithiasis in gallstone pancreatitis. Surgery Gynecology and Obstetrics 164: 252–6
18. Davidson BR, Neoptolemos JP, Leese T, Carr-Locke DL (1988) Biochemical prediction of gallstones in acute pancreatitis: a prospective study of three systems. British Journal of Surgery 75: 213–5
19. Neoptolemos JP, Carr-Locke DL, London N, Bailey I, Fossard DP (1988) ERCP findings and the role of endoscopic sphincterotomy in acute gallstone pancreatitis. British Journal of Surgery 75: 954–60

20. Ostroff JW, Shapiro HA (1989) Complications of endoscopic sphincterotomy. ERCP: Diagnostic and Therapeutic Applications, ed. I. Jacobsen. Elsevier: New York. 61-73
21. Gumaste VV, Dave PB, Waissman D, Messer J (1991) Lipase/amylase ratio. A new index that distinguishes acute episodes of alcoholic from nonalcoholic acute pancreatitis. Gastroenterology 101: 1361-6
22. Pezzilli R, Billi P, Migliola M, Gullo L (1993) Serum amylase and lipase concentrations and lipase/amylase ratio in assessment of etiology and severity of acute pancreatitis. Digestive Disease and Science 38: 1265-9
23. Sadowski DC, Todd JK, Sutherland LR (1993) Biochemical models as early predictors of the etiology of acute pancreatitis. Digestive Disease and Science 38: 637-43
24. Jaakkola M, Sillanaukee P, Lof K, Koivula T, Nordback I (1994) Blood tests for detection of alcoholic cause of acute pancreatitis. Lancet 343: 1328-9
25. Lin A, Feller ER (1990) Pancreatic carcinoma as a cause of unexplained pancreatitis: report of ten cases. Annals of Internal Medicine 113: 166-7
26. Bernard JP, Sahel J, Giovannini M, Sarles H (1990) Pancreas divisum is a probable cause of acute pancreatitis: a report of 137 cases. Pancreas 5: 248-54
27. Lans JI, Geenen JE, Johansen JF, Hogan WJ (1992) Endoscopic therapy in patients with pancreas divisum and acute pancreatitis: a prospective, randomized, controlled clinical trial. Gastrointestinal Endoscopy 38: 430-4
28. Goldberg PB, Long WB, Oleaga JA, Mackie JA (1980) Choledochocele as a cause of recurrent pancreatitis. Gastroenterology 78: 1041-5
29. Venu RP, Geenen JE, Hogan W, Stone J, Johnson GK, Soergel K (1989) Idiopathic reccurent pancreatitis: an approach to diagnosis and treatment. Digestive Diseases and Science 34: 56-60
30. LeBovics E, Heier SK, Rosenthaw B (1986) Sphincter of Oddi motility: developments in physiology and clinical application. American Journal of Gastroenterology 81: 736-43
31. Khuroo MS, Zargar SA, Yattoo GN, Koul P, Khan BA, Dar MY, Alai MS (1992) Ascaris-induced pancreatitis. British Journal of Surgery 79: 1335-8
32. Lee MJ, Choi TK, Lai EC, Wong KP, Ngan H, Wong J (1986) Endoscopic retrograde cholangiopancreatography after acute pancreatitis. Surgery, Gynecology and Obstetrics 163: 354-8
33. Neoptolemos JP, London NJM, Carr-Locke DL (1993) Assessment of main pancreatic duct integrity by endoscopic retrograde pancreatography in patients with acute pancreatitis. British Journal of Surgery 80: 94-9
34. Gebhardt CH, Biemann JF, Lux G (1983) The importance of ERCP for the surgical tactic in haemorrhagic pancreatitis (preliminary report). Endoscopy 15: 55-8
35. Von Brambs HJ (1991) Endoskopische retrograde Pankreatographie (ERP) bei akuter alkoholischer und biliarer Pankreatitis. Fortsch Roentgenstr 154: 509-13
36. Gebhardt CH, Kraus D, Schonekas H, Muschweck H (1989) Frueh-ERCP bei akuter Pankreatitis. Leber Magen Darm 3: 125-38
37. Nealon WH, Townsend CM, Thompson JC (1989) Preoperative endoscopic retrograde cholangiopancreatography (ERCP) in patients with pancreatic pseudocyst associated with resolving acute and chronic pancreatitis. Annals of Surgery 209: 532-40
38. Osborne DH, Imrie CW and Carter DC (1981) Biliary surgery in the same admission for gallstone-associated acute pancreatitis. British Journal of Surgery 68: 758-61
39. de Virgilio C, Verbin C, Chang L, Linder S, Stabile BE, Klein S (1994) Gallstone pancreatitis: the role of preoperative endoscopic retrograde cholangiopancreatography. Archives of Surgery 129: 909-13
40. Rijna H, Borgstein PJ, Meuwissen SGM, de Brauw LM, Wildenborg NP, Cuesta MA (1995) Selective preoperative endoscopic retrograde cholangiopancreatography in laparoscopic biliary surgery. British Journal of Surgery 82: 1130-3
41. Hernandez CA, Lerch MM (1994) Sphincter stenosis and gallstone migration through the biliary tract 341: 1371-3
42. Lerch MM, Weidenbach H, Hernandez CA, Preclik G, Adler G (1994) Pancreatic outflow obstruction as the critical event for human gallstone induced pancreatitis. Gut 35: 1501-3
43. Sarkany RPE, Moreland BH (1985) Enhancement of the autocatalytic activation of trypsinogen to trypsin by bile and bile acids. Biochemica et Biophysica Acta 839: 262-7
44. Runzi M, Saluja A, Lerch MM, Dawra R, Nishino H, Steer ML (1993) Early ductal decompression prevents the progression of biliary pancreatitis: an experimental study in the opossum. Gastroenterology 105: 157-64

45. Hirano T, Manabe T (1993) A possible mechanism for gallstone pancreatitis: repeated short-term pancreaticobiliary duct obstruction with exocrine stimulation in rats. Proceedings of the Society for Experimental Biology and Medicine 202: 246–52
46. Nowak A, Nowakowska-Duzawa E, Rybicka J (1990) Urgent endoscopic sphincterotomy vs conservative treatment in acute biliary pancreatitis-a prospective, controlled trial. Hepato-Gastroenterology 37 ((Suppl II)): A5 (Abstract)
47. Nowak A, Nowakowska-Dulaw E, Marek TA, Rybicka J (1995) Final results of the prospective, randomized, controlled study on endoscopic sphincterotomy versus conventional treatment in acute biliary pancreatitis. Gastroenterology 108: A380 (Abstract).
48. Fan ST, Lai CS, Mok FPT, Lo CM, Rheng SS, Wong J (1993) Early treatment of acute biliary pancreatitis by endoscopic papillotomy. New England Journal of Medicine 328: 228–32
49. Fan ST, Choi TK, Lai ECS, Wong J (1989) Prediction of severity of acute pancreatitis: an alternative approach. Gut 30: 1591–5
50. Heath DI, Imrie CW (1994) The Hong Kong criteria and severity prediction in acute pancreatitis. International Journal of Pancreatology 15: 179–85
51. Folsch UR, Nitsche R, Ludtke R, Hilgers RA, Creutzfeldt W, et al (1995) Controlled randomised multicentre tial of urgent endoscopic papillotomy for acute biliary pancreatitis. Gastroenterology
52. Kozarek RA, Ball TJ, Patterson DJ, Brandabur JJ, Raltz SL (1995) Endoscopic approach to pancreas divisum. Digestive Diseases and Sciences 40: 1974–81
53. Kozarek RA, Patterson DJ, Ball TJ, Traverso LW (1989) Endoscopic placement of pancreatic stents and drains in the management of pancreatitis. Annals of Surgery 209: 261–6
54. Kozarek RA, Ball TJ, Patterson DJ, Freeny PC, Ryan JA, Traverso LW (1991) Endoscopic transpapillary therapy for disrupted pancreatic duct and peripancreatic fluid collections. Gastroenterology 100: 1362–70
55. Kochhar R, Goenka MK, Nagi B, Singh K (1995) Pancreatic ascites and pleural effusion treated by endoscopic pancreatic stent placement. Indian Journal of Gastroenterology 14: 106–7
56. Barthet M, Sahel J, Bodiou-Bertei C, Bernard JP (1995) Endoscopic transpapillary drainage of pancreatic pseudocysts. Gastrointestinal Endoscopy 42: 208–13
57. Welbourn, CRB, Beckly DE, Eyre-Brook IA (1995) Endoscopic sphincterotomy without cholecystectomy for gallstone pancreatitis. Gut 37: 119–20
58. Winslet MC, Neoptolemos JP (1991) The place of endoscopy in the management of gallstones. Clinics in Gastroenterology 5: 99–129

II
Functional Methods

Appropriate Use of Serum Pancreatic Enzymes for the Diagnosis of Acute Pancreatitis

F. Carballo · J. E. Domínguez-Muñoz

Introduction

The aim of this chapter is to discuss the progress in the biological diagnosis of acute pancreatitis that has been made over the last 10 years. Although many important contributions have been reported on this topic during this time, major problems remain. In order to discuss these unresolved problems, this article begins with a description of the clinical setting in which acute pancreatitis is usually diagnosed. In this way, the concept of degree of clinical suspicion for the disease will be defined. Thereafter, the main concepts for the evaluation of diagnostic tests will be discussed.

Diagnostic Process

A first consideration for the study of tests to be applied in the diagnosis of acute pancreatitis is the definition of the setting in which the diagnosis is made. Biochemical methods are an appropriate first step for the diagnosis of acute pancreatitis, since increased serum levels of pancreatic enzymes are included in the definition of acute pancreatitis according to the Revised Marseille Classification [1]. However, a clinical suspicion of the disease is required before biological diagnostic methods are applied. The clinical suspicion of acute pancreatitis is based on the presence of acute abdominal pain. If the acute episode is painless or the patient is unable to express symptoms, the clinician will not suspect acute pancreatitis and will not request any enzyme determination. In these circumstances, diagnosis of acute pancreatitis fails, although pancreatitis is in fact present. In relation to this description, the clinical setting in which pancreatic enzymes play a role is the examination of a patient with acute abdominal pain. In the absence of this typical presentation, a high degree of clinical suspicion of the disease is the key to a correct diagnosis. An important question is currently whether the degree of clinical suspicion is similar in different patients in the presence of a typical clinical picture. The answer is clearly no, because clinical suspicion does not only depend on symptoms. Patient characteristics and presence of associated factors, such as alcohol consumption or gallstone disease, are important complementary information for the diagnosis. In this context, it is important to note the need for a high degree of clinical expertise in arriving at a clinical suspicion of acute pancreatitis.

In summary, the clinician suspects the presence of acute pancreatitis, according to a reasoning that is not always evident. He or she establishes a subjective probability of disease before applying any diagnostic test. This pre-test probability is not usually quantified, but its measurement is indispensable to appropriately evaluate the impact of tests, thus changing the probability of disease.

With the aim of obtaining an objective measure of the pre-test probability of acute pancreatitis, our team performed a study based on a prospective series of 285 consecutive diagnostic evaluations in the emergency unit. Acute pancreatitis was suspected in all the patients studied. The criterium to include a patient in the study was the blind request from the clinician to determine serum amylase. Acute pancreatitis was finally confirmed in 47 % of the patients. Consequently, we can consider 50 % to be a good estimation of the pre-test probability. This probability refers to the habitual setting of the diagnostic process for acute pancreatitis and represents the incidence of acute pancreatitis among patients in whom the disease is suspected in the described setting.

When pancreatic enzymes are used to diagnose acute pancreatitis, the clinician tries to change the pre-test probability to a higher one, the post-test probability of disease. A perfect test is defined by post-test probability of 100 % when the result is positive together with a post-test probability of 0 % for a negative result. The post-test probability of disease depends on the quality of the test in terms of sensitivity and specificity, but also on the pre-test probability.

To assess the quality of different tests, well-designed studies should be performed. Most published data about the sensitivity and specificity of pancreatic enzymes for the diagnosis of acute pancreatitis were obtained from studies that were not adequately designed. Some useful rules should be applied in the design of diagnostic studies:

- The study must be done in the same clinical setting in which the evaluated test will be further applied; this includes the analysis of the whole spectrum of the disease.
- It is important to avoid the inclusion of only patients with certain special characteristics, since the results obtained will be only applicable to this special group of subjects.
- Recruitment of patients must be correct. Patients must be included either consecutively or by random sampling. Controls should be identical to patients except for the absence of the disease. Ideally, controls should be patients with abdominal pain in whom acute pancreatitis is suspected, but in whom a different final diagnosis is made.
- Tests must be always evaluated by applying their best cutoff points.
- Finally, as previously remarked, a clear definition of the pre-test and post-test probabilities of disease is very important for the clinical application of a test.

Selection of Enzymatic Diagnostic Tests

Determination of serum amylase is the most frequently used test for the biological diagnosis of acute pancreatitis. Even though it is used worldwide in clinical practice, this test is not a perfect gold standard, since it is not organ specific. In addition, serum amylase activity can be normal in some patients with acute alcoholic pancreatitis and in patients examined too late after onset. However, if the optimal cutoff point for amylase is applied and the patient is evaluated in the habitual clinical setting, amylase can be an excellent test [2]. In our experience, the optimal cutoff point for amylase estimated by ROC curves is twice the upper limit of normal. With this cutoff point, serum amylase shows a very good sensitivity (91%) and specificity (96%) for the diagnosis of acute pancreatitis. Thus the probability of disease for a positive results is very high, changing from a pre-test probability of 50% to a post-test one of 95%. In addition, the post-test probability of disease for a negative result (less than twice the upper limit of normal) is only 9% also starting out from a pre-test probability of 50%. If the normal upper limit is applied as the cutoff point, the sensitivity of serum amylase for the diagnosis of acute pancreatitis is logically high (96%), but the specificity is very low (60%).

Lipase is more pancreas specific than amylase, although other organs such as the stomach are also able to synthesize it. Determination of serum lipase has, however, some methodological problems, including limited reproducibility and high interassay variability [3]. Rapid determination of pancreatic isoamylase is based on a selective inhibition of S-isoamylase. This test can be applied in the emergency setting and is very useful for the differential diagnosis of hyperamylasemia. The fraction P3 of amylase, which physiologically is not present in blood, appears to be a very sensitive and specific parameter for the diagnosis of acute pancreatitis [4]. Determination of P3 amylase is, however, based on gel agarose electrophoresis, which cannot be applied in the emergency room. Amylase electrophoresis is especially useful for the differential diagnosis of hyperamylasemia, including macroamylasemia.

With the aim of evaluating the most appropriate serum pancreatic enzyme for the diagnosis of acute pancreatitis, our group performed a prospective comparative study by determining serum amylase, lipase, and P-isoamylase. All rules mentioned above were taken into account [5]. Patients and controls were 300 consecutive patients coming to the emergency unit in whom acute pancreatitis was suspected. A pre-test probability of disease of 50% was considered according to the results shown above. Table 1 shows the resulting sensitivity, specificity, and post-test probability of disease for positive and negative test results. The best figures for positive test results are obtained with amylase and P-isoamylase, and for negative test results with lipase. However, differences among tests are not significant, and figures obtained with all tests are in fact very similar. Therefore, all tests are adequate for the diagnosis of acute pancreatitis, and the choice will depend on local availability.

Obviously, other possibilities for the biological diagnosis of acute pancreatitis can be considered. Thus Le Moine published very good results with trypsin activity [6]. The practical application of these results is the diagnosis of alco-

Table 1. Sensitivity, specificity, and post-test probabilities of three different biological methods for the diagnosis of acute pancreatitis [5]

Method	Sensitivity (%)	Specificity (%)	Post-test probability (%) Positive	Negative
Amylase	91	95	95	9
P-Amylase	92	95	95	7
Lipase	98	88	89	2

holic pancreatitis, including patients with low levels of amylase. A second example is the determination of pancreas-specific protein (PSP). Cheng reported a very high specificity for PSP in the diagnosis of acute pancreatitis, with a sensitivity of 100% [7]. However, it should be remarked that Cheng also obtained very good results for amylase.

We conclude with the title of the Steinberg's paper published in 1985 [8]: "Amylase, the king, is dead. Long live amylase." Amylase can still be used today. Its determination is easy, cheap, and generally available, and its limitations are very well known. If amylase cannot provide a good result in a specific setting, another diagnostic strategy should be used, including new enzymatic determinations (P-amylase, lipase) and morphological methods. Nevertheless, between biological diagnosis and the final diagnosis of acute pancreatitis, clinical expertise is indispensable.

References

1. Gyr KE, Singer MV, Sarles H (eds) Revised classification of pancreatitis – Marseille 1984: proceedings of the second international symposium on the classification of pancreatitis. Excerpta Med Int Congr Ser 624: xxiii
2. Steinberg WM, Goldstein SS, Davis ND, Shamma's J, Anderson K (1985) Diagnostic assays in acute pancreatitis – a study of sensitivity and specificity. Ann Intern Med 102: 576–580
3. Lessinger JM, Ferard G (1994) Plasma pancreatic lipase activity: from analytical specificity to clinical efficiency for the diagnosis of acute pancreatitis. Eur J Clin Chem Clin Biochem 32: 377–381
4. Leclerc P, Forest JC (1983) Variations in amylase isoenzymes and lipase during acute pancreatitis, and in other disorders causing hyperamylasemia. Clin Chem 29: 1020–1023
5. Carballo F, Domínguez E, García A, García J, De la Morena J (1988) Diagnosis of acute pancreatitis: comparative study of enzymatic test. Gastroenterol Int 1: 670
6. Le Moine O, Devaster JM, Deviere J, Thiry P, Cremer O, Ooms HA (1994) Trypsin activity. A new marker of acute alcoholic pancreatitis. Dig Dis Sci 39: 2634–2638
7. Chen CC, Wang SS, Chao Y et al (1994) Serum pancreas-specific protein in acute pancreatitis. Its clinical utility in comparison with serum amylase. Scand J Gastroenterol 29: 87–90
8. Steinberg WM (1985) Amylase (the King) is dead: long live amylase. Arch Pathol Lab Med 109: 973–974

Identification of the Etiological Factor in Acute Pancreatitis

H.-U. Schulz

Introduction

Nearly 100 years ago, Opie [1] described gallstones impacted in the ampulla of Vater as a cause of acute pancreatitis under circumstances of a common channel formed by the common bile duct and the duct of Wirsung. In the same year, Halsted [2] suggested that retrojection of bile into the pancreas was the underlying pathophysiological event linking preampullary gallstone lodgement with consecutive acute pancreatitis. It was only during the past few decades that it became clear that biliary lithiasis and microlithiasis are responsible for about half of all cases of the disease [3–6]. Alcoholism is another major etiological factor in acute pancreatitis [7–9]. Taken together, biliary tract disease and alcoholism account for about 80% of pancreatitis etiologies in Western countries (Table 1). In contrast, other causes such as drugs, hyperparathyroidism, pregnancy, and scorpion stings are rare [7]. Acute pancreatitis following diagnostic or therapeutic procedures is increasingly observed [10–15].

Since it became apparent nearly 10 years ago that early endoscopic retrograde cholangiopancreatography (ERCP) and sphincterotomy may cure gallstone pancreatitis [16, 17], the reliable identification of those patients who have gallstone pancreatitis was and continues to be increasingly important. Several methods have been proposed for the identification of the etiological factor in acute pancreatitis. Biochemical markers of biliary tract disease [18–22] and of alcoholism [23–25], imaging procedures of the biliary tree [26–28], duodenal bile crystal analysis [29], and combinations of all of the above [30–32] can be applied for this purpose.

Table 1. Etiological factors causing acute pancreatitis

Factor	Percentage
Biliary Tract Disease	20–80
Alcoholism	20–60
Post-ERCP	1–15
Postoperative	1–10
Others	1– 5

ERCP, endoscopic retrograde cholangiopancreatography.

Biochemical Markers

Many markers have been described to distinguish biliary from nonbiliary pancreatitis biochemically. However, the rapidity of changes in these biochemical markers make frequent serial testing imperative for an accurate diagnosis [22]. Since in most studies the markers were determined only once or twice daily, much controversy exists concerning sensitivity, specificity, positive and negative predictive values, and the best cutoff for each of the parameters. This dilemma has not yet been resolved, even by combinations of markers. Kazmierczak et al. [22] recently stated that a distinction must be made between admission and peak values of the biochemical markers. This holds true for markers of both biliary tract disease and alcoholism.

Biochemical Markers of Biliary Tract Disease

To identify biliary tract disease as the cause of acute pancreatitis, several serum markers have been proposed [18–22, 33]. These include pancreatic enzymes such as amylase and lipase, liver enzymes such as alanine aminotransferase (ALT; also called ALAT and glutamic-pyruvic transaminase GPT) and aspartate aminotransferase (AST; also called ASAT and glutamine-oxaloacetic transaminase, GOT), as well as the classical markers of cholestasis, bilirubin, alkaline phosphatase (ALP, AP), and gamma glutamyl transferase (γ-GT). Due to the frequently long interval between onset of pain and admission of patients to hospital, the rapidity of changes of serum levels in these biochemical parameters, and the infrequent sampling of blood, all these markers are far from perfect. In a recent meta-analysis, Tenner et al. [21] found that ALT is the best individual marker of biliary tract disease in acute pancreatitis, with a positive predictive value of 95% in cases of threefold or higher elevated levels. AST is described as being nearly equivalent to ALT, whereas ALP and amylase are of lesser and bilirubin, lipase, and γ-GT are of limited value [21–23]. Because of observations that patients with gallstone pancreatitis had high serum amylase levels, whereas patients with alcoholic pancreatitis had high serum lipase levels, the ratio of lipase to amylase was introduced to discriminate between acute episodes of biliary and alcoholic pancreatitis [34]. At a cutoff of 3, this ratio reliably distinguished between biliary and nonbiliary causes of pancreatitis and was nearly as good a marker as ALT [22]. The clinical utility of the lipase to amylase (L/A) ratio is still under investigation, however, as some investigators have found this measure not useful for establishing the etiology of acute pancreatitis [19, 20, 35–37]. In a recent review, Gumaste [38] stated that:

(a) a L/A ratio of less than 2 is unlikely to indicate acute alcoholic pancreatitis;
(b) a high ratio ($>$ 3) is highly suggestive of acute alcoholic pancreatitis; and
(c) a ratio between 2 and 3 appears to be a grey zone of nonspecificity.

The recent data from the literature concerning the clinical utility of biochemical markers of biliary tract disease in acute pancreatitis are summarized in Table 2.

Table 2. Biochemical markers indicative of biliary cause of acute pancreatitis

Marker	Value
Peak ALT	> 150 U/l
AST	> 100 U/l
Peak L/A ratio	< 2
Admission L/A ratio	< 2
Alkaline phosphatase	> 300 U/l
Serum amylase	> 4000 U/l
(Bilirubin, γ-GT)	

The order in the table represents a rank order of clinical utility of these parameters [19, 21–23, 38].
Alt, alanine aminotransferase; AST, aspartate aminotransferase; L/A, lipase–amylase; γ-GT, gamma glutamyl transferase.

Biochemical Markers of Alcoholism

As for biliary tract disease, many biochemical markers have been described for the identification of alcoholism (Table 3). Traditionally, the erythrocyte mean corpuscular volume (MCV), serum γ-GT, and the AST/ALT ratio are used for this purpose [39]. These latter parameters are characterized by a sensitivity ranging from only 20% to 80% and a specificity of 85%–95% [39]. A better marker seems to be the admission serum trypsin activity. At a cutoff of 150 U/l, there was no overlap between patients with alcoholic pancreatitis (range, 165–853 U/l), nonalcoholic pancreatitis (range, 42–98 U/l), alcoholic controls (range, 40–122 U/l), and healthy controls (range, 15–143 U/l) [25]. The small number of patients included in this study ($n = 32$) requires confirmation of these interesting results in a greater trial, however. As already mentioned, an L/A ratio of more than 3 was found to be highly indicative of an alcoholic cause of acute pancreatitis [38]. A newly developed marker of alcoholism, carbohydrate-deficient transferrin (CDT), has been evaluated recently for its value in detecting alcoholism as the cause of acute pancreatitis. In comparison to the classical indicators of alcoholism, MCV and γ-GT, and to the L/A ratio, CDT has been found to be more sensitive and specific. At a cutoff over 17 U/l, the specificity of CDT was 100% and the sensitivity was 75% in detecting an alcoholic cause of acute pancreatitis [24]. Due to its long half-live of about 14 days, serum levels remain elevated for a longer period than those of all other markers. However, it is time-consuming and expensive to determine. Nevertheless, this parameter seems to be the most sensitive and most specific one for the detection of an alcoholic cause of acute pancreatitis.

Biliary Tract Imaging Procedures

In addition to the biochemical markers, many imaging procedures are available for the identification of biliary tract disease as the etiological factor of acute pancreatitis. Oral or iv cholangiography [30] and biliary scintigraphy are rarely applied to this indication. Instead, ultrasonography (US), computed tomogra-

Table 3. Biochemical markers indicative of alcoholic pancreatitis

Marker	Value
Serum CDT	> 15 U/l
Peak L/A ratio	> 3
Admission L/A ratio	> 3
Admission serum trypsin activity	> 150 U/l
AST/ALT ratio	> 2
MCV	> 95 fl
(γ-GT)	

The order in the table does not represent a rank order of clinical utility of these parameters [24, 25, 38, 39].
CDT, carbohydrate-deficient transferrin; L/A, lipase–amylase; AST/ALT, aspartate–alanine aminotransferase; MCV, mean corpuscular volume of erythrocytes; γ-GT, gamma-glutamyl transferase.

phy (CT), and ERCP are widely and successfully used. The use of newly developed techniques such as endoscopic ultrasonography (EUS) and magnetic resonance cholangiopancreatography (MRCP) is currently limited to special centers.

Ultrasonography. US is generally the test of choice for the detection of cholelithiasis; however, it gives only indirect evidence in support of a biliary genesis of acute pancreatitis. US detects 50%–70% of the patients with biliary pancreatitis on initial scanning [18, 30, 31, 40]. Although accuracy improves to about 90% within the first week, in terms of urgent treatment other diagnostic techniques are needed [18].

Computed Tomography. CT is valuable for visualization of the morphological severity of the pancreatitis attack, but is of limited value in detecting its cause. CT is less accurate than ERCP in detecting gallbladder stones, common bile duct stones, and intrahepatic and/or extrahepatic dilatation of the biliary tree [31].

Endoscopic techniques such as ECRP and EUS have advantages over the methods mentioned above in detecting biliary lithiasis and microlithiasis. In 50 patients with acute pancreatitis, ERCP detected 100% of common bile duct stones, 70% of gallbladder stones, and 75% of dilated intrahepatic bile ducts [41]. Even in acute pancreatitis, this procedure can be performed without increased risk [16, 17, 41]. Due to its high sensitivity and low risk, ERCP is now the gold standard for the identification of a biliary cause of acute pancreatitis. In addition, it can easily be combined with a sphincterotomy, which, in turn, may cure biliary pancreatitis [16, 17, 26]. EUS is helpful in identifying microlithiasis in patients with "idiopathic" pancreatitis [32]. The sensitivity of this method can be further increased by combination with ERCP [32] and biliary [32] or duodenal [29] bile crystal analysis. Once the endoscope has been placed, bile or duodenal juice can easily be aspirated for microscopic investigation. In the hands of an experienced investigator, EUS is at least as sensitive as ERCP, and its use may prevent inappropriate invasive explorations of the common bile duct [42]. There are, however, no controlled studies as yet demonstrating a clear advantage of EUS against ERCP or other techniques in detecting biliary disease as the cause of acute pancreatitis.

Magnetic Resonance Cholangiopancreatography. MRCP is a new technique which yields results comparable with those of ERCP [27, 28, 43]. In contrast to ERCP, this method is fully noninvasive and it does not require any endoscopy or contrast medium. For these reasons, this technique may be superior to ERCP and EUS and perhaps may become the method of choice for screening of the biliary tract in patients with acute pancreatitis in the future. If a positive result is found on MRCP, an endoscopy is then required to perform sphincterotomy. The tendency of MRCP to overestimate bile duct stenosis is of relevance in chronic pancreatitis, but not in acute pancreatitis.

Conclusions

To identify the etiological factor in cases of established acute pancreatitis, laboratory tests and imaging procedures can be applied. There is, however, no single parameter or technique with absolute reliability. ERCP is the current gold standard for the detection of a biliary cause of acute pancreatitis. In addition, this method offers the opportunity of taking the pressure off the ductal system quickly by sphincterotomy, which can be curative in most cases of biliary pancreatitis. Methods with comparable accuracy but which are less invasive, such as EUS or MRCP, will perhaps replace ERCP as a first-line measure in the future. As far as the biochemical markers of biliary tract disease and of alcoholism are concerned, there is much controversy in the literature on the sensitivity, specificity, positive and negative predictive values, and best cutoff levels for most of the parameters. Serum ALT and AST seem to be highly suggestive of biliary pancreatitis when elevated threefold or higher. In current daily practice, all patients presenting with an acute abdomen should be evaluated by history and thorough clinical investigation. Once the diagnosis of acute pancreatitis has been established, an early ERCP should be performed in cases where there is evidence of biliary tract disease given by history, clinical examination (jaundice, Courvoisier's sign), laboratory tests (e.g., threefold elevated ALT or AST), X-ray of the abdomen (calculi), or US (calculi, biliary obstruction). The value of promising new methods such as EUS, MRCP, serum CDT, and trypsin activity analysis remains to be established.

References

1. Opie EL (1901) The etiology of acute hemorrhagic pancreatitis. Johns Hopkins Hosp Bull 121-122-123: 182-188
2. Halsted WS (1901) Retrojection of bile into the pancreas, a cause of acute hemorrhagic pancreatitis. Johns Hopkins Hosp Bull 121-122-123: 179-182

3. Acosta JM, Ledesma CL (1974) Gallstone migration as a cause of acute pancreatitis. N Engl J Med 290: 484–487
4. Peracchia A, Gafa M, Sarli L, Lupi M, Longinotti E (1985) Biliary microlithiasis and acute pancreatitis. Int Surg 70: 315–318
5. Ros E, Navarro S, Bru C, Garcia-Puges A, Valderrama R (1991) Occult microlithiasis in "idiopathic" acute pancreatitis: prevention of relapses by cholecystectomy or ursodeoxycholic acid therapy. Gastroenterology 101: 1701–1709
6. Lee SP, Nicholls JF, Park HZ (1992) Biliary sludge as a cause of acute pancreatitis. N Engl J Med 326: 589–593
7. Ranson JHC (1984) Acute pancreatitis: pathogenesis, outcome and treatment. Clinics Gastroenterol 13: 843–863
8. Wilson JS, Lorsten MA, Pirola RC (1989) Alcohol-induced pancreatic injury. Int J Pancreatol 4: 109–125, 233–250
9. Singh M, Simsek H (1990) Ethanol and the pancreas: current status. Gastroenterology 98: 1051–1062
10. Nordback I, Airo I (1988) Post-ERCP acute necrotizing pancreatitis. Ann Chir Gyn 77: 15–20
11. Stanten R, Frey CF (1990) Pancreatitis after endoscopic retrograde cholangiopancreatography. Arch Surg 125: 1032–1035
12. Ammann RW, Deyhle P, Butikofer E (1973) Fatal necrotizing pancreatitis after peroral cholangiopancreatography. Gastroenterology 64: 320–323
13. Kishimoto W, Nakao A, Takagi H, Hayakawa T (1989) Acute pancreatitis after transcatheter arterial embolization (TAE) for hepatocellular carcinoma. Am J Gastroenterol 84: 1396–1399
14. Donelly S, Levy M, Prichard S (1988) Acute pancreatitis in continuous ambulatory peritoneal dialysis (CAPD). Periton Dial Int 8: 187–190
15. Thompson JS, Bragg LE, Hodgson PE, Rikkers LF (1988) Postoperative pancreatitis. Surg Gynecol Obstet 167: 377–380
16. Neoptolemos JP, Carr-Locke DL, London NJ, Bailey IA, James D, Fossard DP (1988) Controlled trial of urgent endoscopic retrograde cholangiopancreatography and endoscopic sphincterotomy versus conservative treatment for acute pancreatitis due to gallstones. Lancet II: 979–983
17. Fan ST, Lai ECS, Mok FPT, Lo CM, Zheng SS, Wong J (1993) Early treatment of acute biliary pancreatitis by endoscopic papillotomy. N Engl J Med 328: 228–232
18. Millat B, Fingerhut A, Gayral F, Zazzo JF, Brivet F (1992) Predictability of clinicobiochemical scoring systems for early identification of servere gallstone-associated pancreatitis. Am J Surg 164: 32–38
19. Sadowski DC, Todd JK, Sutherland LR (1993) Biochemical models as early predictors of the etiology of acute pancreatitis. Dig Dis Sci 38: 637–643
20. Pezzilli R, Billi P, Miglioli M, Gullo L (1993) Serum amylase and lipase concentrations and lipase/amylase ratio in assessment of etiology and severity of acute pancreatitis. Dig Dis Sci 38: 1265–1269
21. Tenner S, Dubner H, Steinberg W (1994) Predicting gallstone pancreatitis with laboratory parameters: a meta-analysis. Am J Gastroenterol 89: 1863–1866
22. Kazmierczak SC, Catrou PG, Van Lente F (1995) Enzymatic markers of gallstone-induced pancreatitis identified by ROC curve analysis, discriminant analysis, logistic regression, likelihood ratios, and information theory. Clin Chem 41: 523–531
23. Tenner SM, Steinberg W (1992) The admission serum lipase:amylase ratio differentiates alcoholic from nonalcoholic acute pancreatitis. Am J Gastroenterol 87: 1755–1758
24. Jaakkola M, Sillanaukee P, Löf K, Koivula T, Nordback I (1994) Blood test for detection of alcoholic cause of acute pancreatitis. Lancet 343: 1328–1329
25. LeMoine O, Devaster JM, Deviere J, Thiry P, Cremer M, Ooms HA (1994) Trypsin activity: a new marker of acute alcoholic pancreatitis. Dig Dis Sci 39: 2634–2638
26. Lai ECS, Lo CM (1994) Acute pancreatitis: the role of ERCP in 1994. Endoscopy 26: 488–492
27. Outwater EK, Gordon SJ (1994) Imaging the pancreatic and biliary ducts with MR. Radiology 192: 19–21
28. Laubenberger J, Büchert M, Schneider B, Blum U, Hennig J, Langer M (1995) Breath-hold projection magnetic resonance-cholangio-pancreaticography (MRCP): a new method for the examination of the bile and pancreatic ducts. Magnet Reson Med 33: 18–23
29. Neoptolemos JP, Davidson BR, Winder AF, Vallance D (1988) Role of duodenal bile crystal analysis in the investigation of "idiopathic" pancreatitis. Br J Surg 75: 450–453

30. Goodman AJ, Neoptolemos JP, Carr-Locke DL, Finlay DBL, Fossard DP (1985) Detection of gall stones after acute pancreatitis. Gut 26: 125–132
31. Schölmerich J, Gross V, Johannesson T, Brobmann G, Rückauer K, Wimmer B, Gerok W, Farthmann EH (1989) Detection of biliary origin of acute pancreatitis: comparison of laboratory tests, ultrasound, computed tomography, and ERCP. Dig Dis Sci 34: 830–833
32. Pages P, Buscail L, Moreau J, Berthelemy P, Frexinos J, Escourrou J (1995) Contribution of endoscopic ultrasonography (EUS), ERCP, biliary microscopy and pancreatic function test to the diagnosis of idiopathic acute pancreatitis. Digestion 56: 308
33. Winslet M, Hall C, London NJM, Neoptolemos JP (1992) Relation of diagnostic serum amylase levels to aetiology and severity of acute pancreatitis. Gut 33: 982–986
34. Gumaste VV, Dave PB, Weissman D, Messer J (1991) Lipase/amylase ratio: a new index that distinguishes acute episodes of alcoholic from nonalcoholic acute pancreatitis. Gastroenterology 101: 1361–1366
35. Lankisch PG, Petersen M (1994) Lipase/amylase ratio: not helpful in the early etiological differentiation of acute pancreatitis. Z Gastroenterol 32: 8–11
36. King LG, Seelig CB, Ranney JE (1995) The lipase to amylase ratio in acute pancreatitis. Am J Gastroenterol 90: 67–69
37. Delternre P, Ghilain JM, Maisin JM, Schapira M, Henrion J, Heller FR (1995) Le rapport L/A permet-il d'identifier les pancréatitis aiguës alcooliques? Acta Gastro-Enterol Belg LVIII: 222–229
38. Gumaste VV (1995) Lipase/amylase ratio: a review. Pancreas 10: 210–212
39. Arndt T, Gressner AM, Kropf J (1994) Labordiagnostik und Kontrolle des Alkoholabusus – ein Plädoyer für Carbohydrate-deficient transferrin (CDT). Med Welt 45: 247–257
40. Schölmerich J, Johannesson T, Brobmann G, Wimmer B, Thiedemann B, Groß V, Gerok W, Farthmann EH (1989) Die Sonographie bei der akuten Pankreatitis – Diagnose, Ätiologieabklärung und Prognoseabschätzung. Ultraschall 10: 290–294
41. Schölmerich J, Lausen M, Lay L, Salm R, Rückauer K, Gross V, Roth M, Leser HG, Farthmann EH (1992) Value of endoscopic retrograde cholangiopancreatography in determining the cause but not course of acute pancreatitis. Endoscopy 24: 244–247
42. Prat F, Amouyal G, Pelletier G, Fritsch J, Choury AD, Buffet C, Etienne JP (1996) Prospective controlled study of endoscopic ultrasonography and endoscopic retrograde cholangiography in patients with suspected common-bileduct lithiasis. Lancet 347: 75–79
43. Takehara Y, Ichijo K, Tooyama N, Kodaira N, Yamamoto H, Tatami M, Saito M, Watahiki H, Takahashi M (1994) Breath-hold MR cholangiopancreatography with a long-echo-train fast spin-echo sequence and a surface coil in chronic pancreatitis. Radiology 192: 73–78

Exocrine Pancreatic Function During and Following Acute Pancreatitis

J. E. Domínguez-Muñoz · P. Malfertheiner

Exocrine Pancreatic Function During Acute Pancreatitis

The state of exocrine pancreatic function during acute pancreatitis is an important aspect of the disease due to its therapeutical implications. In fact, for a long time one of the mainstays of the treatment of acute pancreatitis has been the inhibition of pancreatic secretion in order to put the gland to rest, and many therapeutical studies have focussed on this concept.

More than a decade ago, some studies in animals demonstrated that both basal and stimulated pancreatic secretion are markedly decreased during experimental acute pancreatitis [1–5]. More recently, Niederau and coworkers [6] confirmed this finding in several animal models. They showed that basal pancreatic secretion during acute pancreatitis was reduced to values between 27 % and 45 % normal basal values and that stimulated pancreatic secretion decreased to values below 5 % of normal stimulated secretion [6]. The clinical implication of these findings in experimental studies is that, since pancreatic secretion is already markedly reduced in the context of acute pancreatitis, pharmacological inhibition of that secretion does not make sense.

Very few studies have reported on pancreatic function during acute pancreatitis in humans. In a therapeutical clinical study with cimetidine and glucagon, Regan and coworkers found normal basal secretion of trypsin in two of three patients with acute pancreatitis [7]. Very recently we studied exocrine pancreatic secretion in the early phase of human acute pancreatitis by means of a standard duodenal intubation perfusion technique [8]. Four of the eight patients studied suffered from necrotizing pancreatitis. We found that exocrine pancreatic secretion was normal in all but one patient (Fig. 1). This patient with reduced secretion suffered from a second attack of necrotizing pancreatitis and had undergone surgical resection of the necrotic tail of the pancreas during the course of the first attack; therefore, the amount of viable acinar tissue was presumed to be critically reduced to maintain normal secretion. Moreover, we found that interdigestive exocrine pancreatic secretion during human acute pancreatitis mantains a normal cyclical pattern (Fig. 2), supporting the fact that factors regulating interdigestive pancreatic secretion also function normally. The clinical implication of this finding is that pharmacological inhibition of pancreatic secretion can be attempted. However, this therapeutical measure does not have any influence on the clinical course of acute pancreatitis.

Fig. 1. Exocrine pancreatic secretion of amylase and trypsin within an interdigestive cycle in the early phase of acute pancreatitis. Data are shown as individual values (patients with acute pancreatitis) and median and range (healthy subjects). (From [8])

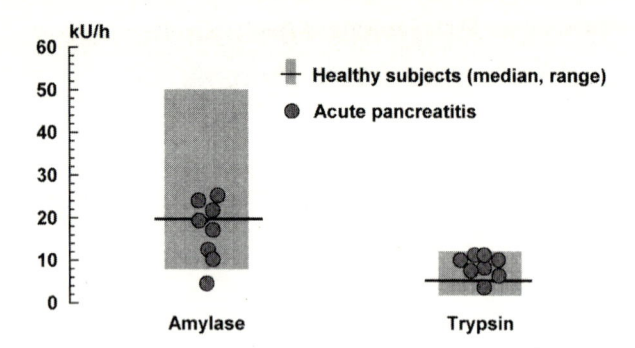

Exocrine Pancreatic Function Following Acute Pancreatitis

Several problems limit the study of the functional sequelae following acute pancreatitis:

The first is that we usually do not know how pancreatic function was before acute pancreatitis occurred. Therefore, it is usually not possible to differentiate between functional alterations that occur as a consequence of acute pancreatitis, in the context of chronic pancreatitis, or as age-related changes. If chronic changes within the pancreas are excluded by imaging methods, the next problem is to define how long after the acute attack the functional impairment can be considered to be caused by acute pancreatitis.

Several factors define the frequency, severity, and duration of exocrine pancreatic dysfunction following acute pancreatitis: first, the severity of the attack, i.e., edematous pancreatitis, necrotizing pancreatitis (and extent of necrosis), and second, the etiology of the disease, mainly alcoholic or nonalcoholic pancreatitis (biliary and other etiologies). A third factor is, of course, the test used to study pancreatic function since most indirect tests are unable to detect mild functional alterations. More than 10 years ago, two studies already demonstrated that exocrine pancreatic function can be abnormal even 3 years after acute pancreatitis and that it can return to normal later on (Table 1) [9, 10]. More recently, authors have reported conflicting data, ranging from studies showing pathological function in as many as 50 % of patients even 3 years after

Fig. 2. Cyclic interdigestive exocrine pancreatic secretion of amylase in a patient with acute pancreatitis and a healthy subject

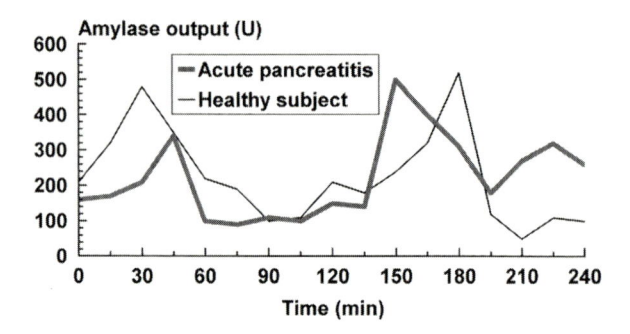

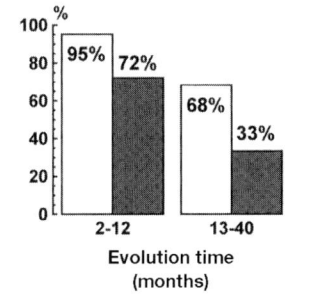

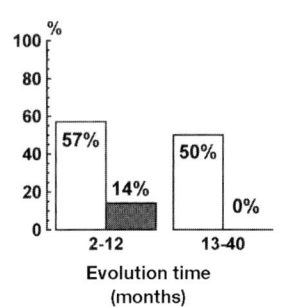

Table 1. Proportion of patients with impaired exocrine pancreatic function after acute pancreatitis (AP); number of patients with impaired function/total number of patients

Author (reference)	Recovery phase	4 weeks after AP	2–6 months after AP	7–12 months after AP	1–3 years after AP	3–4 years after AP
Mitchell [9]	100% (30/30)	75% (6/8)	40% (4/10)	40% (8/20)	0% (0/5)	–
Angelini [10]	–	–	–	36% (4/11)	20% (1/5)	0% (0/5)
Arenas [14]	54% (14/26)	18% (2/11)	–	–	–	–
Büchler [11]	–	–	–	70% (42/60)	50% (17/34)	–
Garnacho [15]	100% (19/19)	100% (19/19)	53% (10/19)	42% (8/19)	–	–
Glasbrenner [12]	79% (23/29)	10% (3/29)	–	–	–	–

AP, acute pancreatitis.

the acute episode [11] to studies showing a normal function in 90% of patients 4 weeks after acute pancreatitis [12]. These differences basically respond to the proportions of patients with necrotizing pancreatitis and alcoholic etiology included in the different studies as well as to the pancreatic function test applied.

Most of the patients with necrotizing pancreatitis have impaired exocrine pancreatic function during the first year of evolution that, contrary to patients with edematous pancreatitis, seldom returns to normal later on (Fig. 3) [11]. Similarly, patients with alcoholic pancreatitis, unlike those with biliary disease, sometimes do not normalize pancreatic function even after an episode of edematous pancreatitis (Fig. 3) [11]. Very recently, Bozburk and coworkers also found that most patients have an exocrine pancreatic insufficiency (most mild-moderate) even 18 months after an episode of acute necrotizing pancreatitis (Fig. 4) [13].

Fig. 3. Frequency of impaired exocrine pancreatic function after acute pancreatitis according to the severity and etiology of the disease. *Left*, necrotizing pancreatitis; *right*, edematous pancreatitis. *White bars*, alcoholic etiology; *shaded bars*, biliary etiology. (Data from [10])

Fig. 4. Proportion of patients with normal exocrine pancreatic function, mild-moderate, and severe insufficiency 18 months after an episode of acute necrotizing pancreatitis. (Data from [13])

Fig. 5. Proportion of patients with impaired exocrine pancreatic function after acute pancreatitis. Summary of all the data reported in the literature considered

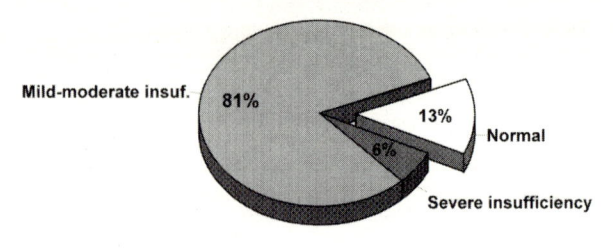

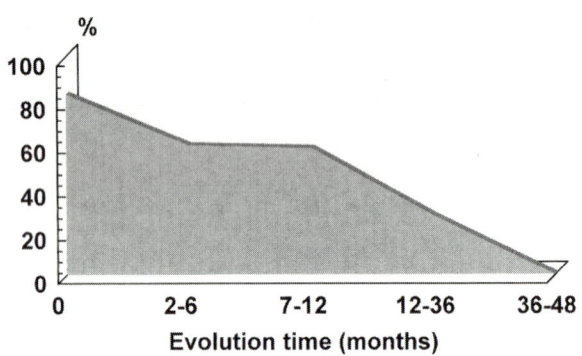

In summary, exocrine pancreatic function is frequently impaired following acute pancreatitis, mainly following episodes with parenquimal necrosis and those of alcoholic etiology. This functional impairment tends to return to normal several months after the acute attack. Functional recovery is possible even 3 years after acute pancreatitis (Fig. 5).

References

1. Adler G, Hupp T, Kern HF (1979) Course and spontaneous regression of acute pancreatitis in the rat. Virchows Arch (A) 382: 32–47
2. Gilliland L, Steer ML (1980) Effects of ethionine on digestive enzyme synthesis and discharge by mouse pancreas. Am J Physiol 239: G418–26
3. Kioke K, Steer ML, Meldolesi J (1982) Pancreatic effects of ethionine: blockade of exocytosis and appearance of crinophagy and autophagy precede cellular necrosis. Am J Physiol 242: G297–307
4. Evander A, Hederström E, Hultberg B, Ihse I (1982) Exocrine pancreatic secretion in acute experimental pancreatitis. Digestion 24: 159–67
5. Saluja A, Saito I, Saluja M, et al (1985) In vivo rat pancreatic cell function during supramaximal stimulation with caerulein. Am J Physiol 259: G702–10
6. Niederau C, Niederau M, Lüthen R, Strohmeyer G, Ferrell LD, Grendell JH (1990) Pancreatic exocrine secretion in acute experimental pancreatitis. Gastroenterology 99: 1120–7
7. Regan PT, Malagelada JR, Go VLW, Wolf AM, DiMagno EP (1981) A prospective study of the antisecretory effects of cimetidine and glucagon in human acute pancreatitis. Mayo Clin Proc 56: 499–503
8. Domínguez-Muñoz JE, Pieramico O, Büchler M, Malfertheiner P (1995) Exocrine pancreatic secretion in the early phase of acute pancreatitis. Scand J Gastroenterol 30: 186–191
9. Mitchell CJ, Playforth MJ, Kelleher J, McMahon MJ (1983) Functional recovery of the exocrine pancreas after acute pancreatitis. Scand J Gastroenterol 18: 5–8

10. Angelini G, Pederzoli P, Caliar S, et al (1984) Long-term outcome of acute necrohemorrhagic pancreatitis. Digestion 30: 131–7
11. Büchler M, Hauke A, Malfertheiner P (1987) Follow up after acute pancreatitis: Morphology and function. In: Beger HG, Büchler M, eds. Acute pancreatitis. Springer-Verlag: Berlin-Heidelberg 367–74
12. Glasbrenner B, Büchler M, Uhl W, Malfertheiner P (1992) Exocrine pancreatic function in the early recovery phase of acute oedematous pancreatitis. Eur J Gastroenterol Hepatol 4: 563–7
13. Bozkurt T, Maroske D, Adler G (1995) Exocrine pancreatic function after recovery from necrotizing pancreatitis. Hepatogastroenterology 42: 55–8
14. Arenas M, Pérez-Mateo M, Graells ML, Sillero C, Vázquez N (1986) Valoración de la función pancreática exocrina mediante el test del PABA en pacientes con pancreatitis aguda. Rev Esp Enf Ap Dig 70: 43–8
15. Garnacho J, Aznar A, Corrochano MD, et al (1989) Evolución de la función exocrina del páncreas tras la pancreatitis aguda. Factores pronósticos. Rev Esp Enf Ap Dig 76: 19–24

Endocrine Pancreatic Function During and Following Acute Pancreatitis

J. E. Domínguez-Muñoz · P. di Sebastiano · P. Malfertheiner

Endocrine Pancreatic Function During Acute Pancreatitis

The metabolic response during acute pancreatitis may depend on the one hand on acute stress, which is similar to that seen in other diseases such as sepsis or clinical situations such as surgical interventions, and on the other hand on damage to the Langerhans's islets related to pancreatic inflammation. Hyperglycemia develops rather often in the early phase of acute pancreatitis, mainly in patients with severe disease [1-3]. This hyperglycemia could thus be the result of a hyperglucagonemia secondary to stress or the result of decreased synthesis and release of insulin secondary to the damage of pancreatic β-cells [4-7].

The endocrine response to hyperglycemia in acute pancreatitis is clearly different from that observed in other clinical situations associated with acute stress [4]. In fact, although hyperinsulinemia has been reported in patients with acute pancreatitis as a response to hyperglycemia, plasma insulin levels are clearly lower than expected for glucose levels [4, 7]. Therefore, it could be hypothesized that a relative endocrine pancreatic insufficiency occurs during acute pancreatitis. However, insulin release in patients with acute pancreatitis increases significantly after intravenous infusion of alanine [6], suggesting that the relative pancreatic endocrine insufficiency observed during acute pancreatitis is due to inhibition of insulin release in response to hyperglycemia rather than to impairment of the synthesis and storage of the hormone within the pancreatic β cells.

Serum basal levels of glucagon are increased during the early phase of acute pancreatitis in spite of hyperglycemia. Moreover, this increase is higher than expected of a simple response to stress [4]. Several factors may be involved in the production of hyperglucagonemia during acute pancreatitis, such as alteration of pancreatic α cells in association with the disease and high levels of circulating catecholamines.

In summary, relative hypoinsulinemia and hyperglucagonemia probably are, together with the elevated levels of catecholamines and cortisol, the most important factors involved in the pathogenesis of hyperglycemia observed during acute pancreatitis.

Increased glucagon release together with relatively decreased insulin release was described by Solomon and coworkers after the intravenous infusion of arginine in patients with acute pancreatitis [5]. However, if the response to arginine is compared not to healthy subjects but to other patients in a similar stress situ-

Fig. 1a–c. Plasma levels of **a** glucose, **b** insulin and **c** glucagon in response to intravenous administration of arginine in patients with acute pancreatitis (*gray line*) and patients under surgical stress (*black line*). Arginine was injected continuously for the first 30 min. (Data from [8])

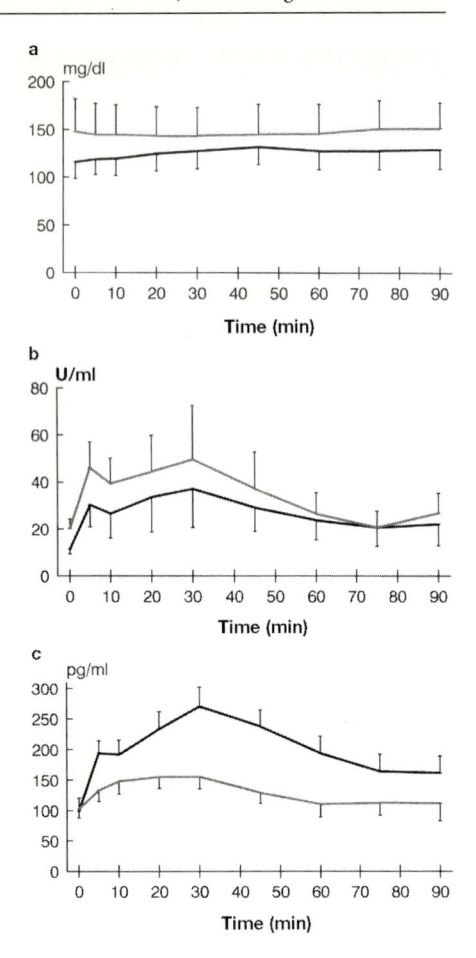

ation (e.g., surgical stress), patients with acute pancreatitis show similar insulin release and significantly decreased glucagon release (Fig. 1) [8]. Furthermore, insulin and glucagon release demonstrate similar behavior based on serum glucose levels in patients with acute pancreatitis and patients after surgical intervention [8].

Similar to exocrine pancreatic function, endocrine pancreatic function during acute pancreatitis depends basically on the severity of the disease, mainly on the presence and extent of pancreatic necrosis. Different severity degrees of the disease and different control populations explain the discrepancies observed among the studies hitherto reported on endocrine function in the early phase of acute pancreatitis.

Table 1. Proportion of patients with impaired endocrine pancreatic function after acute pancreatitis (AP; number of patients with impaired function/total number of patients

Author (reference)	2–6 months after AP	1–2 years after AP	2–3 years after AP	3–4 years after AP
Angelini [9]	64 % (9/14)	44 % (8/18)	67 % (6/9)	40 % (2/5)
Büchler [10]	35 % (19/55)		30 % (9/30)	

Endocrine Pancreatic Function Following Acute Pancreatitis

Endocrine pancreatic function usually follows a parallel evolution to exocrine pancreatic function after resolution of acute pancreatitis. However, the number of studies focussing on endocrine pancreatic function after acute pancreatitis are very limited. Endocrine pancreatic function tends to return to normal a few months after acute edematous pancreatitis, independent of etiology [9, 10]. The situation is different following acute necrotizing pancreatitis, in which alteration of endocrine pancreatic function as glucose intolerance or even manifest diabetes mellitus persists in more than 50 % of patients [9–11]. The persistent alteration of endocrine pancreatic function occurs more frequently in cases of alcoholic than biliary pancreatitis [9, 11]. Table 1 summarizes the data hitherto reported in this respect by using the oral glucose tolerance test as a method for exploring endocrine pancreatic function.

In patients after acute pancreatitis and normal oral glucose tolerance test, the curves of insulin and C-peptide following 100 g of oral glucose were found to be significantly higher than those in controls, whereas no difference was found regarding the curves of pancreatic glucagon [12]. Therefore, a normal response to glucose after recovery from an attack of acute pancreatitis is maintained at the cost of increased insulin secretion [12]. These findings have recently been confirmed in an experimental model of acute pancreatitis, in which serum glucose concentrations in postpancreatitic rats were similar to those in the control rats whereas basal as well as stimulated insulin release tended to be higher in postpancreatitic rats than in control rats [13].

Similar to exocrine pancreatic function, endocrine pancreatic function usually returns to normal within the first 12 months after acute pancreatitis; functional recovery later on is rare but possible, mainly in patients who suffered from biliary pancreatitis with moderately extended pancreatic necrosis.

References

1. Ranson JHC (1982) Etiology and prognostic factors in human acute pancreatitis: a review. Am J Gastroenterol 77: 633–63
2. Imrie CW, Benjamin IS, McKay AJ, Mackenzie I, O'neill J, Blumgart LH (1978) A single centre double blind trial of Trasylol therapy in primary acute pancreatitis. Br J Surg 65: 337–341
3. Fan ST, Choi TK, Lai ECS, Wong J (1989) Prediction of severity of acute pancreatitis: An alternative approach. Gut 30: 1591–1595
4. Drew SI, Joffe B, Vinik A, Seftel H, Singer F (1978) The first 24 hours of acute pancreatitis. Am J Med 64: 795–803
5. Solomon SS, Duckworth WC, Jallepalli P, Bobal MA, Iyer R (1980) The glucose intolerance of acute pancreatitis: Hormonal response to arginine. Diabetes 29: 22–26
6. Dunowitz M, Hendler R, Spiro HM, et al (1975) Glucagon secretion in acute and chronic pancreatitis. Ann Intern Med 83:778–781
7. Day JL, Knight M, Condon JR (1972) The role of pancreatic glucagon in the pathogenesis of acute pancreatitis. Clin Sci 43: 597–603
8. Domínguez-Muñoz JE, Uhl W, Lohr C, DiSebastiano P, Büchler M, Malfertheiner P (1992) Endocrine pancreatic response to arginine stimulation during the early phase of human acute pancreatitis. Gastroenterology 102: A263
9. Angelini G, Pederzoli P, Caliari S, et al (1984) Long-term outcome of acute necrohemorrhagic pancreatitis. Digestion 30: 131–137
10. Büchler M, Hauke A, Malfertheiner P (1987) Follow-up after acute pancreatitis: Morphology and function. In: Beger HG, Büchler M, eds. Acute pancreatitis. Springer-Verlag: Berlin-Heidelberg 367–374
11. Doepel M, Erikson J, Halme L, Kumpulainen T, Hockerstedt K (1993) Good long-term results in patients surviving severe acute pancreatitis. Br J Surg 80: 1583–6
12. Stastna R, Karasova L, Svacek J, Petrasek R, Winkler L, Lanska V, Skala I (1990) Endocrine pancreatic secretion in patients after acute pancreatitis. Pancreas 5: 358–60
13. Otsuki M, Nakano S, Tachibana I (1994) Treatment with cholecystokinin receptor antagonist loxiglumide enhances insulin response to intravenous glucose stimulation in postpancreatitic rats. Regul Pept 52: 85–95

III
Prognostic Evaluation

Pathophysiological Determinants of Severity of Acute Pancreatitis

R. Lüthen · C. Niederau

Although the mortality rate in acute pancreatitis has significantly decreased within the last decade, mostly due to the improvement of intensive care treatment, there is still the need for an early prognosis of the severity of acute pancreatitis. Such early prognosis is desirable, since mild, edematous pancreatitis mostly takes a benign course and requires neither costly diagnosis (computed tomography (CT) scan) nor intensive care treatment. On the other hand, necrotizing acute pancreatitis often takes a severe course and does need early and repeated imaging procedures, laboratory tests, and intensive care treatment. Thus, early prognosis of the severity of acute pancreatitis is required in order to offer the patient the appropriate care and to save costly resources. Although several prognostic scores, such as Acute Physiology and Chronic Health Evaluation (APACHE) II and the Ranson score, and laboratory markers e.g. polymorphonuclear (PMN) elastase, C-reactive protein (CRP), trypsinogen activation peptide (TAP), are available, other pathophysiological determinants of the severity of acute pancreatitis are sought.

Epidemiologic data indicate that the mortality rate associated with acute pancreatitis is not correlated with a certain etiology. Gallstone-induced pancreatitis, alcohol-induced pancreatitis, idiopathic pancreatitis, and postoperative pancreatitis all carry a comparable mortality rate of 4.5%–7.2%. Endoscopic retrograde cholangiopancreatography (ERCP)-induced pancreatitis has a slightly lower mortality rate. When the mortality rate associated with acute pancreatitis is based on the number of deaths, there is a peak in a younger age group (31–40 years). However, when pancreatic deaths are based on the number of subjects, there is an almost linear increase with age. Thus age seems to be a risk factor for mortality associated with acute pancreatitis. The number of patients with pancreatic necrosis on CT scan does not differ among the age groups and therefore does not account for the different mortality rates. It is well known from the literature that systemic complications such as initial shock or organ failure and mortality associated with acute pancreatitis are closely related. Multiorgan failure in particular, carries a high mortality rate of more than 40%. However, these organ failures are more likely to be consequences than individual pathophysiological determinants in the course of acute pancreatitis. Among the systemic complications of acute pancreatitis, sepsis might be a single pathophysiological determinant of the course of the disease. A prediction of septic complications in acute pancreatitis, however, is not possible as yet. Its occurrence may be related to the amount of pancreatic necrosis, certain bacterial species in the colon, or defects in the immune system.

As edematous pancreatitis tends to take a more benign course and necrotizing pancreatitis is more likely to take a severe course, it would be desirable to identify factors that cause the transition of edematous pancreatitis to severe necrotizing pancreatitis. The clinical setting does not supply sufficient answers to this question. Most studies on aggressive and defensive factors are done after the initiation of acute pancreatitis. Thus, one cannot differentiate between predisposing factors, byproducts, and consequences of the disease. Similarly, the experimental setting does not contribute significant information in this field, because little work has been done in this regard. There is experimental evidence that a combination of several noxious factors and a reduction of defensive factors aggravate pancreatitis. It is conceivable that combined actions of several noxious factors such as proteases, active digestive enzymes, ischemia, and direct toxic effects (certain drugs, alcohol, bile salts) increase the severity of pancreatitis. On the other hand, hampered protection due to reduction of antiproteases, ATP depletion, or reduction of levels antioxidants (e.g., glutathione) could also increase the severity of pancreatitis. There are several predisposing factors which may reduce the defensive potential of the pancreas: alcohol, malnutrition, liver cirrhosis, and other accompanying diseases, and possibly immune dysfunction.

Glutathione is one of the important cellular defense systems which protects against oxidant stress and maintains cellular structure and function. Recent work from our laboratory has shown that the pancreatic tissue level of reduced glutathione is significantly reduced in several animal models of acute pancreatitis. Conversely, the pancreatic tissue level of oxidized glutathione is elevated during the early course of experimental pancreatitis. Additional evidence for the important role of glutathione in acute pancreatitis was gathered in experiments which showed that injection of glutathione precursors such as glutathione monoethylester or L-2-oxothiazolidine-carboxylate ameliorated the course of an experimental pancreatitis. Furthermore, histological and biochemical changes similar to a mild acute pancreatitis were induced by complete depletion of pancreatic glutathione without employing any other standard experimental model of acute pancreatitis.

The delicate balance between pancreatic digestive proteases on the one hand and protease inhibitors on the other could also be a factor that causes the transition of an edematous pancreatitis to severe necrosis. It has been shown by other investigators using in vitro assays and by our own laboratory using an immunohistochemistry method that trypsinogen activation occurs in the early phase of acute pancreatitis. These experiments were based on the fact that during the activation process of trypsinogen rendering enzymatically active trypsin, a cleavage peptide (TAP) is formed. A polyclonal antibody that specifically labels TAP has been raised and well characterized. It was shown in experimental work from our laboratory that positive labeling of TAP occurs within 1 h after injection of one supramaximal dose of the cholecystokinin (CCK) analogue cerulein and is located at the apical side of the acinus cell, possibly along the late stages of the secretory pathway. Uncontrolled intracellular liberation of enzymatically active digestive enzymes might influence the course of the acute pancreatitis.

Other pathophysiological factors that might influence the severity of acute pancreatitis are circulating proteases, lipases and phospholipases, inflammatory mediators e.g., tumor necrosis factor (TNF), interleukin (IL)-6 and IL-8, PMN, and their products (e.g., H_2O_2, elastase) and complement products (C3 and C4). It is hypothesized that the activation of inflammatory cells and mediators during the course of acute pancreatitis can be divided into two phases. In the early phase, a massive release of free radicals and inflammatory mediators with subsequent activation of inflammatory cells takes place. In the late phase in complicated disease, insufficient or improperly controlled function of inflammatory cells and mediators might contribute to the further course of the disease.

It has been shown by other investigators that ischemia leads to a very mild pancreatitis. It is also known that cerulein hyperstimulation in animal models causes a mild edematous pancreatitis. However, when both experimental models (ischemia plus cerulein hyperstimulation) are combined, a necrotizing pancreatitis ensues. Thus interactions of several noxious and protective factors might be involved in the conversion of edematous to necrotizing pancreatitis.

In summary, pathophysiological determinants of severity of acute pancreatitis can possibly be divided into certain mechanisms acting at different stages. The severity of the pancreatic autodigestion will certainly influence the degree of pancreatic necrosis and hemorrhage. Initiation of the inflammatory cascade of mediators causes systemic damage to extrapancreatic organs and influences morbidity and mortality in patients with acute pancreatitis. In the later stages of the disease, bacterial infection of pancreatic necrosis often leads to sepsis and multiorgan failure.

Clinical Value of Multifactorial Classification in the Prognostic Evaluation of Acute Pancreatitis

G. Uomo · G. Manes · P. G. Rabitti

Introduction

Acute pancreatitis (AP) presents a broad clinical spectrum ranging from a mild self-limiting disease to a potentially fatal illness with multiple organ failure [1–4]. The development of pancreatic necrosis in patients with AP results in an increase in clinical severity and in mortality risk compared to acute edematous/interstitial pancreatitis [5]. The terms *severe AP* [6] and *necrotizing AP* [7] are broadly synonymous because the necrotic destruction of pancreatic parenchyma is the major determinant of the severity of the disease. Despite improvements in diagnosis and treatment, necrotizing AP is still associated with a high mortality rate. Several factors influence the clinical course and final outcome of the disease [3, 8–9]: the presence of systemic complications, the extent of intrapancreatic and extrapancreatic necrosis, the infection of necrosis, and/or fluid collections.

All clinicians dealing with AP soon learn that one of the main characteristics of the disease is its unforeseeable outcome. The need for an objective prognostic assessment of patients with AP is of paramount importance for at least two reasons [3]. Firstly, early identification of the risk of life-threatening complications allows appropriate application of monitoring and therapeutic intervention, which can also spare the use (or abuse) of invasive and otherwise costly measurements in mild cases [2, 10]. Secondly, objective means to stratify the various populations of patients with AP appear to be necessary for the evaluation of proposed treatments (i.e., in controlled clinical trials involving different centers) [11]. In accordance with Ranson [3], an ideal prognostic method should have several characteristics:

1. Objectivity
2. Accuracy
3. Simplicity
4. Availability at diagnosis
5. Noninvasiveness
6. Quantitativeness
7. Independence with regard to etiology
8. Independence with regard to patient's preexisting disease
9. Complication specificity
10. Usefulness for disease course monitoring

None of the means of assessment of severity currently available fulfils all these characteristics. However, one characteristic of primary importance is that the prognostic indicators must be detected with the first 24 h, this being the crucial time period in severe cases [12].

Prognostic Assessment by Means of Clinical Evaluation

A number of early clinical findings have been reported as having prognostic value. Increasing age, fever, tachypnoea, tetany, Grey-Turner's and Cullen's signs, abdominal mass, prolonged paralytic ileus, detectable intra-abdominal mass, obesity, and cardiovascular collapse are all correlated with a severe outcome [2, 3, 8, 10, 13, 14], but all are either not present in many patients with severe disease or take a long time to assess. Furthermore, of these findings, only age, fever, and body mass index can be objectively quantified. Using clinical assessment alone, McMahon et al. [15], Corfield et al. [16], and Heath and Imrie [13] reported the percentage of patients with severe disease correctly classified on admission as 39%, 34%, and 64%, respectively. These data confirm that the discriminating ability of clinical assessment alone is not satisfactory. In contrast, a reevaluation of the clinical criteria arises from their integration with other (biochemical, instrumental) indexes in various multifactorial prognostic systems that will be discussed below.

Prognostic Assessment by Means of Single Serum Markers

Single serum factors reported to be of early prognostic value in AP include the following:

- Hematocrit [17]
- White blood cell count [2, 18]
- Coagulation factors [19]
- Blood glucose and/or urea [18]
- Complement activation factors [20]
- C-reactive protein [21]
- Amylase [18]
- Phospholipase A_2 [22]
- Polymorphonuclear (PMN) elastase [23]
- Calcium [24]
- Arterial hypoxemia [2, 18]
- Acidosis [18]
- Liver function [2, 18]
- Methalbumin [18, 25]
- Ribonuclease [26]
- α_1-Protease inhibitor [21, 27]
- α_2-Macroglobulin [27, 28]
- Trypsinogen activation peptides [29]

- Interleukin-6 [30]
- Pancreatitis-associated protein [31]
- Tumor necrosis factor (TNF) receptor antagonists [32]
- Neopterin [33]

Most of these serum markers have not yet confirmed their initial validity in further studies; in many instances, they have been correlated with the necrotic process of AP rather than with clinical findings; in other cases, clinical evaluation involves only a small number of patients. Furthermore, some measurements such as C-reactive protein or ribonuclease levels serve as diagnostic rather than prognostic parameters [3]. Finally, the presence of concomitant diseases (often observed in AP) may influence serum levels of these factors, independent of the severity of AP. An ideal single serum prognostic marker would be a serum component that is easy to assay and reflects with sensitivity and specificity the extent of pancreatic damage and the presence of complications. Unfortunately, however, we have by no means achieved this goal.

In summary, most single serum markers do not enable clinicians to identify patients at risk. As for the clinical data, such single factors became valid prognostically when integrated into multifactorial systems.

Multifactorial Scoring System

Ranson and Glasgow Scoring System

Ranson's 11 objective prognostic factors have been available since 1974 [34] and are still in use today (Table 1). These signs were developed from a statistical analysis of the relationship between early measurements and overall morbidity and mortality of AP. Of the 11 signs, five are measured at the time of admission (all, except age, reflect the intensity of the inflammatory process) and six are determined within the first 48 h of admission (all reflect serious systemic complications). In 1979, Ranson [35] modified this prognostic system for patients with gallstones (Table 1). In both assessment systems, a severe attack is predicted by the presence of three or more positive factors: with three to five positive signs mortality is 10–20%; with six or more positive signs, the mortality rate is greater than 50 % [3]. Patients with more than three Ranson signs have a higher incidence of systemic complications and a higher likelihood of pancreatic necrosis than those with fewer than three signs [36]. Karimgani et al. [37] reported Ranson scores significantly higher among patients affected by necrotizing AP with sterile necrosis and fatal outcome than among those who survive.

Modified Glasgow criteria have been proposed by Osborne et al. [38] and widely used in Great Britain. This scoring system is quite similar to Ranson's (Table 2). On the whole, Glasgow criteria are as accurate as Ranson's score with reported overall sensitivity of 61 %–100 % and specificity of 85 %–92 % [3, 15–16]. Thus, Ranson's and Glasgow scores continue to be helpful in assessing severity, but some important limitations must be kept in mind when these

Table 1. The original (A) and modified (B) Ranson criteria for severity assessment in acute pancreatitis

	A	B
On admission		
Age (years)	>55	>70
White blood cells	>16 000/mm³	>18 000/mm³
Blood glucose	>180 mg/dl	>220 mg/dl
LDH	>350 IU/l	>400 IU/l
AST	>120 IU/l	>250 IU/l
During initial 48 h		
Fall in hematocrit	>10 %	>10 %
Serum calcium	<8 mg/dl	<8 mg/dl
Increase in blood urea	>5 mg/dl	>5 mg/dl
Base deficit	>4 mEq/l	>5 mEq/l
Fluid sequestration	>6000 ml	>6000 ml
Arterial pO$_2$	<60 mmHg	/

A severe attack is predicted by the presence of three or more positive criteria.

assessment systems are used. Inherent disadvantages include the following [11, 39–41]: (a) too many factors and values might be checked; (b) assessment of severity usually takes 48 h to complete, and within that period some patients may already have recovered or others may already have experienced severe complications; (c) Ranson's score is most helpful at the extremes (i.e., zero to two positive signs for prediction of mild attacks or six or more positive signs for prediction of severe forms), but less helpful in large numbers of patients with three to five positive signs; (d) some of the parameters in both scoring systems could be influenced by the treatment given during the 48-h period; (e) repetitive assessment to monitor the patient is impossible because these systems only include data from an early phase of AP; (f) it is uncertain whether these criteria are useful in patients with nonalcoholic, nonbiliary AP.

Table 2. The modified Glasgow criteria for severity prediction in acute pancreatitis

Criterion	Value
Arterial pO$_2$	<60 mmHg
Serum albumin	<3.2 g/dl
Serum calcium	<8 mg/dl
White blood cells	>15 000/mmc
AST	>200 IU/l
LDH	>600 IU/l
Blood glucose	>180 mg/dl
Blood urea	>45 mg/dl

A severe attack is predicted by the presence of three or more positive criteria.
AST, aspartate aminotransferase; LDH, lactate dehydrogenase.

Nonspecific Illness Scoring Systems

The APACHE (Acute Physiology and Chronic Health Evaluation) II illness grading system [42] awards points of severity on the basis of the extent of abnormality of several physiological variables and, in addition, includes points for age and chronic disease (Table 3). Recent studies have suggested that APACHE II is more accurate than Ranson and Glasgow systems in evaluating and monitoring the course of AP: Wilson et al. [43], utilizing as a cutoff a score of 9, reported a sensitivity of 82% and specificity of 76% in distinguishing mild and severe attacks of AP; Larvin and McMahon [44], utilizing a cutoff value of 10 points, found a sensitivity of 72% and specificity of 92%. Other studies gave disappointing results [11, 36]. In general, an APACHE II score at admission of 7 or less predicts a mild attack of AP, whereas scores greater than 7 usually reflect a more severe attack [13, 41]. Thus measurement of APACHE II score is useful as early assessment of AP severity; after 48 h it appears that the accuracy of APACHE II and Ranson's and Glasgow scores are approximately equal (70%–80%) [45]. In patients with necrotizing AP with sterile necrosis [37], APACHE II scores were significantly higher at admission among those with a fatal outcome (mean score, 14.5) than those who survived (mean score 6.5). The advantages of this assessment method are that it can be employed at any time during the patient's hospitalization and may be of value in assessing patients whose initial management may not be well documented; a major disadvantage is its complexity. SAPS (Simplified Acute Physiology Score) is a prognostic system that is less complex, but its sensitivity is lower than that of the APACHE II scoring system [13, 46].

In 1989, using a multivariate analysis on 16 admission analytes in 203 patients with AP, Fan et al. [39] were able to identify two parameters (blood urea >7.4 mmol/l, glucose >11 mmol/l) that could predict patients with fatal or nonfatal complications with a sensitivity of 75% and specificity of 80.3%. Positive results of these very simple criteria (Hong Kong criteria) were not subsequently confirmed by Heath and Imrie [13] (sensitivity of 33% and specificity of 83%) nor by ourselves [47] (sensitivity of 28.5% and specificity of 87.5%) (Table 4). Recently, Talamini et al. [48] showed that the association of a serum creatinine level of more than 2 mg/dl with pathological chest X-rays (pleural effusions and/or densifications) at admission gave a reliable prediction of death from AP. Results of this article, if confirmed, appear to be worthy of note because the study utilizes simple routine tests also available in minor hospital centers.

Complications-Specific Prognostic Criteria

Local and systemic complications greatly influence the outcome of AP. Multiorgan system failure (MOSF) and infection of necrotic pancreatic tissue have become the most important complications and cause of death and morbidity from AP [6]. In order to evaluate specific therapeutic measures, it may be helpful to have early measurements that predict these complications.

Table 3. The APACHE II Severity of Disease Classification System

Physiological variable	High abnormal range +4	+3	+2	+1	0	Low abnormal range +1	+2	+3	+4
Rectal temperature (C)	≥41	39–40.9		38.5–39.9	36–38.4	34–35.9	32–33.9	30–31.9	≤29.9
Blood pressure (mmHg)	≥160	130–159	110–129		70–109		50–69		≤49
Heart rate	≥180	140–179	110–139		70–109		55–69	40–54	≤39
Respiratory rate (nonventilated or ventilated)	≥50	35–49		25–34	12–24	10–11	6–9		≤5
Oxygenation (mmHg) $FiO_2 > 0.5/AaDO_2$	>500	350–499	200–349		<200				
$FiO_2 < 0.5/PaO_2$					$PO_2 > 70$	PO_2 61–70	PO_2 55–60	$PO_2 < 55$	
Arterial pH	≥7.7	7.6–7.69		7.5–7.59	7.33–7.49		7.25–7.32	7.15–7.24	<7.15
Serum Na⁺ (mmol/l)	≥180	160–179	155–159	150–154	130–149		120–129	111–119	≤110
Serum K⁺ (mmol/l)	≥7	6–6.9		5.5–5.9	3.5–5.4	3–3.34	2.5–2.9		<2.5
Serum creatinine (mg/100 ml); double point score for ARF	≥3.5	2–3.4	1.5–1.9		0.6–1.4		<0.6		
Hematocrit (%)	≥60		50–59.9	46–49.9	30–45.9		20–29.9		<20
WBC (×10³/mm³)	≥40		20–39.9	15–19.9	3–14.9		1–2.9	<1	
Glasgow coma score (GCS): score = 15 minus actual GCS.									

Total acute physiology score (APS): sum of 12 individual variable points.
APACHE II score is given by the *sum* of the APS, chronic health points, and age points (age <44, zero; 45–54, 2 points; 55–64, 3 points; 65–74, 5 points; and >75, 6 points). Chronic health points are assigned if the patient has a history of severe organ system insufficiency or is immunocompromised as follows: for nonoperative or emergency postoperative patients, 5 points; and for elective postoperative patients, 2 points. Organ insufficiency or immunocompromised state must be evident before hospital admission [42].
FiO₂, fraction of inspired oxygen; WBC, white blood cells; ARF, acute renal failure.

Table 4. Sensitivity, specificity, positive predictive value (VP + ve), negative predictive value (VP − ve), and efficiency of various prognostic indexes in 53 patients suffering from necrotizing acute pancreatitis

		CT	SPC	MGC	HK
Sensitivity	(%)	90.4	76.1	76.1	28.5
Specificity	(%)	77.7	84.3	43.7	87.5
VP + ve	(%)	75	76.1	47	60
VP − ve	(%)	91.3	84.3	73.6	65.1
Efficacy	(%)	85.1	81.1	56.6	64.1

Patients were divided into two groups: (a) 21 cases with severe prognosis (deaths or multicomplicated outcome) and (b) 32 cases with lighter prognosis [47].
CT, computed tomography [52]; SPC, simple prognostic criteria [48]; MGC, modified Glasgow criteria [38]; HK, Hong Kong criteria [39].

Tran et al. [11] utilized the organ-specific MOSF scoring system for the evaluation of severity in patients with AP. Organ system failure was defined as the dysfunction of one or more of the seven evaluated organ systems listed in Table 5; the MOSF score was defined as the sum of failing organ systems during the same day, and varied from 0 to 7. Severity resulted as significantly increased with the number of organ systems involved, and virtually all patients with severe outcome (local complications or death) had a MOSF score of 4 or more. Accuracy in prediction of severity for a score of more than 1 is 88% on admission and 90% at 48 h.

Table 5. Multi-Organ-System-Failure (MOSF) scoring system for the evaluation of severity in patients with acute pancreatitis [11]

Organ system	Criteria
Cardiovascular	Mean arterial pressure ≤ 50 mmHg, need for volume loading and/or vasoactive drug to maintain systolic blood pressure above 100 mmHg Heart rate ≤ 50 beats/min; ventricular tachycardia/fibrillation; cardiac arrest; acute myocardial infarction
Pulmonary	Respiratory rate ≤ 5 min or ≥ 50 min. Mechanical ventilation for 3 or more days or fraction of inspired $O_2 > 0.4$ and/or positive end-expiratory pressure > 5 mmHg
Renal	Serum creatinine ≥ 3.5 mg/dl; dyalisis/ultrafiltration
Neurological	Glasgow coma scale ≤ 6 (in absence of sedation)
Hematological	Hematocrit ≤ 20%; leukocyte count ≤ 3000/mm^3; thrombocyte count ≤ 50 000/mm^3; disseminated intravascular coagulation
Hepatic	Total bilirubin ≥ 3 mg/dl in the absence of hemolysis; ALT > 100 U/l
Gastrointestinal	Stress ulcer requiring transfusion of more than 2 units of blood per 24 h. Acalcolous cholecystitis; necrotizing enterocolitis; bowel perforation

ALT, alanine aminotransferase.

Table 6. The prognostic criteria for pancreatic sepsis in acute pancreatitis [3]

	Risk of sepsis if positive (%)
Admission	
WBC $> 16\,000/mm^3$	29
Blood glucose > 240 mg	36
LDH > 500 IU	40
48 hours	
Increase of blood urea > 5 mg	65
Calcium < 7.6 mg	52
Fluid sequestration > 6000 ml	29
Base deficit > 7 mEq/l	28
Laparotomy	30
Pancreatic drains	85

Agarwal and Pitchumoni [49] have also stressed the importance of organ system failure in determining the severity of AP. These authors proposed a system called "Simplified Prognostic Criteria" based on failure of cardiac (blood pressure < 90 mmHg and/or tachycardia $> 130/\text{min}$), pulmonary ($pO_2 < 60$ mmHg), renal (urinary output < 50 cc/h), and metabolic (calcium < 8 mg/dl, albumin < 3.2 g/dl) functions. Results are inferior to those obtained with MOSF score. In our experience (Table 4) the simplified prognostic criteria give a sensitivity of 76.1 % and a specificity of 84.3 %.

Attempts to predict infection of necrosis in AP without imaging techniques or percutaneous sampling have been performed by Ranson [3]. Starting from a large series of patients (558 cases), the author identified some prognostic criteria (Table 6) indicating the risk of sepsis; interestingly, the incidence of death from sepsis correlated well with the number of criteria considered positive.

Computed Tomography

There have been a number of prospective studies that have evaluated usefulness of computed tomography (CT) scan as a means of severity assessment in AP [8, 13, 47, 50–51]. Revision of CT grading of AP and CT classification in defining severity of the disease [52] are beyond the purpose of this article which addresses *multifactorial* prognostic evaluation of AP. However, we can bring to mind and note that enhanced CT scan is currently the gold standard in identification of pancreatic necrosis and its quantification. In the absence of air in the retroperitoneum, the usefulness of CT as a predictor of necrosis infection remains controversial even if there is some evidence [53–54] that the extent of necrosis correlates well with the risk of pancreatic sepsis. Clinical value of CT in decision-making processes may be increased by associating CT findings with multifactorial scoring systems. In our experience [47], the association of CT score according to Balthazar [52] with simple Hong Kong criteria [39] yields an overall accuracy of 90.3 % in discriminating the most severe forms within a group of patients suffering from necrotizing AP.

Conclusions

Accurate early evaluation of the severity of AP is an important goal since prompt intensive care is required for patients with severe forms. Attempts to identify pancreatic necrosis may be helpful but are less direct than attempts to predict the clinical course [3]. Several grading systems have been proposed that include clinical, radiological, and biochemical parameters. Those that proved helpful were sometimes complex and generally time-consuming. An ideal prognostic system should be eminently practical and should be applied early in the clinical course using information routinely collected by clinicians. Assessment of severity should also enable the clinician to prevent systemic complications or minimize their impact and to identify pancreatic necrosis and distinguish sterile from infected necrosis [45]. The results of multifactorial prognostic systems show that it is now possible to recognize most patients with severe AP within a few hours of admission. Although the accuracy of early assessment of the severity of AP has undoubtedly improved over the past few years, whether this leads to the improvement of treatment and to a decrease in mortality still remains open to discussion and clarification.

References

1. Kloppel G, Maillet G (1993) Pathology of acute and chronic pancreatitis. Pancreas 8: 659–670
2. Blamey SL, Imrie CW, O'Neill J, Gilmour WH, Carter DC (1984) Prognostic factors in acute pancreatitis. Gut 25: 1340–1346
3. Ranson JHC (1994) Stratification of severity for acute pancreatitis. In: Bradley EL (ed) Acute Pancreatitis: Diagnosis and Therapy. Raven Press, New York, pp 13–20
4. Malfertheiner P, Kemmer TP (1991) Clinical picture and diagnosis of acute pancreatitis. Hepato-Gastroenterol 38: 97–100
5. Uomo G, Visconti M, Manes G, Calise F, Laccetti M, Rabitti PG (1996) Nonsurgical treatment of acute necrotizing pancreatitis. Pancreas 12: 142–148
6. Bradley EL (1993) A clinically based classification system for acute pancreatitis. Arch Surg 128: 586–590
7. Beger HG, Kreutzberger W, Bittner R, Block S, Büchler M (1985) Results of surgical treatment of necrotizing pancreatitis. World J Surg 9: 972–979
8. Pitchumoni CS, Agarwal N, Jain NK (1988) Systemic complication of acute pancreatitis. Am J Gastroenterol 83: 597–606
9. Rau B, Pralle U, Uhl W, Schoenberg MH, Beger HG (1995) Management of sterile necrosis in instances of severe acute pancreatitis. J Am Coll Surg 181: 279–288
10. Malfertheiner P, Dominguez-Munoz JE (1993) Prognostic factors in acute pancreatitis. Int J Pancreatol 14: 1–8
11. Tran DD, Cuesta MA (1992) Evaluation of severity in patients with acute pancreatitis. Am J Gastroenterol 87: 604–608
12. de Beaux AC, Palmer KR, Carter DC (1995) Factors influencing morbidity and mortality in acute pancreatitis: an analysis of 279 cases. Gut 37: 121–126
13. Heath DI, Imrie CW (1991) The diagnosis and assessment of severity in acute pancreatitis. In: Pancreatic Disease. Progress and Prospect, Johnson CD and Imrie CW (eds), Springer-Verlag, London, pp 263–285
14. Funnell IC, Bornman PC, Weakley SP, Terblanche J, Marks IN (1993). Obesity: an important prognostic factor in acute pancreatitis. Br J Surg 80: 484–486
15. McMahon MJ, Playforth MJ, Pickford IR (1980) A comparative study of methods for the prediction of severity of attacks of acute pancreatitis. Br J Surg 67: 22–25
16. Corfield AP, Cooper MJ, Williamson RCN et al (1985) Prediction of severity in acute pancreatitis: a prospective comparison of three prognostic indices. Lancet 2: 403–406

17. Gray SH, Rosenman LD (1965) Acute pancreatitis. Arch Surg 91: 485-488
18. Ranson JHC, Pasternack BS (1977) Statistical methods for quantifying the severity of clinical acute pancreatitis. J Surg Res 22: 79-91
19. Goodhead B (1969) Vascular factors in the pathogenesis of acute hemorrhagic pancreatitis. Ann R Coll Surg Engl 45: 80-97
20. Lasson A, Laurell AB, Ohlsson K (1984) The correlation between complement activation protease inhibitors and clinical course in acute pancreatitis in man. Scand J Gastroenterol 19 (suppl 4): 1-10
21. Dominguez-Munoz JE, Carballo F, Garcia MJ et al (1993) Monitoring of serum proteinase-antiproteinase balance and systemic inflammatory response in prognostic evaluation of acute pancreatitis. Dig Dis Sci 38: 507-513
22. Nevalainen TJ (1988) Phospholipase A2 in acute pancreatitis. Scand J Gastroenterol 23: 897-904
23. Uhl W, Büchler M, Malfertheiner P et al (1991) PMN-elastase in comparison with CRP, antiproteases, and LDH as indicators of necrosis in human acute pancreatitis. Pancreas 6: 253-259
24. Trapnell JE (1966) The natural history and prognosis of acute pancreatitis. Ann R Coll Surg 38: 265-287
25. Lankish PG, Koop H, Otto J et al (1978) Evaluation of methalbumin in acute pancreatitis. Scand J Gastroenterol 13: 975-978
26. Warshaw AL, Lee KH (1979) Serum ribonuclease elevations and pancreatic necrosis in acute pancreatitis. Surgery 86: 227-234
27. Büchler M, Malfertheiner P, Schoentensack C et al (1986). Sensitivity of antiproteases, complement factors and C-reactive protein in detecting pancreatic necrosis: results of a prospective study. Int J Pancreatol 1: 227-235
28. Wilson C, Heads A, Shenkin A et al (1989). C-reactive protein, antiproteases and complement factors as objective markers of severity in acute pancreatitis. Br J Surg 76: 177-181
29. Gudgeon AM, Heath DI, Hurley P et al (1990) Trypsinogen activation peptides assay in the early prediction of severity of acute pancreatitis. Lancet 335: 4-7
30. Viedma JA, Perez-Mateo M, Dominguez-Munoz JE, Carballo F (1992) Role of interleukin-6 in acute pancreatitis: comparison with C-reactive protein and phospholipase A2. Gut 33: 1264-1267
31. Iovanna JL, Keim V, Nordback I et al (1994) Serum levels of pancreatitis-associated protein as indicators of the course of acute pancreatitis. Gastroenterology 106: 728-734
32. Exley AR, Leese T, Holliday MP, Swann RA, Cohen J (1992) Endotoxaemia and serum tumor necrosis factor as prognostic markers in severe acute pancreatitis. Gut 33: 1126-1128
33. Uomo G, Spada OA, Manes G et al (1996) Neopterin in acute pancreatitis. Scand J Gastroenterol 31: 1032-1036
34. Ranson JHC, Rifkind KM, Roses DF, Fink SD, Eng K, Spencer FC (1974) Prognostic signs and the role of operative management in acute pancreatitis. Surg Gynecol Obstet 139: 69-81
35. Ranson JHC (1979) The timing of biliary surgery in acute pancreatitis. Ann Surg 189: 654-662
36. Demmy TL, Burch JM, Feliciano DV, Mattox KL, Jordan GL (1988) Comparison of multiple-parameter prognostic systems in acute pancreatitis. Am J Surg 156: 492-496
37. Karimgani I, Porter KA, Langevin RE, Banks PA (1992) Prognostic factors in sterile pancreatic necrosis. Gastroenterology 103: 1636-1640
38. Osborne DH, Imrie CW, Carter DC (1981) Biliary surgery in the same admission for gallstone-associated acute pancreatitis. Br J Surg 68: 758-761
39. Fan ST, Choi TK, Lai ECS, Wong J (1989) Prediction of severity of acute pancreatitis: an alternative approach. Gut 30: 1591-1595
40. Wiliamson RCN (1984) Early assessment of severity in acute pancreatitis. Gut 25: 1331-1339
41. Banks PA (1991) Predictors of severity in acute pancreatitis. Pancreas 6 (suppl): 7-12
42. Knaus WA, Draper EA, Wagner DP, Zimmerman JE (1985) APACHE-II: a severity of disease classification system. Crit Care Med 13: 818-829
43. Wilson C, Heath DI, Imrie CW (1990) Prediction of outcome in acute pancreatitis: a comparative study of APACHE II, clinical assessment and multiple factor scoring systems. Br J Surg 77: 1260-1264
44. Larvin M, McMahon MJ (1989) APACHE-II score for assessment and monitoring of acute pancreatitis. Lancet 2: 201-204

45. Banks PA (1994) Acute pancreatitis: medical and surgical management. Am J Gastroenterol 89 (suppl 8): 78–85
46. Dominguez-Munoz JE, Carballo F, Garcia MJ et al (1993) Evaluation of the clinical usefulness of APACHE II and SAPS systems in the initial prognostic classification of acute pancreatitis: a multicenter study. Pancreas 6: 682–686
47. Uomo G, Rabitti PG, Laccetti M et al (1995) Prognostic assessment of necrotizing acute pancreatitis: results of a prospective study. Presse Med 24: 263–266
48. Talamini G, Bassi C, Falconi M et al (1996) Risk of death from acute pancreatitis. Int J Pancreatol 19: 15–24
49. Agarwal N, Pitchumoni CS (1986) Simplified prognostic criteria in acute pancreatitis. Pancreas 1: 69–73
50. Balthazar EJ, Ranson JHC, Nadich DP et al (1985) Acute pancreatitis: prognostic value of CT. Radiology 156: 767–772
51. Moulton JS (1991) The radiologic assessment of acute pancreatitis and its complications. Pancreas 6 (suppl): 13–22
52. Balthazar EJ, Robinson DL, Megibow AJ, Ranson JHC (1990) Acute pancreatitis: value of CT in establishing prognosis. Radiology 174: 331–336
53. Vesentini S, Bassi C, Talamini G, Campedelli A, Pederzoli P (1993) Positive comparison of C-reactive protein level, Ranson score and contrast-enhanced computed tomography in the prediction of septic complications of acute pancreatitis. Br J Surg 80: 755–757
54. Laccetti M, Rabitti PG, Manes G, Picciotto FP, Esposito P, Uomo G (1993) Relationship between the extent of pancreatic necrosis and sepsis in acute pancreatitis. Eur J Gastroent Hepatol 5: 871–873

Biochemical Markers in the Early Prognostic Evaluation of Acute Pancreatitis

J. E. Domínguez-Muñoz · P. Malfertheiner

Introduction

Acute pancreatitis is a heterogeneous disease that ranges from a mild and self-limited illness to a very severe and rapidly progressive condition leading to multiple organ failure and eventually to death. About 80% of patients develop a mild disease, whereas the remaining 20% suffer from a severe illness and about one fourth of them die. Any clinical decision making regarding treatment for acute pancreatitis must be based, therefore, on a proper prognostic evaluation. The classical method of identifying severity in acute pancreatitis is the application of different score systems, which are described in a previous chapter. Recently, several single biological markers for the prognostic evaluation of acute pancreatitis are attracting special attention. Compared with multifactorial classifications, single biological markers have the advantage that, besides being applicable to the clinical routine, they allow the classification of the acute pancreatitis according to severity even at the time of admission to hospital, and furthermore they are useful for close and continuous monitoring of the disease. Biochemical parameters for the early prognostic evaluation of acute pancreatitis can be classified in markers of necrosis, markers of protease activation and markers of inflammatory response [1].

Markers of Necrosis

It is well known that the presence of circulating methemalbumin indicates hemorrhagic pancreatitis. In fact, methemalbumin results from the complex of circulating albumin and hematin released by the protease-mediated hydrolysis of hemoglobin. The specificity of this marker in the diagnosis of necrohemorrhagic pancreatitis is thus high, but its sensitivity is limited [2, 3]. In a more recent study, the prognostic value of methemalbumin in patients with acute pancreatitis was similar to that of the classical scoring systems [4].

Pancreatic ribonuclease is an intracellular enzyme which is released only in association with cellular death, so that an increase of the serum levels of this enzyme indicates pancreatic necrosis [5, 6]. Similar to methemalbumin, circulating pancreatic ribonuclease is a specific marker for necrotizing pancreatitis, but its sensitivity is low, limiting its clinical use.

Markers of Protease Activation

An interesting approach in the prognostic evaluation of acute pancreatitis is the quantification of the amount of trypsinogen activated by determining trypsinogen activation peptide (TAP) in urine. TAP is generated by pathological intrapancreatic trypsinogen activation (activation of a molecule of trypsinogen results in a molecule of trypsin and a molecule of TAP) and is liberated into the peritoneal cavity and circulation, it is cleared by the kidney and excreted in the urine. A high TAP concentration in peritoneal fluid indicates pancreatic necrosis with an accuracy similar to that of contrast enhanced computed tomography [7] (Table 1). A high renal elimination of TAP is observed from the very beginning of acute pancreatitis in patients with severe disease. According to the study of the group of Glasgow, an urinary TAP concentration higher than 2 nmol/l indicates severe pancreatitis with an accuracy of 85%–90% [8]. The differentiation between mild and severe acute pancreatitis is however possible only during the first 12 h of disease. In a recent study, Tenner and coworkers confirmed the high accuracy of a urinary TAP concentration higher than 10 nmol/l in the prognostic evaluation of acute pancreatitis, but again only during the first 24 h of disease [9]. This finding, together with the fact that determination of TAP requires an enzyme immunoassay, limits the clinical applicability of this marker for the prognostic evaluation of acute pancreatitis.

Markers of Inflammatory Response

The major progress over the last years in the prognostic evaluation of acute pancreatitis has been based on the knowledge of the pathophysiological events occurring in the early phase of the disease (Fig. 1). Whatever etiological factor might initially trigger acute pancreatitis, oxygen free radicals will be released from the damaged acinar cells. These oxygen free radicals contribute to activate pancreatic proteases and to yield chemotactic substances for inflammatory cells [10–12]. Activated neutrophils and macrophages also release oxygen free rad-

Table 1. Sensitivity and specificity of biochemical markers for the prognostic evaluation of acute pancreatitis. Figures represent the lowest and highest value reported in the literature

Marker	Sensitivity (%)	Specificity (%)
TAP	85–100	86–90
Protease inhibitors	70–85	70–80
Proteolytic systems	73–79	73–75
Phospholipase A	42–80	78–89
PMN elastase	88–92	80–100
IL-6	80–93	67–92
CRP	73–95	71–86

Variability in sensitivity and specificity values depends primarily on differences in diagnostic criteria for severity, time elapsed from onset of acute pancreatitis to prognostic evaluation, and number of patients studied.
PMN, polymorphonuclear; IL-6, interleukin-6; CRP, C-reactive protein; TAP, trypsinogen activation peptide.

Biochemical Markers in the Early Prognostic Evaluation of Acute Pancreatitis 111

Fig. 1. Pathophysiological events and release of mediators in severe acute pancreatitis. O_2-FR, O_2 free radicals; PF_4, platelet factor 4; TXA_2, thromboxane, A_2; PG, prostaglandins; LT, leukotrienes; PAF, platelet activating factor; NO nitric oxide; MOF, multiorgan failure

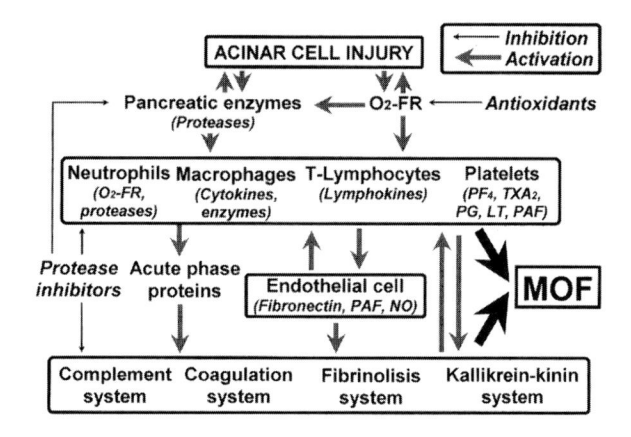

icals together with enzymes and cytokines, which play a major role in the inflammatory process. All these factors, together with mediators released by lymphocytes, platelets and endothelial cells are able to activate the different proteolytic systems (complement, coagulation, fibrinolysis and kallikrein-kinin). The final result will be the development of multiorganic failure. The severity of acute pancreatitis is closely related to the intensity of this inflammatory response. Therefore, quantification of any of these mediators in blood will indicate how intense is the inflammatory reaction and thus how high the risk is of developing severe acute pancreatitis.

Antiproteases

In blood, active proteases are immediately inhibited by circulating antiproteases, basically α_2-macroglobulin (AMG). The protease–AMG complex is thereafter cleared by the reticuloendothelial system. AMG is thus consumed during acute pancreatitis, mainly in patients with severe disease (Fig. 2) [13–15]. A decrease of serum AMG of more than 25 mg/dl within the first 48 h of disease is an index of severe acute pancreatitis with an accuracy of 70%–80% [13] (see table 1). As serum AMG reflects the pathophysiological events occurring during acute pancreatitis (protease–antiprotease balance), serial determination might be useful for monitoring the disease.

Similar accuracy can be obtained with the determination of the serum levels of α_1-protease inhibitor (API). This antiprotease behaves as a positive acute-phase reactant during acute pancreatitis; furthermore, it is not consumed as it transfers the protease molecule to AMG to be cleared. Serum API levels, therefore, increase more markedly in severe cases of acute pancreatitis (Fig. 3) [13–15].

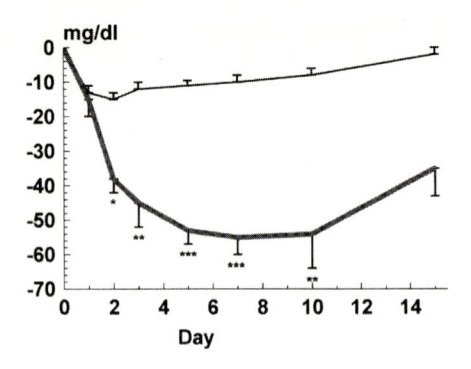

Fig. 2. Serum levels of α_2-macroglobulin in mild (*solid line*) and severe (*shaded line*) acute pancreatitis. Value at time of admission to hospital (between 2 and 12 h from onset of symptoms) was considered as 0, and variations of serum concentrations from this basal value are shown. *$p < 0.05$; **$p < 0.01$; ***$p < 0.001$. (From [13])

Proteolytic Cascades

The different proteolytic systems that participate in the inflammatory process (complement, coagulation, fibrinolysis and kallikrein-kinin systems) show extensive and complex interactions with plasma protease inhibitors, inflammatory cells, feedback mechanisms, cytokines, hormones and endotoxins. Once any of the proteolytic systems is activated, the remaining systems will also be activated. There is a great deal of biochemical evidence of the activation of proteolytic systems in acute pancreatitis in humans, the intensity of that activation being correlated with the severity of the disease.

During acute pancreatitis, active pancreatic proteases, neutrophil proteases, endotoxins, plasmin and kallikrein among other factors are able to split complement factors C1, C3 and C5 to produce biologically active fragments that mediate a marked inflammatory reaction and aggravate the course of the disease (see Fig. 1). Serum levels of complement factors in acute pancreatitis are the result of the balance between consumption due to activation, which predominates during the early phase of the disease, and synthesis due to acute phase reaction, which predominates later on (Fig. 4) [13]. Consumption of complement factors is more marked in severe than in mild acute pancreatitis and, in fact, low serum levels of C3 and C4 have been repeatedly reported in patients

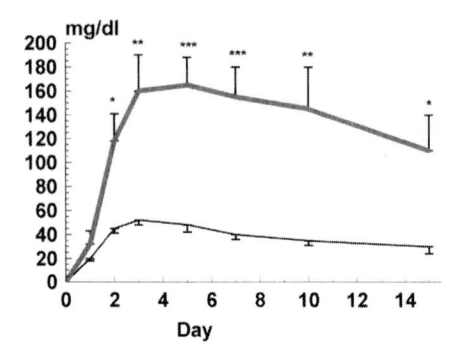

Fig. 3. Serum levels of α_1-protease inhibitor in mild (*solid line*) and severe (*shaded line*) acute pancreatitis. Value at time of admission to hospital (between 2 and 12 h from onset of symptoms) was considered as 0, and variations of serum concentrations from this basal value are shown. *$p < 0.05$; **$p < 0.01$; ***$p < 0.001$. (From [13])

Fig. 4. Serum levels of complement factor C3 in mild (*solid line*) and severe (*shaded line*) acute pancreatitis. Value at time of admission to hospital (between 2 and 12 h from onset of symptoms) was considered as 0 and variations of serum concentrations from this basal value are shown. $*p<0.05$; $**p<0.01$; $***p<0.001$. (From [13])

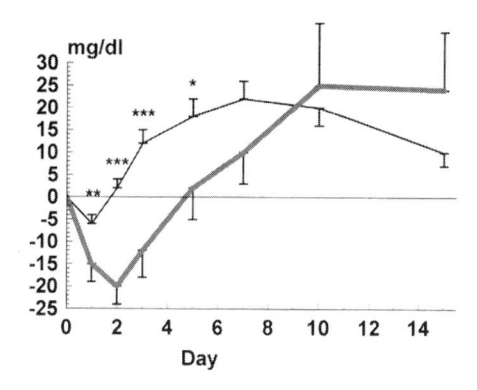

with severe desease [13, 16, 17]. The accuracy of serum levels of complement factors in the early prognostic evaluation of acute pancreatitis is, however, limited (see Table 1).

Coagulation, fibrinolysis and kallikrein-kinin systems may also be activated in acute pancreatitis. In this context, decreased circulating levels of antithrombin III and C-peptide [18], plasminogen-activator inhibitor and α_2-plasmin inhibitor [18, 19] and prekallikrein and kininogen [20] have been described in patients with severe acute pancreatitis. However, the clinical utility of these factors in the prognostic classification of acute pancreatitis has not been evaluated.

Cell-Mediated Inflammatory Response

One of the earliest events in the pathogenesis of acute pancreatitis is the infiltration into the pancreatic interstitium of activated neutrophils and macrophages, which release a great amount of active inflammatory mediators. Among the substances released by the activated neutrophils, elastase is the best studied and probably the most relevant from a clinical point of view. This enzyme is able to degrade all the components of the extracellular matrix, to hydrolyze a large number of key plasma proteins, such as immunoglobulins, complement proteins, coagulation and fibrinolysis factors, and even to attack intact cells [21]. Plasma concentrations of polymorphonuclear (PMN) elastase rise from the very onset of acute pancreatitis in patients who subsequently develop a severe form of the disease (Fig. 5) [22, 23]. The relationship between plasma levels of PMN elastase and the grade of severity of acute pancreatitis is so close that this test has an accuracy for the early prognostic evaluation of the disease higher than 90% [22]. Neutrophils synthesize and release many other active substances, among them interleukin (IL)-1β that is a potent inducer of IL-6 in peripheral blood monocytes [24].

Determination of the circulating levels of IL-6 also has a high accuracy in the prognostic evaluation of acute pancreatitis [25–27], and a high correlation between circulating IL-6 and PMN-elastase has been reported in these patients [25].

Fig. 5. Plasma levels of polymorphonuclear (PMN) elastase in mild (*solid line*) and severe (*shaded line*) acute pancreatitis. $*p < 0.05$; $***p < 0.001$. (From [22])

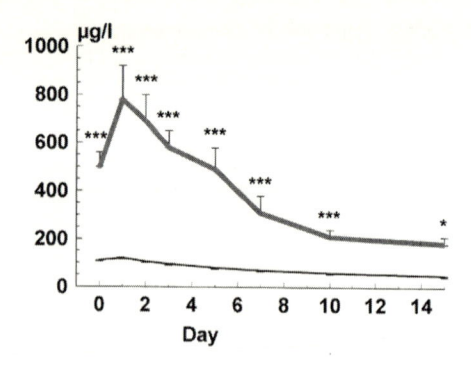

Phospholipase A_2, a marker of phagocytic activity in inflammation and necrosis, is involved in the pathophysiological process of severe acute pancreatitis. The monocyte-macrophage system is thought to be the major source of active phospholipase A in plasma. This enzyme has been implicated in the development of pancreatic necrosis and pulmonary failure during acute pancreatitis [28] and its plasma activity correlates with the severity of the disease [25, 28, 29]. The accuracy of the plasma phospholipase A activity for the assessment of severity in acute pancreatitis is around 80%, but its determination is methodologically cumbersome and, therefore, difficult to use routinely in clinical practice.

The measurement of other circulating PMN or monocyte mediators should provide similar prognostic information in patients with acute pancreatitis. The clinical applicability of all these parameters depends on the development of new biochemical assays which are easily applicable in the clinical routine.

Acute-Phase Proteins

The increase of acute-phase reactants, such as C-reactive protein (CRP), during acute pancreatitis is a consequence of stimulated hepatic synthesis of these proteins mediated mainly by IL-6. The elevation of CRP im serum occurs, therefore, with delay with respect to neutrophil and monocyte mediators [13, 25-27, 30]. This increase is much higher in patients with severe than with mild pancreatitis (Fig. 6). The clinical utility of serum CRP levels for predicting severity in acute pancreatitis is thus similar to that of circulating cell mediators (IL-6, PMN elastase), although not as early but 48-72 h after the onset of the disease [13, 16, 17, 25-27, 30, 31] (see Table 1). The clinical applicability of serum CRP in the prognostic evaluation of acute pancreatitis is facilitated by the availability of biochemical methods for its determination.

Fig. 6. Serum levels of C-reactive protein in mild (*solid line*) and severe (*shaded line*) acute pancreatitis. **$p < 0.01$; ***$p < 0.001$. (From [13])

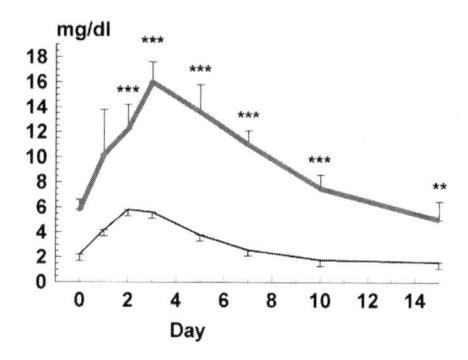

Prognostic Evaluation of Acute Pancreatitis: Guidelines

Early prognostic evaluation of acute pancreatitis is unfortunately not accompanied by therapeutic measures that, if applied early, can improve the clinical outcome of the disease. Early prognostic evaluation of acute pancreatitis assists however in selecting patients that should be closely monitored from the onset of the disease enabling early treatment and even prevention of systemic complications of the disease. Moreover, evaluation of prognostic factors in acute pancreatitis are useful in the classification of patients to be included in clinical trials.

Table 1 summarizes the sensitivity and specificity of the different biochemical markers in the prognostic classification of acute pancreatitis. Among them, TAP, PMN elastase, IL-6 and CRP are generally found to be the most accurate markers. TAP has the drawback of being useful only at the very beginning of the disease. Furthermore, TAP as well as IL-6 require an enzyme immunoassay for quantification, which makes the application in the clinical routine as emergency parameter difficult. CRP and PMN elastase appear, therefore, to be the most valuable markers in acute pancreatitis. Circulating concentrations of these two parameters usually increase before the severity of the disease is clinically evident and if a determined cutoff is reached (CRP > 120 mg/l, PMN elastase > 250 µg/l) further explorations, i.e., contrast enhanced computed tomography (CT), and close monitoring of vital functions become necessary. On the other hand, low levels of both biochemical factors may spare further investigations; a careful clinical evaluation is, however, always required. The guidelines we propose for the early prognostic evaluation of acute pancreatitis are summarized in Fig. 7.

Fig. 7. Guidelines for the prognostic evaluation of acute pancreatitis. Determination of polymorphonuclear (*PMN*) elastase and C-reactive protein (*CRP*) over the first 72 h. *CT*, computed tomography

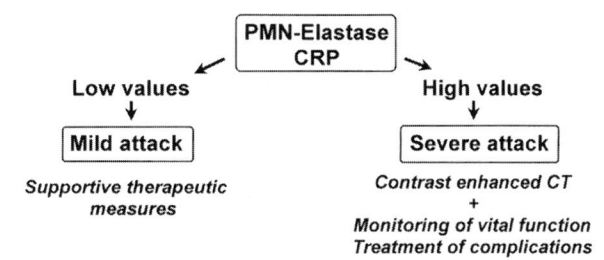

References

1. Malfertheiner P, Domínguez-Muñoz JE (1993) Prognostic factors in acute pancreatitis. Int J Pancreatol 14: 1-8
2. McMahon MJ, Playforth MJ, Pickford R (1980) A comparative study of methods for the prediction of severity of attacks of acute pancreatitis. Br J Surg 67: 22-25
3. Ranson JHC, Rifkind KM, Roses DF, et al (1974) Objective early identification of severe acute pancreatitis. Am J Gastroenterol 61: 443-451
4. Lankisch PG, Schirren CA, Otto J (1989) Methemalbumin in acute pancreatitis: An evaluation of its prognostic value and comparison with multiple prognostic parameters. Am J Gastroenterol 84: 1391-1395
5. Warshaw AL, Lee KH (1979) Serum ribonuclease elevations and pancreatic necrosis in acute pancreatitis. Surgery 86: 227-234
6. Kemmer TP, Malfertheiner P, Büchler M, Kemmer ML, Ditschuneit H (1991) Serum ribonuclease activity in the diagnosis of pancreatic disease. Int J Pancreatol 8: 23-33
7. Heath DI, Wilson C, Gudgeon AM, Jehanli A, Shenkin A, Imrie CW (1994) Trypsinogen activation peptides (TAP) concentrations in the peritoneal fluid of patients with acute pancreatitis and their relation to the presence of histologically confirmed pancreatic necrosis. Gut 35: 1311-1315
8. Gudgeon AM, Heath DI, Hurley P, et al (1990) Trypsinogen activation peptides assay in the early prediction of severity of acute pancreatitis. Lancet 335: 4-8
9. Tenner S, Fernández del Castillo C, Warshaw AL, et al (1995) Urinary trypsinogen activation peptide predicts severity in acute pancreatitis. Gastroenterology 108 (Abstract)
10. Sanfey H, Bulkley GB, Cameron JL (1984) The role of oxygen derived free radicals in the pathogenesis of acute pancreatitis. Ann Surg 200: 405-413
11. Dormandy TL (1983) An approach to free radicals. Lancet 2: 1010-1014
12. Ernster L (1988) Biochemistry of reoxygenation injury. Crit Care Med 16: 947-953
13. Domínguez-Muñoz JE, Carballo F, García MJ, et al (1993) Monitoring of serum proteinase-antiproteinase balance and systemic inflammatory response in the prognostic evaluation of acute pancreatitis: Results of a prospective multicenter study. Dig Dis Sci 38: 507-512
14. McMahon MJ, Bowen M, Mayer AD, Cooper EH (1984) Relation of α_2-macroglobulin and other antiproteinases to the clinical features of acute pancreatitis. Am J Surg 147: 164-170
15. Büchler M, Uhl W, Malfertheiner P (1987) Biochemical staging of acute pancreatitis. In: Beger HG, Büchler M, eds. Acute pancreatitis. Springer-Verlag: Berlin-Heidelberg 143-153
16. Büchler M, Malfertheiner P, Schötensack C, Uhl W, Beger HG (1986) Sensitivity of antiproteases, complement factors and C-reactive protein in detecting pancreatic necrosis. Results of a prospective clinical study. Int J Pancreatol 1: 227-235
17. Wilson C, Heads A, Shenkin A, Imrie CW (1989) C-reactive protein, antiproteases and complement factors as objective markers of severity in acute pancreatitis. Br J Surg 76: 177-181
18. Lässon A, Ohlsson K (1988) Systemic involvement in pancreatic damage: coagulation and fibrinolysis. Int J Pancreatol 3: 579-586
19. Hesselvik JF, Blombäck M, Brodin B, Maller R (1989) Coagulation, fibrinolysis and kallikrein systems in sepsis: Relation to outcome. Crit Care Med 17: 724-733
20. Lässon A, Ohlsson K (1984) Changes in the kallikrein-kinin system during acute pancreatitis in man. Thrombos Res 35: 27-41
21. Janoff A (1985) Elastase in cell injury. Ann Rev Med 36: 207-216
22. Domínguez-Muñoz JE, Carballo F, Garcia MJ, et al (1991) Clinical usefulness of polymorphonuclear elastase in predicting the severity of acute pancreatitis: Results of a multicentre study. Br J Surg 78: 1230-1234
23. Gross V, Schölmerich J, Leser HG, et al (1990) Granulocyte elastase in assessment of severity of acute pancreatitis: Comparison with acute phase proteins C-reactive protein, α_1-antitrypsin, and protease inhibitor α_2-macroglobulin. Dig Dis Sci 35: 97-105
24. Tosato G, Jones KD (1990) Interleukin-1 induces interleukin-6 production in peripheral blood monocytes. Blood 75: 1305-1310
25. Viedma JA, Pérez-Mateo M, Domínguez-Muñoz JE, Carballo F (1992) Role of interleukin-6 in acute pancreatitis: Comparison with C-reactive protein and phospholipase A. Gut 33: 1264-1267
26. Leser HG, Gross V, Scheibenbogen C, et al (1991) Elevation of serum interleukin-6 concentration precedes acute-phase response and reflects severity in acute pancreatitis. Gastroenterology 101: 782-785

27. Heath DI, Crickshank A, Gudgeon M, Jehanli A, Shenkin A, Imrie CW (1993) Role of interleukin-6 in mediating the acute-phase protein response and potential as an early means of severity assessment in acute pancreatitis. Gut 34: 41–45
28. Büchler M, Malfertheiner P, Schädlich H, Nevalainen TJ, Friess H, Beger HG (1989) Role of phospholipase A_2 in human acute pancreatitis. Gastroenterology 97: 1521–1526
29. Bird NC, Goodman AJ, Johnson AG (1989) Serum phospholipase A_2 activity in acute pancreatitis: an early guide to severity. Br J Surg 76: 731–732
30. Uhl W, Büchler M, Malfertheiner P, Martini M, Beger HG (1991) PMN-elastase in comparison with CRP, antiproteases, and LDH as indicators of necrosis in human acute pancreatitis. Pancres 6: 253–259
31. Mayer AD, McMahon MJ, Bowen M, Cooper EH (1984) C-reactive protein: an aid to assessment and monitoring acute pancreatitis. J Clin Pathol 37: 207–211

Prognostic Evaluation of Acute Pancreatitis: When and How – Consequences for Clinical Management

W. Uhl · R. Vogel · M. W. Büchler

Introduction

The diagnosis of "acute pancreatitis" is established relatively rapidly and reliably by an exact case history, typical clinical symptoms during physical examination, and overall by specific laboratory tests, namely, serum pancreatic enzymes [1–8]. However, a clear differentiation of acute pancreatitis in acute interstitial edematous pancreatitis (clinically mild to moderate course) and necrotizing pancreatitis (clinically severe course, with high morbidity and mortality rates even today) is not possible by means of clinical symptoms and routine clinical laboratory parameters. In particular, serum pancreatic enzymes have been shown not to be able to discriminate between mild and severe courses of acute pancreatitis [1–8]. More recently, carboxylic ester hydrolase (CEH) and human pancreas-specific protein (hPASP) have been introduced as being significantly higher elevated in necrotizing pancreatitis as compared to edematous pancreatitis; however, further investigations are mandatory [9, 10].

The current "gold standard" for the discrimination of the two clinical forms of acute pancreatitis is based on the findings of contrast-enhanced computed tomography (CT) scanning, which has in fact the highest sensitivity, specificity, and accuracy rate for assessing the severity of the disease. It has, however, the disadvantage of being relatively expensive and not always available.

This chapter deals with the prognostic evaluation of acute pancreatitis by means of different score systems, single biochemical parameters, and imaging procedures, and their consequences for clinical management.

Clinical Setting and Multifactorial Score Systems

For the clinician, it is extremely important to evaluate the severity of acute pancreatitis correctly at the beginning because patients with necrotizing pancreatitis may profit from early intensive care measures and if necessary from surgical intervention (e.g., necrosectomy and lavage therapy) [1, 11].

Although clinical signs are suitable for supporting the diagnosis of acute pancreatitis, they are not helpful in evaluating the severity of the illness. The main problem is that the clinical presentation of acute pancreatitis is similar to the phenomenon of a "chameleon", so one may not notice any differences between the two morphological forms by assessing the clinical symptoms at the time of admission to hospital [12].

Table 1. A meta-analysis of clinical assessment and score systems for the evaluation of the severity of acute pancreatitis

	Patients (n)	Sensitivity (%)	Specificity (%)
Clinical assessment:	1253	37	94
Score systems:			
Ranson	747	72	76
Glasgow	1369	63	84
APACHE II	447	65	74

In the past few years, different staging systems for the assessment of the prognosis of acute pancreatitis have evolved [2, 13–21]. The best-known score systems are the Ranson, Glasgow, SAPS (Simplified Acute Physiology Score) [22], and APACHE II Score. In the clinical situation, the APACHE II Score [14, 15] and the Ranson Score [19] are found to be the most commonly used score systems to evaluate the severity of acute pancreatitis (Table 1). However, these multifactorial staging systems have at least four disadvantages:

1. The score systems are extensive and require too many factors for their evaluation.
2. For assessment, a 24- to 48-h observation period is necessary.
3. The parameters measured are mainly influenced by therapeutical measures.
4. These score systems do not include any morphological criteria for interinstitutional comparisons of results.

Besides these multifactorial staging systems, single parameters have been developed, such as serum ribonuclease activity [23, 24], methemalbumin in the blood [25, 26], or the judgement of the color of pancreatic ascites [27]. Yet none of these tests have found widespread use in clinical routine (Table 2).

Other single parameters such as acute phase protein, C-reactive protein (CRP) [28, 30], polymorphonuclear (PMN) elastase [31, 33], phospholipase A_2 (PLA$_2$) [34, 36], and the antiprotease α_1-antitrypsin and α_2-macroglobulin [2,

Table 2. A meta-analysis of single prognostic factors for the evaluation of the severity of acute pancreatitis

Parameters	Sensitivity (%) Mean	Range	Specificity (%) Mean	Range
Blood tests				
Methemalbumin	58	11–88	83	72–92
Ribonuclease acitivity	59	31–92	88	85–92
α_1-Antitrypsin	64	50–73	72	68–78
α_2-Macroglobulin	75	70–82	77	75–84
Complement factors: C3, C4	71	69–73	70	67–73
Phospholipase A_2 activity	78	75–80	84	78–89
PMN elastase	85	80–92	89	80–100
Interleukin-6	85	70–100	87	71–79
C-reactive protein	84	60–100	86	71–100
Urine test				
Trypsinogen activating peptide	80		90	

PMN, polymorphonuclear.

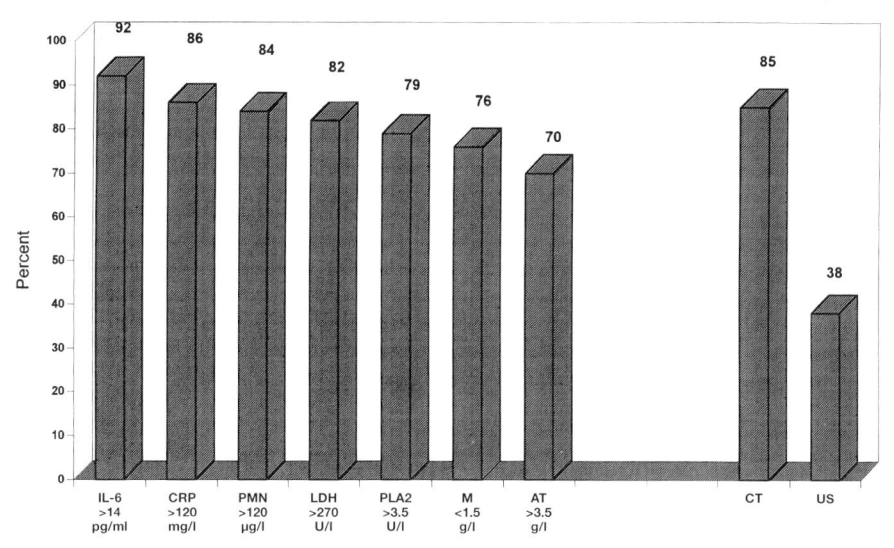

Fig. 1. Overall accuracy rates (sensitivity and specificty) of prognostic single laboratory parameters and imaging procedures for detecting necrotizing pancreatitis. *IL-6*, interleukin-6; *CRP*, C-reactive protein; *PMN*, PMN elastase; *LDH*, Lactate dehydrogenase; PLA_2, phospholipase A_2; *M*, α_2-macroglobulin; *AT*, α_1-antitrypsin; *CT*, contrast-enhanced computed tomography; *US*, ultrasound

28, 37, 38] have been shown to have an impact on detecting severe or necrotizing pancreatitis that is comparable to contrast-enhanced CT scanning (Fig. 1) [1].

Other highly promising markers of necrosis seem to be interleukin-6 [39–42], trypsinogen activating peptide (TAP), and type 1 prophospolipase A_2 activating peptide (PROP) [43–48] in preliminary clinical studies.

Pancreatic Enzymes

In the center of attention of laboratory examinations, detection of different enzymes of the pancreas in the blood and/or urine is found, particularly amylase and/or lipase. Amylase is used more often because of the simplicity and quickness of the method and the long-standing experience in clinical laboratories. Pancreatic enzyme determination is very helpful in the diagnosis of acute pancreatitis, but fails to have any clinical significance for the assessment of the prognosis. However, one may have to take into account that the use of amylase or lipase as diagnostic markers is not in every way recommendable because the sensitivity and specificity of both enzymes are insufficient with time compared to other pancreatic enzymes such as trypsin or elastase-1 [3, 4, 6, 49, 50]. In addition, in the literature certain paradoxical enzyme activities are mentioned [3, 5], namely low amylase activites in necrotizing pancreatitis and high activities in edematous pancreatitis. This phenomenon is probably the result of a

The activation of the whole system can apparently be effected in the classic way (starting with C1 and comprising 11 factors), and also in the alternative way (beginning with C3 by the C3 activator). Active pancreatic and neutrophil proteases, endotoxin, plasmin, and kallikrein can directly activate several complement factors.

In different studies, increased catabolism of complement components has been shown during acute pancreatitis, made visible by reduced serum levels of the factors C3 and C4 [53]. Sensitivity and specificity are approximately 70 % (Table 2). It has to be taken into consideration that the serum levels of the components are dependent on the one hand on catabolism and on the other hand on anabolism, which can vary without any visible mutual interdependence on other mechanisms. However, these parameters did not make a significant difference because of their low clinical relevance.

In this context, decreased levels of antithrombin III, plasminogen activator inhibitor (PAI)-1, α_2-antiplasmin, prekallikrein, and kininogen were measured during severe acute pancreatitis [55]. However, the clinical role of these factors as prognostic parameters still has to be evaluated in the future.

PMN Elastase

The systemic inflammatory response plays an important role during the course of acute pancreatitis. Immigration of PMN granulocytes and macrophages into the inflamed pancreatic and peripancreatic tissue follows immediately after the induction of acute pancreatitis. A very important substance of this inflammatory process is PMN elastase. This enzyme is released by polymorphonuclear granulocytes and has been examined quite thoroughly. In different studies, a correlation between PMN concentrations measured in plasma and the severity of acute pancreatitis has been shown. The accuracy rates of PMN elastase are at approximately 85 % (Figs. 1, 2) [31, 33].

PMN elastase increase takes place before CRP elevation [31, 32, 33], comparable to the behavior of interleukins. In our opinion, the prognostic value is not superior to the results obtained by CRP (Table 2). In addition, there are still methodological problems in adapting the PMN elastase assay to automatic laboratory analyzers.

Plasma Proteinase Inhibitors

One of the central events of the pathogenesis of acute pancreatitis is the local and systemic release of activated proteolytic enzymes. If these enzymes reach the blood circulation during the inflammatory process, more or less specific plasma inhibitors bind to them in order to inactivate them [12, 37, 38, 56].

In systemic circulation, at least six different antiproteases exist, of which α_1-antitrypsin (a polymorphous glycoprotein acting as a specific antienzyme against trypsin and chymotrypsin) and α_2-macroglobulin (also a glycoprotein that binds specifically to plasmin and trypsin) are the most common and important ones. The importance of α_2-macroglobulin seems to be greater because during a reduction to less than 30% of the normal level, activation of different cascade systems such as the coagulation, complement, kallikrein, kinin, and fibrinolytic systems has been observed in vitro.

Several clinical studies have shown that the plasma levels of α_2-macroglobulin are decreased significantly in severe cases of acute pancreatitis in comparison with mild courses [28, 30, 37, 38, 50]. Because of this fact, Ohlsson and Balldin proposed the hypothesis that disruption of the "protease-antiprotease balance" is one of the most important pathogenetic mechanisms in the development of acute pancreatitis. α_1-Antitrypsin, in contrast, is an acute-phase reactant, increasing during acute pancreatitis, especially in severe courses of the disease. However, the prognostic values of both protease inhibitors, α_1-antitrypsin and α_2-macroglobulin, are not much higher than those of the classic scoring systems with sensitivities and specificities of approximately 70%. The determination of serum antiproteases for evaluating the severity of acute pancreatitis is not recommendable due to these low accuracy rates (Table 2).

Phospholipase A$_2$

During the pathogenesis of acute pancreatitis, PLA$_2$ has been claimed to be of utmost importance, especially for the inflammatory process within and outside the pancreas. The activation of other enzymes by PLA$_2$ leads to self-perpetuating pancreatic autodigestion and fat necroses. During this process, it seems that the group of enzymes of PLA$_2$ are extremely important for the development of intra- and extrapancreatic necroses and also for the genesis of systemic organ complications, e.g., by destruction of the surfactant in the lungs by PLA$_2$ [10, 34, 35, 36].

Recent research has shown that at least two different types of secretory PLA$_2$ are present which can be measured in the serum during the course of acute pancreatitis. Type I PLA$_2$ is of pancreatic origin and type II is of unknown origin. The latter is thought to possibly originate from inflammatory cells such as leucocytes or the liver (assuming it is an acute-phase reactant). Clinical studies during the past years have shown that the serum type I PLA$_2$ values do not differ between mild and severe acute pancreatitis. On the contrary, type II PLA$_2$ measured as serum catalytic PLA$_2$ activity has been proved to be a good prognostic marker [34, 35, 36]. It has been shown that between the edematous and necrotizing courses of acute pancreatitis, there is a clear difference in type II PLA$_2$ activities (Table 2, Fig. 1). In addition, a correlation was found between the serum levels and the impairment of pulmonary function [11]. The limiting problem of this marker is the fact that no type II PLA$_2$ assay exists at present for routine clinical use.

Trypsinogen Activating Peptide and Type 1 Prophospholipase A₂ Activating Peptide

Trypsinogen activating peptide (TAP) is a part of trypsinogen consisting of five amino acids (DDDDK) that is released during activation of trypsinogen [43, 44]. In contrast to trypsinogen, TAP is not bound immediately by protease inhibitors but excreted by urine, in which it was first measured by a radioimmunoassay. The results of predicting the course of the disease (mild or severe) in a preliminary study were 80% and 90% for sensitivity and specificity, respectively [44]. In 1994, a test was developed for measuring TAP in the peritoneal fluid, which showed similar results [45]. Recently, the test has also been adapted to measure the parameter in plasma [48].

Type 1 prophospholipase A₂ activating peptide (PROP) is cleaved during the activation of type I PLA₂ and consists of seven amino acids (DSGISPR). The release of PROP seems to be a specific consequence of the activation of granulocytes and seems to be important during detorioration in acute lung impairment [46, 47]. In association with the TAP assay, the additional measurement of PROP could be a new prognostic marker for the future [48], which has still to be proved by prospective clinical studies.

Imaging Procedures

Today, contrast-enhanced computed tomography (CT) is the worldwide "gold standard" for the discrimination of acute interstitial edematous and necrotizing pancreatitis [57, 58, 59, 60, 61]. During the past years, different investigators have confirmed that contrast-enhanced CT is the most important single modality for evaluating patients with acute pancreatitis. In the past, a positive relationship between morphological findings and clinical course and outcome has been demonstrated. This technique also presents the possibility of classifying patients with acute pancreatitis on a morphological basis for interinstitutional comparison.

The main function of dynamic contrast-enhanced CT is to differentiate between perfused and nonperfused tissue in and around the pancreas, representing vital and necrotic tissue, respectively. Furthermore, the findings and scans can be discussed interdisciplinarily in a manner independent of the examiners. For surgeons, this fact is important for developing an accurate preoperative map of the spread of the necroses and for the surgical strategy. Thus, contrast-enhanced CT plays a decisive role in the clinical decision-making process during the course of this acute inflammatory illness (Figs. 1, 3).

Ultrasonography is used chiefly in bedside examinations. In staging acute pancreatitis, this method is certainly less useful than contrast-enhanced CT [28, 62]. The major disadvantage of this imaging procedure is it's limitation regarding a good view into the retroperitoneum in patients with bowel distension and accumulation of intestinal gas due to paralytic ileus, especially in severe acute pancreatitis. However, an ultrasound examination should be performed in all patients in the initial phase at the emergency unit because it may support diffe-

Fig. 3. Algorithm for clinical decision-making in patients with acute pancreatitis. *AP*, acute pancreatitis; *AIP*, acute interstitial edematous pancreatitis; *NP*, acute necrotizing pancreatitis; *ERCP*, endoscopic retrograde cholangiopancreatography; *CT*, computed tomography; *CRP*, C-reactive protein

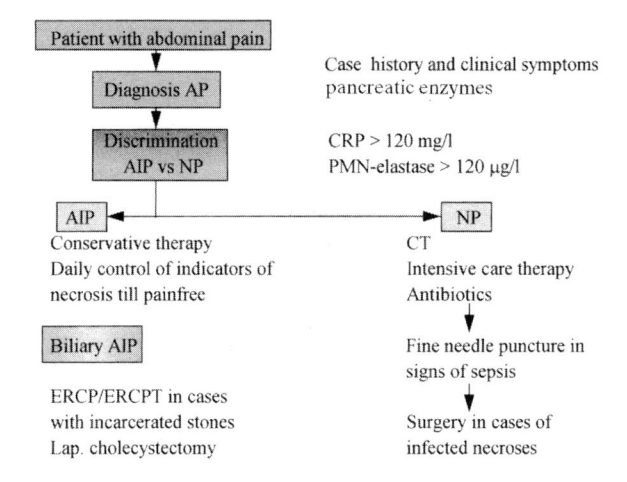

```
Patient with abdominal pain          Case history and clinical symptoms
            ↓                        pancreatic enzymes
      Diagnosis AP
            ↓
      Discrimination                 CRP > 120 mg/l
        AIP vs NP                    PMN-elastase > 120 µg/l
        ↙         ↘
     AIP           NP
Conservative therapy    CT
Daily control of indicators of    Intensive care therapy
necrosis till painfree            Antibiotics
                                       ↓
    Biliary AIP                   Fine needle puncture in
                                  signs of sepsis
ERCP/ERCPT in cases                    ↓
with incarcerated stones          Surgery in cases of
Lap. cholecystectomy              infected necroses
```

rential diagnosis and detection of gallstones as the probable cause of biliary acute pancreatitis.

Consequence for Clinical Management

As mentioned above, there are no problems in diagnosing acute pancreatitis today, which is performed easily by clinical manifestation, history, and overall measurement of serum pancreatic enzymes. The next important step in the management of patients suffering from acute inflammatory disease of the pancreas is the discrimination between acute interstitial edematous and necrotizing pancreatitis. In this respect, the sensitivity and specificity of the markers of necroses (C-reactive protein and PMN elastase) are nearly similar to those of contrast-enhanced CT, so this expensive investigation should be restricted to dealing with special questions concerning those patients with elevated parameters indicating a necrotizing course of the disease (e.g., evaluation of the extent of the necroses; Fig. 3). In cases with acute interstitial edematous pancreatitis, conservative therapy with daily control of indicators of necroses until the patients is painfree is mandatory.

In patients with elevated serum markers of necroses above the cutoff value for strong suspicion of necrotizing pancreatitis, a contrast-enhanced CT scan should be performed as the main basic investigation. These patients should be hospitalized on the ICU or intermediate care ward and treated by maximum intensive care measures for the management of systemic complications and antibiotics penetrating into the pancreas/necroses and covering the germs commonly found in infected pancreatic necroses. This new treatment concept offers the possibility of being more conservative in severe acute pancreatitis in ameliorating the clinical course of the disease and reducing the risk of infection [63, 64, 65]. If the patient presents signs of sepsis in the following course, ultrasound- or CT-guided fine-needle puncture and analysis of the aspirate should be performed. The proof of infected pancreatic necroses is a clear and undisputed indication for surgery, which seems to be the only one in the future.

References

1. Beger HG, Büchler M, Malfertheiner P (1993) Standards in Pancreatic Surgery. Springer Verlag, Berlin, Heidelberg, New York
2. Büchler M (1991) Objectivation of the severity of acute pancreatitis. Hepato-Gastroenterol 38: 101-108
3. Koop H (1984) Serum levels of pancreatic enzymes and their clinical significance. In: Creutzfeld W (Hrsg) Clinics in Gastroenterology. The Exocrine Pancreas. Saunders Company, London 737-762
4. Levitt MD, Eckfeldt JH (1986) Diagnosis of acute pancreatitis. In: Exocrine Pancreas: Biology, Pathobiology, and Disease, Herausgeber: GO VWL; Raven Press, New York 481-502
5. Salt II WB, Schenker S (1976) Amylase – its clinical significance: a review of the literature. Medicine 55: 269-289
6. Tokes PP (1991) Biochemical tests in pancreatic disease. Curr Opinion Gastroenterology 7: 709-713
7. Uhl WH (1987) Wertigkeit differenzierter Enzymanalysen und bildgebender Verfahren für Diagnose und Prognose der akuten Pankreatitis. Dissertation Fakultät für Klinische Medizin der Universität Ulm, Germany
8. Uhl W, Malfertheiner P, Drosdat H, Martini M, Büchler M (1992) Deterination of pancreatic lipase by immuno-activation technology: a rapid test system with high sensitivity and specificity. Int J Pancreatol 12: 253-261
9. Schmid S, Uhl W, Steinle A, Seiler Ch, Büchler MW (1966) Human pancreas-specific protein: A diagnostic and prognostic marker in acute pancreatitis and pancreas transplantation. Int J Pancreatol 19: 165-170
10. Blind PJ, Büchler M, Bläckberg L, Andersson Y, Uhl W, Beger HG, Hernell O (1991) Carboxylic ester hydrolase. A sensitive serum marker and indicator of severity of acute pancreatitis. Int J Pancreatol 8: 65-73
11. Isenmann R, Büchler M, Uhl W, Malfertheiner P, Martini M, Beger HG (1990) Pancreatic necrosis: an early finding in severe acute pancreatitis. Pancreas 8: 358-361
12. Steinberg WM (1990) Predictors of severity of acute pancreatitis. Gastroenterology Clinics of North America 19: 849-861
13. Blamey SJ, Imrie CW, O'Neill J, Gilmour WH, Carter DC (1984): Prognostic factors in acute pancreatitis. Gut 25: 1340-1346
14. Knaus WA, Zimmermann JE, Wagner DP, et al (1981) Apache-acute physiology and chronic health evaluation: A physiologically based classification system. Crit Care Med 9: 591
15. Knaus WA, Draper EA, Wagner DP, Zimmermann JE (1985) Apache II: A severity of disease classification system. Crit Care Med 818-829
16. Corfield AP, Cooper HJ, Williamson RCN, et al (1985) Prediction of severity in acute pancreatitis: prospective comparison of three prognosticating indices. Lancet 2: 403-407
17. Larvin M, McMahon MJ (1989) Apache II score for assessment and monitoring of acute pancreatitis. Lancet 2: 201-205
18. Leese T, Shwa D (1988) Comparison of three Glasgow multifactor prognostic scoring system in acute pancreatitis. Br J Surg 75: 460-462
19. Ranson JHC, Rifkind KM, Roses DF, Fink SD, Eng K, Spencer FC (1974) Prognostic signs and the role of operative management in acute pancreatitis. Surg Gynecol Obstet 139: 69-81
20. Uhl W, Beger HG (1991) Prediction of severity in acute pancreatitis. HPB Surgery 5: 61-64
21. Wilson C, Heath DI, Imrie CW (1990) Prediction of outcome in acute pancreatitis: A comparative study of Apache II, clinical assessment and multiple scoring systems. Br J Surg 77: 1260-1264
22. Le Gall JR, Loirat P, Alperovich A. (1984) A simplified acute physiology score for ICU patients. Crit Care Med 12: 975-977
23. Kemmer TP, Malfertheiner P, Büchler M, Kemmer ML, Ditschuneit H (1991) Serum ribonuclease activity in the diagnosis of pancreatic disease. Int J Pancreatol 8: 23-33
24. Warshaw AL, Lee KH (1979) Serum ribonuclease elevations and pancreatic necrosis in acute pancreatitis. Surgery 76: 177-181

25. Geokas MC, Rinderknecht H, Walberg CB, Weissmann R (1974) Methemalbumin in the diagnosis of acute hemorrhagic pancreatitis. Ann Intern Med 81: 483–486
26. Lankisch PG, Schirren CA, Otto J (1989) Methemalbumin in acute pancreatitis: an evaluation of its prognostic value and comparison with multiple prognostic parameters. Am J Gastroenterol 84: 1391–1395
27. McMahon MJ, Playforth MJ, Pickford IR (1980) A comparative study of methods for the prediction of severity of attacks of acute pancreatitis. Br J Surg 67: 22–25
28. Büchler M, Malfertheiner P, Schoetensack C, Uhl W, Beger HG (1986) Sensitivity of antiproteases, complement factors and C-reactive protein in detecting pancreatic necrosis: results of a prospective study. Int J Pancreatol 1: 227–235
29. Mayer AD, McMahon MJ, Bowen M, Cooper EH (1984) C-reactive protein: an aid to assessment and monitoring of acute pancreatitis. J Clin Pathol 37: 207–211
30. Wilson C, Heads A, Shenkin A, Imrie CW (1989) C-reactive protein, antiproteases and complement factors as objective markers of severity in acute pancreatitis. Br J Surg 76: 177–181
31. Domínguez-Muñoz JE, Carballo F, Garcia MJ, DeDiego JM, Rabago L, Simon MA, De la Morena J (1991) Clinical usefulness of polymorphonuclear elastase in predicting the severity of acute pancreatitis: results of a multicentre study. Br J Surg 78: 1230–1234
32. Gross V, Schölmerich J, Leser HG, Salm R, Lansen M, Schoffal U, Gerok G. (1990) Granulocyte elastase in assessment of severity of acute pancreatitis: comparison with acute phase proteins C-reactive protein, α_1-antitrypsin, and α_2-macroglobulin. Dig Dis Sci 35: 97–105
33. Uhl W, Büchler M, Malfertheiner P, Martini M, Beger HG (1991) PMN-Elastase in compaison with CRP, antiproteases, and LDH as indicators of necrosis in human acute pancreatitis. Pancreas 6: 253–259
34. Büchler M, Malfertheiner P, Schädlich H, Nevelainen TJ, Friess H, Beger HG (1989) Role of phospholipase A_2 in human acute pancreatitis. Gastroenterology 97: 1521–1526
35. Mero M, Schröder T, Tenhunen R, Lempinen M (1982) Serum phospholipase A_2, immunreactive trypsin, and trypsin inhibitors during human acute pancreatitis. Scand J Gastroenterol 17: 413–416
36. Puolakkainen P, Valtanan V, Paananen A, Schröder T (1987) C-reactive protein and serum phospholipase A_2 in the assessment of severity of acute pancreatitis. Gut 28: 764–771
37. Balldin G (1980) On protease-antiprotease imbalance with special reference of the protective role of protease inhibitors in acute pancreatitis. Med Diss Malmö General Hospital, Sweden
38. McMahon MJ, Playforth MJ, Pickford IR (1980) A comparative study of methods for the prediction of severity of attacks of acute pancreatitis. Br J Surg 67: 22–25
39. Heath Di, Cruickshank A, Gudgeon M, Jehanli A, Shenkin A, Imrie CW (1993) Role of interleukin-6 in mediating the acute phase protein response and potential as an early means of severity assessment in acute pancreatitis. Gut 34: 41–45
40. Leser HG, Gross V, Scheibenbogen C (1991) Evaluation of serum interleukin-6 concentration precedes acute-phase response and reflects severity in acute pancreatitis. Gastroenterology 101: 782–785
41. Uhl W, Büchler M, Malfertheiner P, Torab FC, Isenmann R, Beger HG (1992): Interleukin-6: a promising parameter for the early assessment of the severity of acute pancreatitis. Digestion 52: 127
42. Viedma JA, Perez-Mateo M, Dominguez-Muñoz JE, Carballo F (1992) Role of interleukin-6 in acute pancreatitis: comparison with C-reactive protein and phospholipase A. Gut 33: 1264–1267
43. Gudgeon AM, Heath D, Hurley P et al (1988) Trypsinogen activation peptide (TAP) assay in severity assessment of acute pancreatitis. Pancreas 3: 598
44. Gudgeon AM, Heath D, Hurley P et al (1990) Trypsin activation peptides assay in the early prediction of severity of acute pancreatitis. Lancet 335: 4–8
45. Heath DI, Wilson C, Gudgeon AM, Jehanli A, Shenkin A, Imrie CW (1994) Trypsinogen activation peptides (TAP) concentration in the peritoneal fluid of patients with acute pancreatitis and their relation to the presence of histologically confirmed pancreatic necrosis. Gut 35: 1311–1315
46. Rae D, Sumar N, Beechey-Newmann N, Dudgeon M, Hermon-Taylor J (1995) Type 1-phospholipase A_2 propeptide immunoreactivity is released from activated granulocytes. Clin Biochem 28: 71–78
47. Rae D, Porter Joanna, Beechey-Newmann N, Sumar N, Bennett D, Hermon-Taylor J (1994) Type 1-phospholipase A_2 propeptide in acute lung injury. Lancet 344: 1472–73

48. Beechey-Newmann N, Rae D, Sumar N, Hermon-Taylor J (1995) Stratification of severity in acute pancreatitis by assay of trypsinogen and type 1-prophospholipase A_2 activation peptides. Gastroenterol 108: A343
49. Kolars JC, Ellis CJ, Levitt M (1984) Comparison of serum amylase, pancreatic amylase and lipase in patients with hyperamylasemia. Dig Dis Sci 29: 289-293
50. Moeller-Petersen J, Klacke M, Dati F (1986) Evaluation and comparison of cathodic trypsin-like immuno-reactivity, pancreatic lipase and pancreatic isoamylase in the diagnosis of acute pancreatitis in 849 consecutive patients with acute abdominal pain. Clin Chim Acta 157: 151-166
51. Yamamoto K, Pousette Å, Phoebe Ch, Wilson H, El Shanni S, French Ck. (1992) Isolation of a cDNA encoding a human serum marker for acute pancreatitis. J Biol Chem 267: 2575-2581
52. Pousette Å, Fernstad R, Sköldefors H, Carlström K (1988) A novel assay for pancreatic cellular damage: I. Characterization of protein profiles in human pancreatic cytosol and purification and characterization of a pancreatic specific protein. Pancreas 3: 421-426
53. Dominguez-Muñoz JE, Carballo F, Garcia MJ, DeDiego JM, Gea F, Yangüela J, De la Morena J (1993) Monitoring of serum protease-antiprotease balance and systemic inflammatory response in the prognostic evaluation of acute pancreatitis: results of a multicentre study. Dig Dis Sci 38: 507-513
54. Lankisch PG (1981) Serum complement factors in human acute pancreatitis. Hepato-Gastroenterol 28: 261-263
55. Lasson A, Ohlsson K (1988) Systemic involvement in pancreatic damage: coagulation and fibrinoloysis. Int J Pancreatol 3: 579-586
56. Nevalainen TJ (1988) The role of phospholipase A in acute pancreatitis. Scand J Gastroenterol 23: 897-904
57. Block S, Maier W, Clausen C, Bittner R, Büchler M, Malfertheiner P, Beger HG (1986) Identification of pancreas necrosis in severe acute pancreatitis. Gut 27: 1035-1042
58. Beger HG, Büchler M (1989) Management of necrotizing pancreatitis. Gastroenterology 97: 511-512
59. Kivisaari L, Somer K, Standerskjöld-Nordenstam CG, Schröder T, Kivilaakso E, Lempinen M: A new method for the diagnosis of acute hemorrhagic necrotizing pancreatitis using contrast-enhanced CT. Gastrotest Radiol 9: 27-30
60. Balthazar EJ (1989) CT diagnosis and staging of acute pancreatitis. Radiol Clin North Am 27: 19-37
61. Bradley EL, Murphy F, Ferguson C (1989) Prediction of pancreatic necrosis by dynamic pancreatography. Ann Surg 210: 495-504
62. Büchler M, Uhl W, Malfertheiner P (1987) Biochemical staging of acute pancreatitis. In: Beger HG, Büchler M: Acute Pancreatitis. Springer Verlag, Berlin Heidelber New York, 143-153
63. Büchler MW, Malfertheiner P, Friess H, Isenmann R, Vanek E, Grimm H, Schlegel P, Friess T, Berger H.G. (1992) Human pancreatic tissue concentration of bactericidal antibiotics. Gastroenterology 103: 1902-1908
64. Bassi C, Falconi M, Girelli R, Nifosi F, Elio A, Martini N, Pederzoli P (1989) Microbiological findings in severe pancreatitis. Surg Res Commun 5: 1-4
65. Pederzoli P, Bassi C, Vesentini S, Campedelli A. (1993) A randomized multicenter clinical trial of antibiotic prophylaxis of septic complications in acute necrotizing pancreatitis. Surg Gynecol Obstet 176: 480-483

Diagnostic and Prognostic Evaluation of Graft Pancreatitis

S. Benz · U. T. Hopt

Introduction

Simultaneous pancreas kidney transplantation (SPK) is thought to be the optimal therapy for type I diabetes with end-stage renal disease. At present, most centres favor the bladder-drainage technique [1, 2], where the whole pancreas together with a duodenal segment is transplanted. The exocrine secretion is drained into the bladder through a duodenocystostomy (Fig. 1). The only relevant contraindication is severe coronary heart disease. In spite of excellent long-term results, SPK is performed in only a few specialised centres, because the wide range of possible complications [3] require a rather complex postoperative management. At least three main reasons make recipients of an SPK prone to these complications. First, SPK is only indicated at the moment in type I diabetic patients with end-stage renal disease. For this group of patients, it is self-evident that almost all of them suffer from severe late complications of their diabetes. furthermore, the immunogenicity of the pancreas, especially in the first 3 months after transplantation, is far higher than that of an isolated kidney

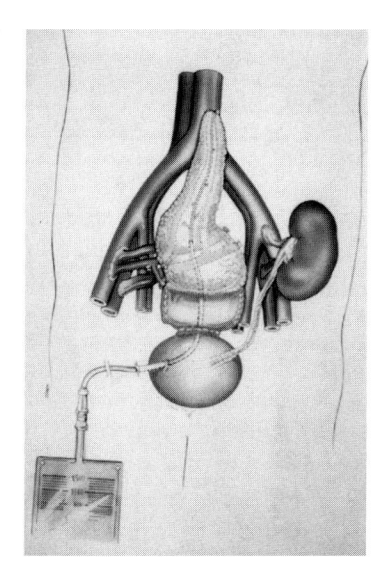

Fig. 1. Technique of simultaneous pancreas/kidney transplantation

graft, which results in a high rate of rejection episodes. In addition, graft pancreatitis can develop in the transplanted pancreas.

Graft pancreatitis can be divided into an early and a late form. The early form, or so-called postimplantation pancreatitis, begins immediately after reperfusion of the pancreas and closely resembles acute genuine pancreatitis. Postimplantation pancreatitis is the subject of this article. The late form is more heterogeneous and comprises graft pancreatitis due to cytomegalovirus (CMV) infection, rejection and inadequate evacuation of the urinary bladder [4].

According to the idea of a common pathway, the pancreas reacts to all sorts of noxious events with the development of acute pancreatitis. Two such well-known events are ischemia and trauma, both of which are present during pancreas transplantation. This explains that a minimal degree of postimplantation pancreatitis can be detected in virtually all pancreas grafts during the first few hours and days after reperfusion of the pancreas. The incidence of a significant postimplantation pancreatitis is reported to be 10%–30%. Graft losses due to postimplantation pancreatitis occur in 0.5%–7.3% [2, 5]. The macroscopic and microscopic appearance is very similar to that of genuine acute pancreatitis. Hence the grading of postimplantation pancreatitis follows the Marseilles classification of acute pancreatitis:

- Grade 0: minimal change (slight deem, scattered fatty necroses)
- Grade I: marked edema, confluent fatty necroses
- Grade II: additional parenchymal necroses

The local and systemic sequelae of genuine acute pancreatitis are well known and often require intensive care treatment and surgery even in otherwise healthy patients. It is therefore obvious that a significant postimplantation pancreatitis can induce severe morbidity in these vulnerable, highly immunosuppressed patients and that an aggressive diagnostic and therapeutic approach is necessary if the life of these patients is not to be jeopardized.

Clinical Signs

Postimplantation pancreatitis usually occurs within the first few days after transplantation. In this early postoperative period, the patients are treated with many pharmacological agents such as antibiotics and immunosuppressives that might veil the clinical picture. Therefore, clinical signs of postimplantation pancreatitis are quite variable and inconsistent. Patients with mild forms of the disease are frequently asymptomatic. Some of them, however, present with right-sided lower abdominal pain and local rebound tenderness that might mimic appendicitis. In more severe cases, the clinical picture resembles that of acute genuine acute pancreatitis, resulting in paralytic ileus, peritonitis, and finally multiorgan failure.

Fig. 2. Acute necrotizing postimplantation pancreatitis

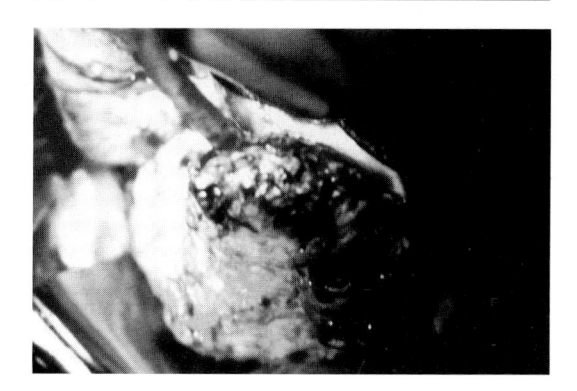

Macroscopic Appearance

The first signs of postimplantation pancreatitis can be seen immediately after reperfusion of the graft. A patchy bluish appearance early after reperfusion is the macroscopic sign of an impaired microcirculation (no reflow phenomenon). Organs that display this aspect are very likely to develop severe postimplantation pancreatitis. In nearly all organs, slight edema with whitish perivascular infiltrations develop within the first 2–3 h after reperfusion. These perivascular infiltrations correspond to perivascular polymorphonuclear leukocyte (PMN) infiltration on histology. Four to six hours after reperfusion, dependent on the degree of the ischemia and reperfusion injury, interlobular and even parenchymal necroses may develop. Thus the macroscopic appearance of the graft indicates quite early on whether edematous or necrotizing postimplantation pancreatitis will develop (Fig. 2). In the case of bacterial infection, the typical findings of infected peripancreatic necroses or peripancreatic abscess formation can be seen on relaparatomy, as in genuine necrotizing pancreatitis.

Histological Findings

The degree of ischemia and reperfusion injury and the evolving pancreatitis can be assessed form biopsies taken after reperfusion of the pancreas graft. On light microscopy, the changes found on histology closely resemble those of acute pancreatitis with interstitial edema, vacuolization of acinar cells, PMN infiltration, and extravasation of erythrocytes. Moreover, the extent of fatty necroses is clearly seen. On electron microscopy, a significant intracellular edema, reduction of zymogen granules, swelling of mitochondria, and a marked dilatation of the endoplasmatic reticulum (Fig. 3) are the most prominent findings [4, 6].

Fig. 3. Acinar cell 4 h after transplantation with vacuolization and dilatation of the endoplasmatic reticulum

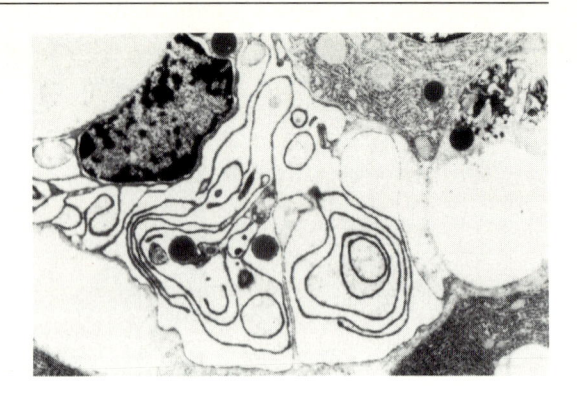

Pancreatic Enzymes

Serum levels of all secretory enzymes are increased during postimplantation pancreatitis and reach peak levels of up to 40-fold (lipase), 20-fold (amylase), 18-fold (p-elastase), and 22-fold (trypsinogen) of normal values. A correlation, however, between serum levels and the degree of pancreatitis can only be demonstrated in the first 24 h after transplantation. In our own series, median amylase levels 24 h after reperfusion reached 3260 U/l in severe (grade II) postimplantation pancreatitis and 1140 U/l in mild (grade 0) forms. In the following 2–3 days, a rapid decrease in amylase serum levels was noted, especially in patients with grade II postimplantation pancreatitis. Thus, beyond 24 h after reperfusion, serum levels of pancreatic enzyme no longer indicate the severity of postimplantation pancreatitis. This corresponds to the findings in genuine acute pancreatitis. In this clinical setting, serum tests are performed with a certain latency after the onset of the disese. It is therefore not surprising that serum amylase levels do not correlate with the severity of the underlying pancreatitis in these patients.

Excocrine Secretion

In simultaneous pancreas kidney transplantation, exocrine secretion is often diverted percutaneousely via a splint in the pancreatic duct in order to protect the duodenocystostomy. In addition, this procedure allows easy monitoring of the exocrine function of the pancreas graft. If no splint is inserted or if it is withdrawn, urinary amylase is used instead to monitor exocrine function.

It is still a matter to debate how the exocrine secretion of the pancreas changes in the case of acute pancreatitis. After pancreas transplantation, however, volume output and enzyme concentration are very sensitive parameters of pancreatic injury. During postimplantation pancreatitis, exocrine secretion is drastically reduced. This can be observed quite long before endocrine insufficiency becomes evident. It has been shown that the exocrine secretion pattern

Fig. 4. Exocrine secretion from graft with different grade of postimplantation pancreatitis

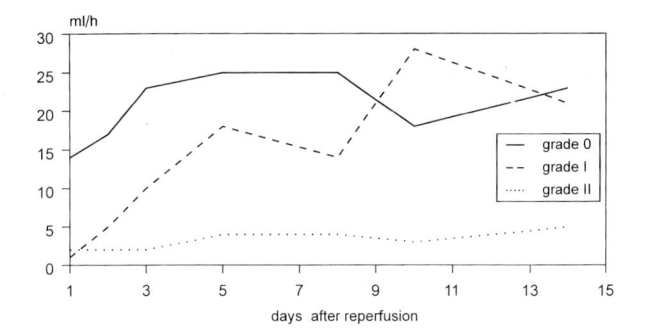

during the first few postoperative days closely correlates with the degree of postimplantation pancreatitis (Fig. 4). Pancreata that produce significant amounts of pancreatic juice in the first few hours after reperfusion will only develop mild signs of postimplantation pancreatitis (grade 0). Similar to acute renal failure, organs with moderate postimplantation pancreatitis (grade I) are characterized by a complete, but reversible exocrine insufficiency lacking pancreatic secretion during the first 2-3 postoperative days. However, they fully recover their exocrine function within the first 2 weeks after transplantation. In patients that develop severe postimplantation pancreatitis, the exocrine secretion does not recover significantly. Endocrine function, however, is preserved in the long term in the majority of patients. Accordingly, in biopsies of these organs there are only few intact acini surrounded by fibrous tissue, but intact islets are found. Besides the characteristic pattern of changes in exocrine secretion during postimplantation pancreatitis, the exocrine secretory capacity is also impaired during acute rejection. In addition, a sudden lack of exocrine secretion is a characteristic sign of impending graft thrombosis. These findings clearly demonstrate that the amount of exocrine secretion, especially in the early postoperative period, is an excellent parameter for monitoring pancreatic integrity.

Pancreatic Enzymes and Leukocytes in the Peritoneal Cavity

In order to remove active pancreatic enzymes and proteases from the peritoneal cavity, some centres use a continuous peritoneal lavage system in the early period after pancreas transplantation. In addition to the therapeutic effect, this allows continuous analysis of the peritoneal effluent and thus monitoring of the pancreas graft. High enzyme levels in the effluent indicate postimplantation pancreatitis, pancreatic fistula, or a leak of the duodenocyctostomy. In this situation, the lavage is continued until enzyme levels become normal. An increased leukocyte count in the peritoneal effluent is usually due to pancreatic or peripancreatic necroses. Especially high levels are seen in the case of bacterial superinfection of these necroses, indicating the need of relaparatomy. In our own series, in all patients with an increased leukocyte count of more that $1000/\mu l$ in the peritoneal effluent, a significant intra-abdominal lesion was found on relaparatomy.

Fig. 5. C-reactive protein (CRP) serum levels in patients with different grades of postimplantation pancreatitis

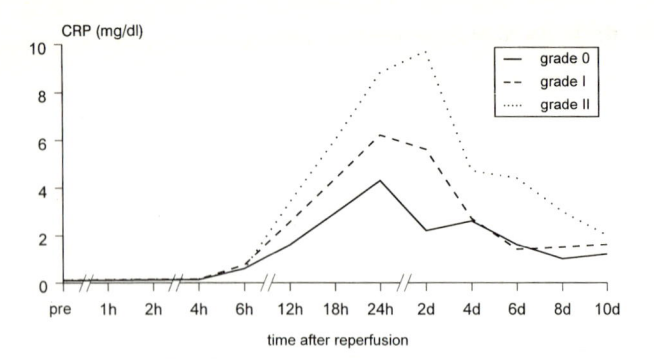

Systemic Inflammatory Reaction

After reperfusion of the pancreas graft, a systemic inflammatory reaction takes place that can be monitored by a set of different markers. As the prototype of the acute-phase proteins, the C-reactive protein (CRP) displays a peak approximately 24 h after reperfusion. As in genuine acute pancreatitis, this peak level correlates well with the degree of postimplantation pancreatitis (Fig. 5). In our own series, peak levels of more than 20 mg/dl were characteristic of the development of postimplantation pancreatitis. CRP levels, however, might be influenced by different protocols of immunosuppression. Therefore, cutoff levels will vary between different centres. Interleukin-6 (IL-6) is known to be a major inductor of CRP synthesis. This cytokine is released from the pancreas graft within the first few seconds after reperfusion. This has clearly been shown by the high levels of up to 574 ng/ml in the venous effluent of the pancreas. Surprisingly, IL-6 levels did not predict the degree of postimplantation pancreatitis. In contrast to the release of IL-6, interleukin-8 (IL-8) release is only encountered in about 30% of recipients. Serum levels of PMN elastase, a marker of granulocyte activation, have been shown to be elevated 24 h after reperfusion as well. A correlation with the degree of postimplantation pancreatitis, however, could not be demonstrated.

Fig. 6. Serum levels of antithrombin III (*AT III*) und thrombin–antithrombin (*TAT*) complexes in a patient with grade II postimplantation pancreatitis. Arrows indicate the time of substitution with 1000 units AT III

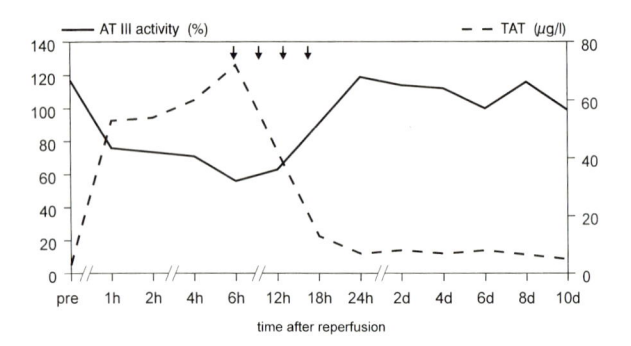

Activation of Plasmatic Cascades

The activation of the kallikrein–kinin system, cascades of coagulation, and fibrinolysis has been described after pancreas transplantation in various papers. Activation markers of coagulation and fibrinolysis (plasmin–antiplasmin complexes, thrombin–antithrombin complexes) show very high levels in the venous effluent of the pancreas immediately after reperfusion. Therefore, it is reasonable to assume that this activation is triggered directly by the pancreas and is related to the ischemia and reperfusion injury. Moreover, after reperfusion a significant consumption of coagulation factors such as antithrombin III, protein C, factor XIII, and prothrombin can be observed. In contrast, fibrinolysis is activated only transiently. This pattern with an ongoing activation of the coagulation system together with a fibrinolytic shutdown leads to a hypercoagulable state that favors graft thrombosis, which is still a major cause of graft loss after pancreas transplantation. The changes described above were found in all patients that have been examined; however, a correlation with the degree of postimplantation pancreatitis could not be shown.

Imaging Methods After Pancreas Transplantation

Contrast-enhanced computed tomography (CT) is considered the gold standard in the diagnosis of acute pancreatitis. It is particularly valuable in grading the disease by revealing pancreatic necroses and peripancreatic exudations. In contrast, CT scanning does not play an essential role in the diagnosis of graft pancreatitis. This is mainly due to the fact that, as discussed above, parameters other than peripancreatic exudations and the degree of necroses are more important in the assessment of postimplantation pancreatitis. In addition, the intraperitoneal position of the graft in the lower abdomen makes visualization of the graft rather difficult. Finally, intravenous contrast dye is contraindicated shortly after simultaneous pancreas/kidney transplantation when kidney function is still impaired.

Although the abdominal ultrasound is not useful in the primary diagnosis of postimplantation pancreatitis, it can be used to check the course of the disease and to detect possible complications such as isolated fluid collections. In this case, transcutaneous drainage can easily be accomplished under ultrasound guidance. The patency of the major pancreatic vessels can be checked by duplex ultrasound, although beginning thrombosis of the splenic vein of the graft might be difficult to identify. Therefore, a negative duplex ultrasound should not postpone relaparatomy when beginning graft thrombosis is suspected.

Magnetic resonance imaging (MRI) is currently being evaluated for its use in graft pancreatitis. Preliminary data suggest it may be able to differentiate between the different forms of graft pancreatitis. However, this issue needs further investigation.

References

1. Hopt UT, Büsing M, Schareck WD, Becker HD (1992) Management der exokrinen Pankreassekretion – ein zentrales Problem der allogenen Pankreastransplantation. Chirurg 63: 186–192
2. Sollinger HW, Ploeg RJ, Eckhoff DE, Stegall MD, Isaacs R, Pirsch JD, D'Alessandro AM, Knechtle SJ, Kalayoglu M, Belzer FO (1993) Two hundred consecutive simultaneous pancreas-kidney transplants with bladder drainage. Surgery 114 (4): 736–743
3. Benz S, Pfeffer F, Büsing M, Becker HD, Hopt UT (1996) Lokale und systemische Komplikationen nach kombinierter Nieren/Pankreas Transplantation. Chir Gastroenterol 12 [suppl]: 44–48
4. Büsing M (1994) Pathophysiologie und Morphologie der Transplantatpankreatitis. Dissertation
5. Grewal HP, Garland L, Novak K, Gaber L, Tolley EA, Gaber AO (1993) Risk factors for postimplantation pancreatitis and thrombosis in pancreas transplant recipients. Transplantation 56: 609–612
6. Büsing M, Hopt UT, Quacken M et al (1993) Morphological studies of graft pancreatitis following pancreas transplantation. Br J Surg 80: 1170–1173
7. Büsing M, Hopt UT, Schareck WD, Becker HD (1992) Pankreastransplantation: Erfolge und Probleme. Z Gastroenterol 30: 431–435
8. Büsing M, Schulz T, Benz S, Pfeffer F, Becker HD, Hopt UT (1996) Pathophysiologie der Frühform der Tansplantatpankreatitis. Chir Gastroenterol 12 [suppl 1]: 111–116
9. Benz S, Keuper H, Kraus M, Pfeffer F, Büsing M, Becker HD, Hopt UT (1995) Local activation of coagulation after reperfusion of human pancreas grafts. Digestion 56(5): 271
10. Nader A, Büsing M, Blumenstock I, Heimburger N, Jochum M, Hopt UT (1993) Coagulation disorders after reperfusion of pancreatic allografts. Transplant Proc 25(4): 1174–1175
11. König M, Luka B, Martin D, Golin U, Büsing M, Heuser L (1996) Bildgebende Verfahren in der Diagnostik nach Pankreastransplantation. Chir Gastroenterol 12 [suppl 1]: 54–60

IV
Guidelines

Acute Pancreatitis: Diagnostic Guidelines for General Practitioners, Clinicians in Community Hospitals and in Specialized Centres

M. Pérez-Mateo

Introduction

The diagnosis of acute pancreatitis is usually established by the presence of abdominal pain and biochemical evidence of pancreatic lesion. Therefore, the general practitioner should be alert to the possibility of acute pancreatitis in any patient with acute abdominal pain. Characteristically, the pain is located in the epigastrium and often radiates to the back and upper quadrants, is steady, dull and boring in quality, and peaks in intensity within 15 min to 6 h after the onset. The pain is frequently more intense when the patient is supine, and patients often obtain relief by sitting with the trunk flexed and knees drawn up. Nausea and vomiting are also frequent presenting complaints.

Clinical findings vary according to the time elapsed since the onset of symptoms. Physical examination usually shows abdominal tenderness and lack of guarding or muscle rigidity, a discrepancy that should suggest the diagnosis of acute pancreatitis. Bowel sounds are usually diminished, but not absent. Low-grade fever, tachycardia and hypotension are fairly common.

Because many patients experience episodic bouts of acute pancreatitis, assessment of former medical history, in particular a previously documented attack of acute pancreatitis is very helpful in establishing the diagnosis. Other conditions that should be investigated include history of cholelithiasis, alcohol abuse, treatment with drugs associated with acute pancreatitis, known hyperlipemia, or familial history of pancreatic inflammatory disease.

When laboratory determination of serum pancreatic enzymes is not easily available to the general practitioner, definitive diagnosis of acute pancreatitis is usually established at the emergency room of the community hospital. Serum levels of amylase and lipase continue to have more diagnostic value than other enzyme tests. The standard diagnostic criteria include a two- to three-fold increase of the upper limit of normality of both enzymes in a patient with abdominal pain [1]. The diagnosis is unequivocal when improvement of the patient's clinical condition is accompanied by progressive normalization of amylase and lipase levels, or there is evidence of the pancreatic origin of hyperamylasemia (amylase isoenzymes).

Conventional chest X-rays and abdominal films are necessary to exclude other causes of acute abdominal pain, such as intestinal perforation, as well as to provide positive evidence of acute pancreatitis (colon cut-off sign). Eventually, calcifications in the pancreatic gland strongly suggest an acute exacerbation of chronic pancreatitis.

When the clinician suspects the diagnosis of acute pancreatitis, several questions should be formulated: (a) whether the diagnosis of acute pancreatitis is correct, (b) what the prognosis is, (c) whether an associated condition can be identified and (d) whether complications are developing.

Confirming the Diagnosis

Increased serum amylase concentrations may be found in other conditions, different from acute pancreatitis, that should be carefully ruled out and some of them surgically treated, i.e. choledocholithiasis, perforated peptic ulcer, mesenteric ischaemia, intestinal obstruction, aneurysm, acute appendicitis. On the other hand, to provide positive evidence to support the diagnosis of pancreatitis, the ultrasonography showing a diffusely edematous gland or the CT scan are extremely helpful, especially in patients seeking medical care late in the course of the disease, in whom laboratory tests are not useful to establish the diagnosis. However, a computed tomography (CT) scan, as a diagnostic procedure should be indicated only when the other diagnostic tests are not conclusive.

By contrast, an incorrect diagnosis of acute pancreatitis may be established when abdominal pain and hyperamylasemia are associated with any of the following [2]: progression of symptoms over more than 48 h; evidence of sepsis within the first 3 days; moderate increase in serum amylase and lipase at the initial laboratory studies; a very severe attack of apparent acute pancreatitis with evidence of chronic pancreatitis, progressive deterioration of the patient's clinical condition despite standard medical treatment for acute pancreatitis; and a normal pancreatic CT scan in a patient with apparently severe acute pancreatitis.

Prognosis

In addition to multiple prognostic criteria developed by Ranson and Imrie, polymorphonuclear elastase (Fig. 1) and C-reactive protein (Fig. 2) are the most helpful biochemical markers for the early prediction of outcome. Increased levels of both parameters on days 1 and 2 closely linked to the occurrence of complications in the course of the disease [3]. On the other hand, pancreatic necrosis can only be detected by abdominal CT examination. Scores of the CT severity index, established according to the degree of pancreatic involvement before and after the administration of contrast medium, show a strong correlation with severity of the disease [4].

Fig. 1. Multiple box and whisker plot of polymorphonuclear elastase (*ELAS-PMN*) during days 1–5 after the stay in hospital. *Broken lines* represent the upper and lower limit (interval 95 %) of the reference group. M, mild acute pancreatitis; S, severe acute pancreatitis

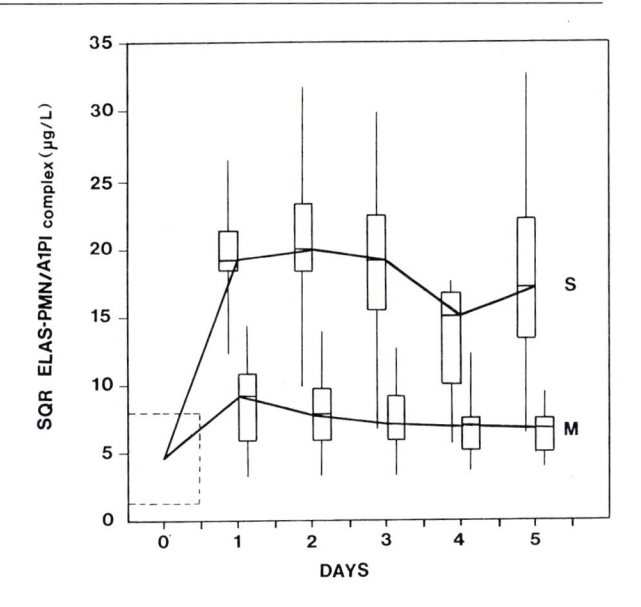

Identification of Associated Conditions

In some cases, the recognition of cholelithiasis by abdominal ultrasound may be difficult due to intestinal gases. Numerous studies have shown that advanced age, female sex, elevated amylase levels and abnormal liver function tests are highly suggestive of a biliary etiology of acute pancreatitis [5]. By con-

Fig. 2. Time course of C-reactive protein (CRP). M, mild acute pancreatitis; S, severe acute pancreatitis

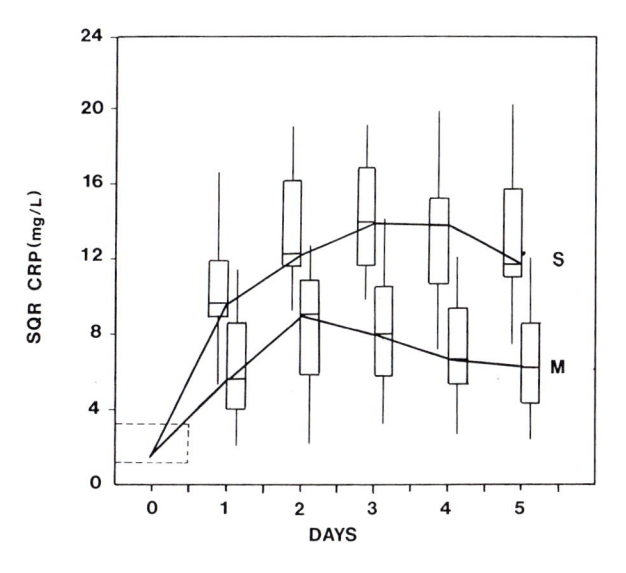

B
Chronic Pancreatitis

I
Chronic Pancreatitis: Clinical Features

Pathomorphological Features of Chronic Pancreatitis

D. E. Bockman

Introduction

Pathomorphological features of chronic pancreatitis become evident in a number of ways. Some are revealed by methods used for diagnosis of the disease. Dilation of the ductal system, strictures, and pseudocysts may be detected during endoscopic retrograde pancreatography (Malfertheiner et al. 1987). Enlargement of the pancreas becomes obvious during investigation by ultrasound or computed tomography.

Direct observation of gross change is possible, of course, during surgical intervention or upon autopsy. More thorough investigation becomes possible with histological and/or ultrastructural observation of tissue from surgical resections (Frey 1973; Beger et al. 1985; Bockman et al. 1988) or autopsy specimens.

The changes that characteristically are present upon direct observation include a gland that is enlarged in whole or in part, and that is more firm than normal due to increased quantities of collagenous connective tissue. Histological examination reveals regressive changes in exocrine parenchyma. Altered acinar tissue is afloat in a sea of fibrosis. Islets of Langerhans frequently are less affected, so they appear in greater proportion in the fibrotic background. Large nerves also are evident among the fibrosis. There may be foci of chronic inflammation.

Some details of the pathomorphological features accompanying chronic pancreatitis are discussed below.

Changes in the Stroma

Fibrosis is an expected component of chronic pancreatitis. In well developed cases the quantity of connective tissue separating the lobules, as well as that surrounding acini within the lobules, is markedly increased. There is, therefore, both interlobular and intralobular fibrosis (Fig. 1).

Fibrosis is generally present throughout the pancreas of patients with chronic pancreatitis. The distribution is, however, not necessarily equal in all parts. Fibrosis may be involved in a prominent enlargement in the head region, a situation that has been referred to as an inflammatory mass in the head of the pancreas (Beger et al. 1985). Less frequently, a relative enlargement can occur in the body and tail.

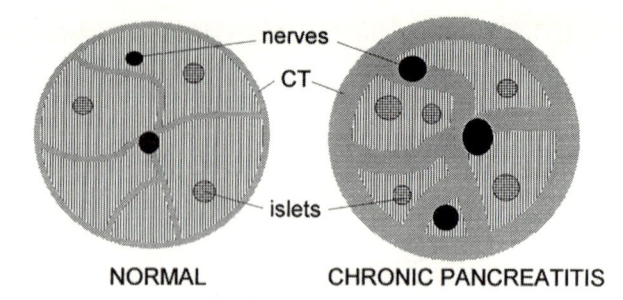

Fig. 1. Some of the pathomorphological changes associated with chronic pancreatitis. Fibrosis is indicated by the increased proportion of connective tissue (*CT*). There is a greater density of nerves that have a mean diameter greater than normal. The concentration of islets of Langerhans is greater in an intermediate stage of progression of the disease

The mechanism for the generation of fibrosis is not completely understood. Fibrosis appears to be a general reaction to changes that occur in the pancreas in a variety of conditions. It occurs in acute pancreatitis (Elsasser et al. 1989, 1992) but is reversed with resolution of the attack, in distinction to the persistent fibrosis of chronic pancreatitis. Fibrosis is prominent in cystic fibrosis and may occur in association with uremia (Avram 1977; Bronson et al. 1982). It commonly occurs with aging, and accompanies pancreatic cancer (Gress et al. 1995). It may be induced experimentally by restriction of outflow through the ductal system (Strombeck et al. 1984; Noda et al. 1987; Karanjia et al. 1994), and by wrapping with cellophane (Rosenberg et al. 1983). Stenting has produced a similar change (Alvarez et al. 1994).

Useful information about fibrogenesis has been derived from studies of transgenic mice that overexpress transforming growth factor alpha. In this experimental model, fibrosis and other changes characteristic of chronic pancreatitis develop routinely. It has been possible to quantify the amount of fibrosis (Fig. 2) and to determine that the enlargement of the gland can be accounted for by the increase in connective tissue (Bockman and Merlino 1992). The extracellular matrix in the pancreas of this model develops increased quantities of collagen types I, III, and IV, and of laminin and fibronectin (Bockman and Merlino 1992; Gress et al. 1994; Schmid et al. 1996).

Fig. 2. Comparison of the proportion of pancreas that is connective tissue in control mice (3.5%) as compared with transgenic mice overexpressing transforming growth factor alpha (*TGFalpha;* 30.5%), as an illustration that the increase in connective tissue can account for the increased size of the pancreas

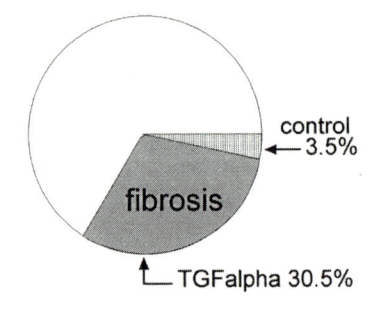

Another growth factor, transforming growth factor beta, is generally more closely associated with induction of fibrosis. Overexpression of this factor, indeed, causes fibrosis in the pancreas of the mice provided with it as a transgene (Lee et al. 1995; Sanvito etal. 1995). Fibroblast proliferation and abnormal deposition of extracellular matrix are observed from birth on. It is interesting that cellular infiltrates of macrophages and neutrophils are found in the pancreas of this model, and that acinar proliferation is inhibited. The possibility that transforming growth factor beta is involved in the development of fibrosis in chronic pancreatitis is heightened by the observation of increased levels of its precursor in mononuclear cells in the pancreas of patients with the disease, and in damaged ducts (Van Laethem et al. 1995). Binding protein for the factor was found in mononuclear cells and in the extracellular matrix around them. Intense signals for transforming growth factor beta 1 were detected in chronic pancreatitis (Van Laethem et al. 1995).

Administration of transforming growth factor beta to mice which have been subjected to multiple courses of caerulein-induced pancreatitis causes pancreatic fibrosis (Van Laethem et al. 1996). Whereas control animals display only mild inflammatory changes after repeated acute pancreatitis, those receiving the growth factor had distinct interlobular and intralobular fibrosis adjacent to inflammatory and necrotic foci.

Although knowledge about the mechanism for induction of fibrosis remains incomplete, these recent observations indicate that growth factors and inflammatory cells must be involved. It is important to determine the initial stimulus for these changes.

The presence of fibrosis in different conditions in the pancreas, and in response to growth factors and experimental manipulation, leads to the supposition that fibrosis in chronic pancreatitis represents a secondary reaction to changes in other components rather than a primary change that initiates the disease. The exact relationship of transforming growth factor alpha to fibrosis, and to transforming growth factor beta, remains to be determined.

Another area of interest is the temporal relationship of the pathomorphological changes associated with chronic pancreatitis, with respect to consumption of alcohol and the appearance of clinical symptoms.

Development of Pathomorphological Changes Before Clinical Symptoms

The development of pancreatic fibrosis has been used as a criterion for the development of pathomorphological changes due to chronic consumption of alcohol. In order to address the question of the relative time of development of pancreatic changes, studies have been conducted that compare the pancreas from chronic alcoholics with that from nonalcoholics. There is good evidence that changes occur before (or in the absence of) clinical symptoms (Bordalo et al. 1977; Pitchumoni et al. 1984; Banciu et al. 1991; Suda et al. 1994).

Pitchumoni and coworkers studied specimens from the pancreas of alcoholics and nonalcoholics obtained by autopsy. Specimens from those who had a clinical diagnosis of pancreatitis or pancreatic cancer were excluded. There was

Fig. 3. Hypothesized chain of events for generation of pathomorphological changes and progression to clinical pancreatitis. At an interval after beginning chronic alcohol intake of a high enough level in certain individuals, pathomorphological changes begin. They progress silently in the interval indicated by "pancreatic damage". At some point, the individual begins to feel pain. Soon after this, the physician diagnoses clinical pancreatitis

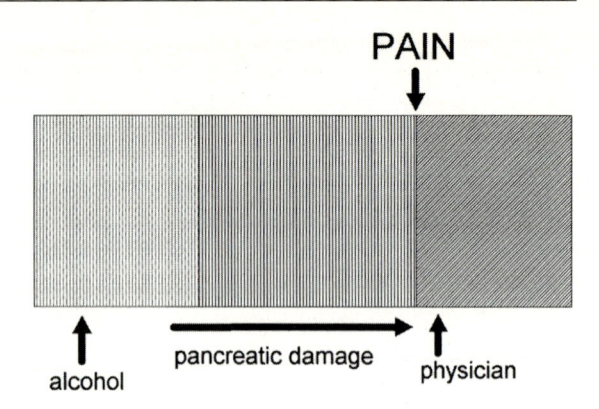

fibrosis in two thirds of the alcoholic group but only in about one third of the nonalcoholic group. In some specimens there was widespread destruction of exocrine parenchyma, tubular complexes, and preservation of islets, in addition to fibrosis. In other words, there were morphological indications of chronic pancreatitis without a clinical disease. Bordalo et al. (1977) reported similar changes in surgical biopsies from chronic alcoholics without clinical pancreatitis. Banciu et al. (1991) reported echographic structural changes in a majority of chronic consumers of alcohol. In most of these patients, who were hospitalized for conditions other than pancreatitis, the changes were interpreted as definitely indicating pancreatic fibrosis.

It is difficult to escape the conclusion, based on these studies, that in some cases chronic alcoholism induces pathomorphological changes in the pancreas for some period of time before the clinical symptoms of pancreatitis are detected. The suggestion is that at an interval after beginning chronic, heavy alcohol consumption in these individuals, changes in the pancreas are initiated. With the passage of time, the changes increase. When the damage progresses to a certain point, the individual experiences pain (Fig. 3). Perhaps soon after the initiation of severe pain, a physician is consulted and clinical pancreatitis is diagnosed.

Chronic Inflammation

A common component in the pancreas of patients with chronic pancreatitis is foci of chronic inflammatory cells. These foci may lie free in the fibrotic stroma, or may be associated closely with pancreatic parenchyma or nerves. Chronic inflammatory cells also may be concentrated in the walls of the ducts.

The inflammatory cell types are varied. The most numerous are lymphocytes. However, macrophages and neutrophils normally are present. Eosinophils and basophils or mast cells may or may not be present in the chronic inflammatory foci (Keith et al. 1985). Some foci may expand to a distinct nodule with a germinal center.

It is perhaps significant that chronic inflammatory foci are a rich source of cytokines. Interaction of the cells may lead to the release of large quantities of biologically active substances. Macrophages, for example, may release a number of factors, including transforming growth factor beta, tumor necrosis factor alpha, and platelet-derived growth factor, which are major factors that may initiate fibrosis (Ridderstad et al. 1991; Thornton et al. 1991). Stimulation of B lymphocytes leads to the production and release of immunoglobulins.

Thus inflammation may be involved in the production of factors that lead to some of the pathomorphological changes observed in chronic panereatitis. The extent of the complex interactions of these substances remains unknown. Some may appear in pancreatic fluids. Some of the interactions almost certainly are destructive of the normal morphology (and therefore function) of the pancreas.

Changes in Ducts

The chronic inflammation and resultant destructive effects that occur in the general exocrine parenchyma and stroma may be observed as well in the major ducts. The epithelium lining the ductal lumen normally is a continuous layer of columnar cells that are attached to each other by tight junctions. The epithelium, therefore, effectively separates the ductal lumen from the underlying pancreatic tissue. A continuous basal lamina underlies the epithelial layer. Beneath this is a layer of connective tissue.

Examination of pancreatic ducts in surgical resections from patients with chronic pancreatitis reveals chronic inflammatory cells in the region immediately subjacent to the epithelial layer. Lymphocytes and plasma cells are prominent (Fig. 4), but macrophages and neutrophils also are present. The capillaries close to the lumen are increased in number, are enlarged, and tend to be packed with erythrocytes and neutrophils.

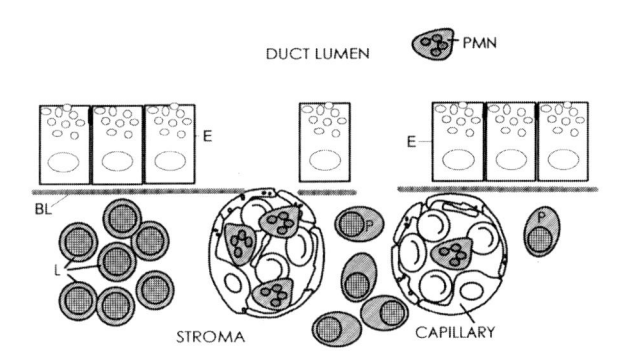

Fig. 4. Pathomorphological changes in the pancreatic duct of a patient with chronic pancreatitis. The epithelial layer (E), is interrupted, as is the basal lamina (BL). Numerous, enlarged capillaries packed with erythrocytes and neutrophils lie close to the duct lumen. Lymphocytes (L) and plasma cells (P) represent some of the inflammatory cells that lie in the connective tissue close to the lumen. A polymorphonuclear neutrophil (PMN) has migrated into the lumen, and will be a component of the pancreatic juice, as will immunoglobulins, albumin, and other substances

The epithelial layer in many cases is discontinuous, and the basal lamina in some places has holes in it (Lederer et al. 1976; Bockman et al. 1994). The result is that the barrier between lumen and underlying tissue is breached. These changes explain to some extent the changes that occur in the pancreatic juice in patients with chronic pancreatitis and, to some extent, in chronic alcoholics without clinical pancreatitis (Bockman et al. 1985).

The loss of the normal barrier in the pancreatic duct, combined with chronic inflammation, provides a mechanism for the addition of immunoglobulins, albumin, and cells to pancreatic juice (Clemente et al. 1971 a, b; Figarella 1976; Brasher et al. 1982), as well as penetration of duct contents into the pancreatic parenchyma. Neutrophils in the pancreatic juice may explain the increase in lactoferrin that has been detected in patients with chronic pancreatitis (Masson et al. 1969; Miyauchi and Watanabe 1978; Hayakawa et al. 1993).

Damage to Nerves

Some of the foci of chronic inflammatory cells in the pancreas of patients with chronic pancreatitis are associated closely with nerves (Frey 1973; Bockman et al. 1988). The stimulus for this association is unknown, but there is evidence that the nerves are damaged in these regions.

Pancreatic nerves are bundles of mostly unmyelinated nerve fibers. The bundle is enclosed by a usually multilayered sheath of epithelioid cells, the perineurium. The layering and tight junctions of the perineurium provide a distinct barrier that separates the inner compartment of the nerve from the surrounding tissue. Nerves normally function with a specialized microenvironment within this inner compartment.

It has been demonstrated that in the region of the chronic inflammatory cells, the perineurium is damaged (Bockman et al. 1988), removing the barrier normally provided by the perineurium and thus altering the specialized microenvironment. Inflammatory cells may invade the nerve (Fig. 5). Some nerve fibers are damaged.

Damage to the nerves serving the pancreas raises the possibility that this is one of the mechanisms that may be involved in the chronic pain often associated with chronic pancreatitis. Because the nerves are mixed, carrying both

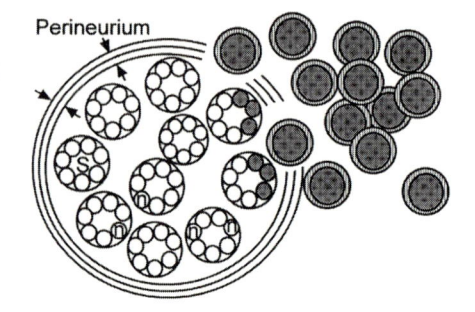

Fig. 5. Damage to a pancreatic nerve as a result of a focus of inflammatory cells. The perineurium has been damaged, decreasing its function as a barrier. Nerve fibers (n) associated with Schwann cells (S) are damaged. Inflammatory cells and biologically active substances may invade the damaged nerve, presumably initiating pain and perhaps alterations in secretion and microcirculation

sensory and motor fibers, it is also possible that nerve damage would affect secretion and control of blood flow as well.

Changes in Exocrine Parenchyma

Progression of chronic pancreatitis involves the regression of exocrine tissue. Both the quantity and the nature of exocrine tissue changes. In advanced cases, areas of exocrine tissue are completely replaced by fibrosis. The transition from normal parenchyma to this condition is accomplished through cell death (apoptosis) and through redifferentiation of acinar cells (Bockman et al. 1982; Bockman 1995).

When the environment of acinar cells is altered beyond a critical point, they are unable to sustain their differentiated state, producing, storing, and secreting enzymes. They revert to a morphology that is indistinguishable from ductular cells. The markers used for distinguishing acinar from ductular cells change. Zymogen granules disappear from acinar cells. Marker enzymes associated with ductules may appear in the altered acinar cells.

During these regressive changes there are areas of accumulated tubules that have the appearance of ductules. These have been termed tubular complexes (Bockman et al. 1982). They result from the redifferentiation of acinar cells to those with the morphology of ductular cells. The developing tubular complexes also incorporate ductular cells and centroacinar cells that were part of the normal architecture.

Further progression of the disease leads to death of these cells as well, with fibrous replacement. The islets of Langerhans, which are more resistant than acinar tissue to destruction, eventually may be destroyed.

References

Alvarez C, Robert M, Sherman S, Reber HA (1994) Histologic changes after stenting of the pancreatic duct. Arch Surg 129: 765–768
Avram MM (1977) High prevalence of pancreatic disease in chronic renal failure. Nephron 18: 68–71
Banciu T, Susan L, Jovin G, Sporea I, Vacariu V (1991) Prevalence of chronic (latent) pancreatitis in hospitalized chronic consumers of alcohol. Rom J Int Med 29: 49–53
Beger HG, Krautzberger W, Bittner R, Büchler M, Limmer J (1985) Duodenum-preserving resection of the head of the pancreas in patients with severe chronic pancreatitis. Surgery 97: 467–473
Bockman DE (1995) Toward understanding pancreatic disease: From architecture to cell signaling. Pancreas 11: 324–329
Bockman DE, Merlino G (1992) Cytological changes in the pancreas of transgenic mice overexpressing transforming growth factor alpha. Gastroenterology 103: 1883–1892
Bockman DE, Boydston WR, Anderson MC (1982) Origin of tubular complexes in human chronic pancreatitis. Am J Surg 144: 243–249
Bockman DE, Singh M, Laugier R, Sarles H (1985) Alcohol and the integrity of the pancreas. Scand J Gastroenterol 20 (suppl 112): 106–113
Bockman DE, Büchler M, Malfertheiner P, Beger HG (1988) Analysis of nerves in chronic pancreatitis. Gastroenterology 94: 1459–1469
Bockman DE, Büchler M, Beger HG (1994) Compromise of barrier function and immunological reaction in pancreatic ducts from patients with chronic pancreatitis. Int J Pancreatol 16: 325

Bordalo O, Goncalves D, Noroñha M, Cristina ML, Salgadinho A, Dreiling DA (1977) Newer concept for the pathogenesis of chronic alcoholic pancreatitis. Am J Gastroenterol 68: 278–285

Brasher GW, Dyck WP, Spiekerman AM (1982) Immunoglobulin characterization of human pancreatic fluid. Am J Dig Dis 20: 454–459

Bronson RT, Strauss W, Wheeler W (1982) Pancreatic ectasia in uremic macaques. Am J Path 106: 342–437

Clemente F, Ribeiro T, Columb E, Figarella C, Sarles H (1971a) Comparaison des proteins de sucs pancreatiques humains normaux et pathologique. Dosage des proteines seriques et mise en evidence d'une protein particuliere dan la pancreatite chronique calcifiante. Biochym Biophys Acta 251: 456–466

Clemente F, Ribeiro T, Figarella C, Sarles H (1971b) Albumine, IgG et IgA dans le suc pancreatique humain normal chez l'adulte. Clin Chim Acta 33: 317–324

Elsasser HP, Adler G, Kern HF (1989) Fibroblast structure and function during regeneration from hormone-induced acute pancreatitis in the rat. Pancreas 4: 169–178

Elsasser HP, Haake T, Grimmig M, Adler G, Kern HF (1992) Repetitive cerulein-induced pancreatitis and pancreatic fibrosis in the rat. Pancreas 7: 385–390

Figarella C (1976) Immunoglobulin characterization. Am J Dig Dis 21: 77

Frey CF (1973) Ninety-five percent pancreatectomy. In Carey LC, ed, The Pancreas. St Louis, Mosby, pp 202–229

Gress TM, Muller-Pillasch F, Lerch MM, Friess H, Büchler M, Beger HG, Adler G (1994) Balance of expression of genes coding for extracellular matrix proteins and extracellular matrix degrading proteases in chronic pancretitis. Zeitschrift Gastroenterol 32: 221–225

Gress TM, Muller-Pillasch F, Lerch MM, Friess H, Büchler M, Adler G (1995) Expression and in-situ localization of genes coding for extracellular matrix proteins and extracellular matrix degrading proteases in pancreatic cancer. Int J Cancer 62: 407–413

Hayakawa T, Kondo T, Shibata T, Murase T, Harada H, Ochi K, Tanaka J (1993) Secretory component and lactoferrin in pure pancreatic juice in chronic pancreatitis. Dig Dis Sci 38: 7–11

Karanjia ND, Widdison AL, Leung F, Alvarez C, Lutrin FJ, Reber HA (1994) Compartment syndrome in experimental chronic obstructive pancreatitis: effect of decompressing the main pancreatic duct. Brit J Surg 81: 259–264

Keith RG, Keshavjee SH, Kerenyi NR (1985) Neuropathology of chronic pancreatitis in humans. Can J Surg 28: 207–211

Lederer P, Stolte M, Tulusan H. (1976) Oberflächengestaltung des Gangbaums der gesunden und kranken Bauchspeicheldrüse. Virchows Archiv A; 372: 109–121

Lee MS, Gu D, Feng L, Curriden S, Arnush M, Krahl T, Furushanthaiah D, Wilson C, Loskutoff DL, Fox H et al (1995) Accumulation of extracellular matrix and developmental dysregulation in the pancreas by transgenic production of transforming growth factor-beta 1. Am J Pathol 147: 42–52

Malfertheiner P, Büchler M, Stanescu A, Ditschuneit H (1987) Pancreatic morphology and function in relationship to pain in chronic pancreatitis. Int J Pancreatol 2: 59–66

Masson PL, Heremans JF, Schonne E (1969) Lactoferrin, an iron-binding protein in neutrophilic leukocytes. J Exp Med 130: 643–658

Miyauchi J, Watanabe Y (1978) Immunocytochemical localization of lactoferrin in human neutrophils. An ultrastructural and morphometrical study. Cell Tiss Res 247: 249–258

Noda A, Shibata T, Ogawa Y, Hayakawa T, Kameya S, Hiramatsu E, Watanabe T, Horiguchi Y (1987) Dissolution of pancreatic stones by oral trimethadione in a dog experimental model. Gastroenterology 93: 1002–1008

Pitchumoni CS, Glasser M, Saran RM, Panchacharam P, Thelmo W (1984) Pancreatic fibrosis in chronic alcoholics and nonalcoholics without clinical pancreatitis. Am J Gastroenterol 79: 382–388

Ridderstad A, Abedi-Valugerdi M, Moller E (1991) Cytokines in rheumatoid arthritis. Ann Med 23: 219–223

Rosenberg L, Brown RA, Duguid WP (1983) A new model for the development of duct epithelial hyperplasia and the initiation of nesidioblastosis. J Surg Res 35: 63–72

Sanvito F, Nichols A, Herrera PL, Huarte J, Wohlwend A, Vassalli JD, Orci L (1995) TGF-beta 1 overexpression in murine pancreas induces chronic pancreatitis and, together with TNF-alpha, triggers insulin-dependent diabetes. Biochem Biophys Res Comm 217: 1279–1286

Schmid RM, Menke A, Bachem MG, Lührs H, Adler G (1996) Characterization of the extracellular matrix, acinar and ductal cells in transgenic mice expressing TGF-α in the exocrine pancreas. Gastroenterology 110: A429

Strombeck DR, Wheeldon E, Harrold D (1984) Model of chronic pancreatitis in the dog. Am J Vet Res 45: 131–136

Suda K, Shiotsu H, Nakamura T, Akai J, Nakamura T (1994) Pancreatic fibrosis in patients with chronic alcohol abuse: Correlation with alsoholic pancreatitis. Am J Gastroenterol 89: 2060–2062

Thornton SC, Por SB, Penny R, Richter M, Shelley L, Breit SN (1991) Identification of the major fibroblast growth factors released spontaneously in inflammatory arthritis as platelet derived growth factor and tumor necrosis factor-alpha. Clin Exp Immunol 86: 79–86

Van Laethem JL, Deviere J, Resibois A, Rickaert F, Vetongen P, Ohtani H, Cremer M, Miyazono K, Robberecht P (1995) Localization of transforming growth factor beta 1 and its latent binding protein in human chronic pancreatitis. Gastroenterology 108: 1873–1881

Van Laethem JL, Robberecht P, Resibois A, Deviere J (1996) Transforming growth factor beta promotes development of fibrosis after repeated courses of acute pancreatitis in mice. Gastroenterology 110: 576–582

Pathophysiological Events in Chronic Pancreatitis: The Current Concept

C. Beglinger

Introduction

Chronic pancreatitis is characterized by recurrent or persistent abdominal pain with destruction and permanent loss of exocrine pancreatic parenchyma. The irreversible morphological changes in the pancreas may lead to a progressive or permanent loss of exocrine and endocrine pancreatic function [1].

The main features of chronic pancreatitis are exocrine pancreatic insufficiency, endocrine pancreatic insufficiency, and pain.

It is generally accepted that prolonged ingestion of large amounts of alcohol is a major risk factor for the development of chronic pancreatitis [2]. The effect of alcohol on the exocrine pancreas depends on (1) the amount of alcohol ingestion and (2) dietary factors such as the extent of fat and/or protein-rich diets. The critical amount of daily alcohol consumption is 40 g/day in women and 80 g/day in men with an exposition interval of at least 5 years [3]. Besides alcohol and dietary factors, several other pathogenetic influences have been proposed such as nicotine abuse, genetic factors, and a lack of trace elements (zinc, copper, selenium).

Hypotheses

The mechanisms that induce chronic pancreatitis, however, remain unclear. Three major hypotheses have emerged in recent years:

1. Duct obstruction
    - Disturbed regulation: changes in juice composition
    - Protein plugs
    - Pancreatic stone protein
2. Toxic-metabolic destruction
    - Alcohol, metabolites
3. Free radicals

Duct Obstruction

A large amount of experimental evidence, most of it generated in animals, suggests that the primary event after prolonged and chronic alcohol consumption is a disturbance in the regulation of acinar cell function with subsequent changes in juice composition; these changes can induce protein plugs and/or pancreatic stone protein formation. The biochemical events during this process are not clear, but formation of a specific stone protein has been proposed [4-7]. Apart from obstruction, a disrupted diffusion barrier and an increased permeability between the interstitial and ductal compartments may contribute to modifications in juice composition, thereby promoting diffusion of active enzymes into the tissue [6, 7]. Pancreatic stone protein, also known as lithostatin, belongs to a group of naturally occurring proteins [8-10]. Under certain experimental conditions, lithostatin can inhibit $CaCO_3$ crystal growth; whether this effect is of clinical relevance is not clear. Furthermore, the reduced production of lithostatin observed in chronic pancreatitis is unclear. Finally, the suggestion that a genetically determined reduction in lithostatin production might cause susceptibility to increased alcohol toxicity would make a nice hypothesis, but experimental support is insufficient. The main conclusion of this paragraph is therefore that morphologic changes are secondary to secretory changes.

Toxic-Metabolic Destruction

This hypothesis is largely derived from histopathological changes observed in histologic sections of patients with chronic pancreatitis and is contrary to the hypothesis described above [11-13]. According to this hypothesis, toxic compounds such as alcohol induce intrapancreatic changes such as lipid depositions which over time can lead to fibrosis and atrophy. In this model, pancreatic insufficiency develops as a consequence of irreversible tissue changes: Based on this hypothesis, the secretory changes are secondary to morphologic changes.

Free Radicals

Apart from the two main hypotheses described above, an alternative concept has been developed on the basis of disrupted hepatic detoxification [14-15]. In this concept, an excess of free radicals circulate in the body with a variety of toxic metabolites produced (oxidative stress). These metabolites may generate the cascade of events that can induce an inflammatory response in the pancreas (Fig. 1).

Unfortunately, the oxidative stress hypothesis is not supported by many experimental data.

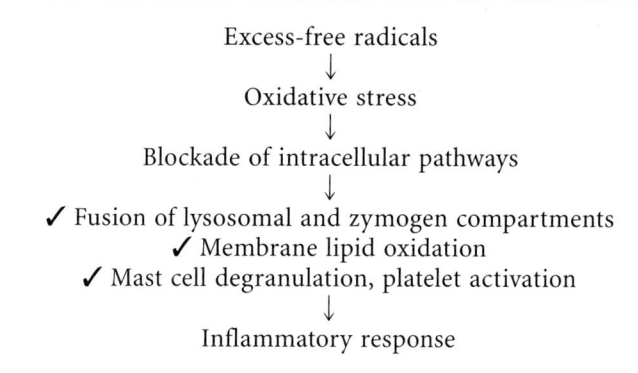

Excess-free radicals
↓
Oxidative stress
↓
Blockade of intracellular pathways
↓
✓ Fusion of lysosomal and zymogen compartments
✓ Membrane lipid oxidation
✓ Mast cell degranulation, platelet activation
↓
Inflammatory response

Fig. 1. Cascade of events occurring in the free radicals' hypothesis of development of chronic pancreatitis. (From [14, 15])

Conclusion

The pathophysiology of chronic pancreatitis is most likely a multifactorial event. Alcohol is the most important etiologic factor, but the mechanisms involved in the development of the disease remain unclear, and a number of questions remain to be elucidated.

References

1. Sarles H, Bernard JP, Johnson C (1989) Pathogenesis and epidemiology of chronic pancreatitis. Annu Rev Med 40: 453–468
2. Devaux MA, Lechêne de la Porte P, Johnson C, Sarles H (1990) Structural and functional effects of long-term alcohol administration on the dog exocrine pancreas submitted to two different diets. Pancreas 5: 200–209
3. Frezza M, di Padova C, Pozzato G, Terpin M, Baraona E, Lieber CS (1990) High blood alcohol levels in women. The role of decreased gastric alcohol dehydrogenase activity and first-pass metabolism. N Engl J Med 323: 95–99
4. Sahel J, Sarles H (1979) Modifications of pure human pancreatic juice induced by chronic alcohol consumption. Dig Dis Sci 24: 897–905
5. Renner IG, Rinderknecht H, Valenzuela JE, Douglas AP (1980) Studies of pure pancreatic seretions in chronic alcoholic subjects without pancreatic insufficiency. Scand J Gastroenterol 15: 241–244
6. Reber HA, Roberts C, Way LW (1979) The pancreatic duct mucosal barrier. Am J Surg 137: 128–134
7. Layer P, Hotz J, Schmitz-Moormann HP, Goebell H (1982) Effects of experimental chronic hypercalcemia on feline exocrine pancreatic secretion. Gastroenterology 82: 309–316
8. Yamadera K, Moriyama T, Makino I (1990) Identification of immunoreactive pancreatic stone protein in pancreatic stone, pancreatic tissue, and pancreatic juice. Pancreas 5: 255–260
9. Hoops TC, Rindler MJ (1991) Isolation of the cDNA encoding glycoprotein-2(GP-2), the major zymogen granule membrane protein. Homology to uromodulin/Tamm-Horsfall protein. J Biol Chem 266: 4257–4263
10. Fukuoka SI, Freedman SD, Scheele GA (1991) A single gene encodes membranebound and free forms of GR-2, the major glycoprotein in pancreatic secretory (zymogen) granule membrances. Proc Natl Acad Sci USA 88: 2898–2902

11. Bordalo O, Goncalves D, Noronha M, Cristina ML, Salgadinho A, Dreiling DA (1977) Newer concept for the pathogenesis of chronic alcoholic pancreatitis. Am J Gastroenterol 68: 278–285
12. Noronha M, Salgadinho A, Ferreira De Almeida MJ, Dreiling DA, Bordalo O (1981) Alcohol and the pancreas. I. Clinical associations and histopathology of minimal pancreatic inflammation. Am J Gastroenterol 77: 114–119
13. Noronha M, Bordalo O, Dreiling DA (1981) Alcohol and the pancreas. II. Pancreatic morphology of advanced alcoholic pancreatitis. Am J Gastroenterol 76: 120–124
14. Braganza JM (1983) Pancreatic disease: a casualty of hepatic "detoxification"? Lancet 2: 1000–1003
15. Klöppel G, Maillet B (1991) Pseudocysts in chronic pancreatitis: A morphological analysis of 57 resection specimens and 9 autopsy pancreata. Pancreas 6: 266–274

Clinical Presentation and Course of Chronic Pancreatitis

G. Manes · J. E. Domínguez-Muñoz · M. Büchler ·
H. G. Beger · P. Malfertheiner

Introduction

Chronic pancreatitis (CP) is a dynamic, evolutive disease in which a progressive destruction of the pancreatic parenchyma due to inflammation and consequent biosynthesis or large amounts of fibrotic tissue leads to a complete change in the architecture of the gland and impairment of its function.

The typical clinical picture of CP is that of a patients who, after years of alcohol abuse and a history of recurrent abdominal pain, develops steatorrhea and general malnutrition. In this late phase of the disease, the diagnosis is easy, since morphological changes of the pancreas (i.e., calcifications pseudocysts, atrophy) are characteristic and detectable by common imaging procedures. This phase represents only the final stage of an evolutive process of several years.

Pancreatic histology is available only in rare cases. Furthermore, functional and morphological procedures do not provide unequivocal diagnostic information in the early stage of CP. As a consequence, exact knowledge of the clinical natural history of CP is important in order to recognize the disease at an early stage and to answer important questions regarding management.

Clinical course

The three main clinical manifestations of CP are abdominal pain, pancreatic insufficiency (exocrine and endocrine), and local complications. The manifestations may occur together, usually in an advanced stage of the disease, or alone. Each of them is characteristic of an evolutive phase of CP. While abdominal pain is often the first symptom of the disease, it can be further associated with the development of pseudocysts, biliary stenosis, or other local complications; in the end stage of CP, when exocrine pancreatic insufficiency develops, pain usually disappears in the so-called burning out pancreas.

This description of the clinical course of CP corresponds to what Amman et al. [1] described in their classical paper as the early, intermediate, and final stages of CP. In the early stage of CP, inflammation of the pancreas is the predominant feature. Patients suffer from recurrent attacks of abdominal pain with still normal exocrine and endocrine pancreatic function. Diagnosis of CP in this phase is difficult, since morphological findings may be equivocal and pancreatic function tests are still usually normal. The evolution of the disease leads to progressive alteration of the pancreatic architecture with development of ductal stricture and occasionally pseudocysts. In this phase, pain tends to occur more frequently or to be continuous, and pancreatic function becomes abnormal; however, steatorrhea is not yet present. Local complications usually occur in this phase and can influence the clinical presentation of disease. In the terminal stage of CP, the pancreatic gland appears to be totally fibrotic and calcifications are usually present. Exocrine (steatorrhea, malnutrition) and endocrine (diabetes mellitus) insufficiency develops, whereas pain tends to disappear.

This classification has a general didactic value and describes the typical clinical history of a patient with alcoholic CP. Several aspects must, however, be taken into consideration in patients with CP of different etiologies. Typically, the onset of alcoholic CP is characterized by an acute episode of pain occurring during the third or fourth decade of life; after several years of relapsing pain episodes, exocrine and endocrine pancreatic insufficiency and calcifications develop. Pain is the first symptom in about 80%-90% of patients with alcoholic CP, and in 50% of patients the disease begins as an episode of acute pancreatitis. Pain recurs at intervals of months or years and then progressively becomes more frequent until becoming persistent or tends to decrease in intensity and frequency in close relationship to the progressive fibrotic transformation of the pancreas [1-3]. By contrast, in idiopathic CP the clinical features are more variable, and the presence of pain and development of pancreatic calcifications and steatorrhea depends on the age of patients at the onset of disease [4, 5]. Pain is the clinical symptom in almost every patient with early-onset idiopathic CP. In these patients, the disease develops before the age of 35 (median, 20 years), and calcifications and pancreatic insufficiency appear 10-20 years later. Pain appears in only 50% of patients with late-onset idiopathic CP. In these patients, the disease becomes evident at a median age of 55 years, and steatorrhea and/or diabetes mellitus is frequently the first clinical manifestation [4, 5].

Abdominal Pain

Pain is the most important clinical symptom and represents the first clinical manifestation of CP in about 80%-90% of patients. Features of pain are heterogeneous, so that its frequency, duration, severity, and relation to food intake vary. In spite of this variability, in most cases pain evolves during the course of disease following a recurrent scheme, paralleling other clinical features of CP, as above described. Increased intraductal and parenchymal pressure has been proposed as a cause of pain in CP [6-8], in spite of the fact that intensity of pain does not always correlate with pressure level [9] and morphology of the pancreatic duct system [10-13]. Furthermore, intrapancreatic nerves are involved in the inflammatory process that characterizes CP [14] and may be irritated by a variety of agents present in the tissue (histamine, prostaglandins, enzymes). Cumulative experience supportes the hypothesis that pain has a multifactorial etiology; it is likely that in the initial stages of disease, when pain is recurrent and sometimes associated with acute relapse of pancreatitis, inflammation of the gland and inflammatory neural involvement play a major role; later on,

Clinical Presentation and Course of Chronic Pancreatitis

development of parenchymal hypertension and local complications (pseudocysts) are additional factors causing pain. In the final stage of the disease, a marked decrease in the exocrine function is associated with pain relief.

In Fig. 1, the clinical characteristics of 163 patients with CP at the time of the first diagnosis in the gastroenterological and surgical departments of the University of Ulm are reported. In 85% of patients, pain was the main symptom that led to the diagnosis, and only in 15% was the diagnosis suspected on the basis of other manifestations, mainly malnutrition and steatorrhea in patients without pain. In 65% of patients pain was recurrent, and in 30% of patients continuous. The duration from the anamnestically recorded onset of pain and diagnosis was 3.8 years in the first group and 5.8 years in the second. These data confirm the fact that characteristics of pain change in the course of disease, according to the above-mentioned hypothesis.

Local Complications

The most frequent complication in CP is the development of pseudocysts. They occur at some time in the course of the disease in about 25%–70% of cases, according to different studies [15–19]. In about 75% of cases, they develop in patients with alcoholic CP and are usually seen in the fourth to sixth decade of life. They occur more commonly in the body of the pancreas, than in the head or tail. Clinically, most pseudocysts are silent, although in some cases they can produce a continuous abdominal pain. The first clinical manifestation of a

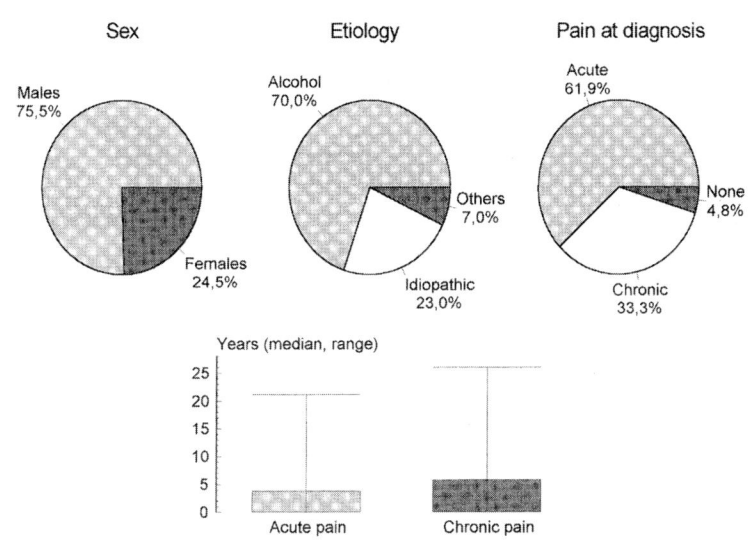

Fig. 1. Clinical characteristics of a series of 163 consecutive patients diagnosed with chronic pancreatitis (CP) at the University of Ulm, Germany

pseudocyst may be due to obstruction of the common bile duct, secondary infection, intraperitoneal rupture or fistula with pancreatic ascites, hemorrhage into the pseudocyst with conversion into a pseudoaneurysm, or hemorrhage from gastric varices secondary to splenic vein obstruction. Uncomplicated spontaneous resolution of chronic pseudocysts is a rare event. The incidence of complications is related to the evolution time and size of the pseudocyst. Hemorrhage, rupture, and secondary infection may occur more frequently than previously appreciated and may represent life-thretening conditions if not promptly recognized and treated.

Cholestatis occurs in about 10%–50% of patients in the course of CP, but only in the minority of cases is it associated with jaundice [20-23]. In most cases, cholestasis is recognized in asymptomatic patients by increased values of biliary enzymes. Development of pseudocyst or of an inflammatory mass of the head of the pancreas is the most frequent cause of cholestasis in CP.

Development of segmental portal hypertension and splenic vein thrombosis are rare complications in the course of CP, usually due to compression of the splenic vein [24]. Since portal hypertension may result in gastric and esophageal varices that can bleed, prompt recognition is mandatory.

Other hemorrhagic complications may occur from pseudoaneurysms that involve the splenic, gastroduodenal, or pancreaticoduodenal arteries. They are usually associated with a pseudocyst, and their rupture usually occurs in the cyst or in the pancreatic duct, resulting in hematemesis and melena [25].

Other rare complications of CP are bowel obstruction [26] due to the direct spread of inflammation from the pancreas to the gut, pancreatic ascites usually due to a leakage from the pancreatic duct or pseudocyst [27], and pancreatic fistula usually following operative or percutaneous drainage [26].

In about 5% of patients, pancreatic cancer develops during the course of CP. In a CP population, the risk of developing a pancreatic cancer is 1.8 and 4.0 times higher than in a normal control population over a period of 10 and 20 years, respectively [28].

The prevalence of local complications in a series of 163 patients with CP followed up at the University of Ulm is reported in Table 1.

Table 1. Complications in the course of chronic pancreatitis

Complication	Patients (%)
Pseudocyst	55
< 6 cm	43
> 6 cm	12
Diabetes mellitus	34
Exocrine insufficiency	18
Cholestasis / jaundice	15
Duodenal stenosis	6
Portal hypertension	4
Ascites	2
Colon stenosis	0.6

Exocrine and Endocrine Pancreatic Insufficiency

Development of exocrine pancreatic insufficiency is a typical feature of the late phase of CP. Steatorrhea and malnutrition are the first symptoms in only about 5%–10% of patients with CP. Steatorrhea occurs when secretion of pancreatic lipase is less than 10% of normal and usually when more than 85% of total exocrine cells are lost [29]. In different studies, the prevalence of steatorrhea in the CP population was reported to the between 10% and 40% [30]. However, current direct and indirect exocrine function tests are able to recognize subclinical impairment of pancreatic function at an even earlier stage of disease. Pancreatic insufficiency develops progressively and parallel to the development of fibrosis and structural changes within the pancreas; this is supported by the close correlation between morphological (endoscopic retrograde pancreatography, ERP; computed tomography, CT) and functional findings (secretin-pancreozymin test, pancreolauryl test) [10, 31]. Pancreatic calcifications are a frequent findings in patients with pancreatic insufficiency, but occasionally they can be revealed before steatorrhea occurs [32].

Endocrine insufficiency, in the form of a latent or overt diabetes, develops frequently in the final stage of CP. Prevalence varies according to the stage of the disease in the different series studied and can be observed in 30%–70% of patients with steatorrhea and calcifications [33]. In our series, exocrine pancreatic insufficiency (steatorrhea) was present in 18% of patients with CP; of these, 69% had pancreatic calcifications and 59% suffered from insulin-dependent diabetes mellitus. In our general CP population, the prevalence of diabetes mellitus was 34%, and 53% of these patients required treatment with insulin.

Prognosis

The prognosis of CP depends on various factors:

- Frequency and intensity of abdominal pain
- Development of exocrine and/or endocrine insufficiency
- Development of complications
- Age of patients at the time of first diagnosis
- Further alcohol consumption after diagnosis

Only 13% of patients die from a condition directly related to CP [34]. However, the mean life expectancy from the onset of symptoms is 37 years for alcoholics and 39 years for nonalcoholics [34]. Ten years after the onset of symptoms, 80% of nonalcoholic CP patients and only 65% of alcoholic CP patients are still alive [34].

Alcohol consumption seems to be the most important determinant of prognosis in CP patients, since it may determine evolution of disease and development of complications as well as the need for surgery. Furthermore, smoking and drinking are common coexisting social habits in western industrialized countries, and malnutrition is a frequent feature in alcoholic subjects. All these factors determine together with CP and its complications the prognosis of these patients.

References

1. Amman R, Akovbiantz A, Largiader F, Schüler G (1984) Course and outcome of chronic pancreatitis. Gastroenterology 86: 820-828
2. Amman RW, Bühler H, Münch R, Freiburghaus AW, Siegenthaler W (1987) Differences in the natural history of idiopathic (nonalcoholic) and alcoholic pancreatitis. Pancreas 2: 368-377
3. The Copenhagen Pancreatic Study Group (1981) An interim report from a prospective epidemiological multicenter study. Scand J Gastroenterol 16: 305-312
4. Layer P, Kalthoff L, Clain JE, DiMagno EP (1985) Nonalcoholic chronic pancreatitis - two diseases? Dig Dis Sci 30: 980
5. Layer P, Yamamoto H, Kalthoff L, Clain JE, Bakken LJ, DiMagno EP (1994) The different courses of early- and late-onset idiopathic and alcoholic chronic pancreatitis. Gastroenteroloy 107: 1481-1487
6. Bradley EL (1982) Pancreatic duct pressure in chronic pancreatitis. Am J Surg 144: 313-315
7. Madesen P, Winkler K (1982) The intraducatal pancreatic pressure in chronic obstructive pancreatitis. Scand J Gastroenterol 17: 553-554
8. Ebbehoj N, Borly L, Madsen P, Svensen LB (1986) Pancreatic tissue pressure and pain in chronic pancreatitis. Pancreas 1: 556-558
9. Manes G, Büchler M, Pieramico O, DiSebastiano P, Malfertheiner P (1994) Is increased pancreatic pressure related to pain in chronic pancreatitis? Int J Pancreatol 15: 113-117
10. Malfertheiner P, Büchler M, Stanescu A, Ditschuneit H (1987) Pancreatic morphology and function in relationship to pain in chronic pancreatitis. Int J Pancreatol 1: 59-66
11. Borman PC, Marks IN, Girdwood AH, et al (1980) Is pancreatic duct obstruction or stricture a major cause of pain in calcific pancreatitis. Br J Surg 76: 425-428
12. Jensen AR, Matzen P, Malchow-Moller A, Christoffersen I: The Copenhagen Pancreatitis Study Group (1984) Pattern of pain, duct morphology, and pancreatic function in chronic pancreatitis. Scand J Gastroenterol 19: 334-338
13. Girdwood AH, Borman PC, Marks IN (1990) Ductal morphology and pain in chronic alcohol-induced pancreatitis. In: Beger HG, Buechler M, Ditschuneit H, Malfertheiner P (eds) Chronic pancreatitis. Springer, Berlin Heidelberg New York, pp 218-219
14. Bockmann DE, Büchler M, Malfertheiner P, Beger HG (1988) Analysis of nerves in chronic pancreatitis. Gastroenterology 94: 1459-1469
15. Aranha GV, Prinz RA, Esguerra AC, Greenlee HB (1983) The nature and course of cystic pancreatic lesions diagnosed by ultrasound. Arch Surg 118: 486-488
16. Crass RA, Way LW (1981) Acute and chronic pancreatic pseudocysts are different. Am J Surg 142: 660-663
17. McConnel DB, Gregory JR, Sasaki TM, Vetto RM (1982) Pancreatic pseudocyst Am J Surg 143: 599-601
18. Bradley ER (1990) Pseudocysts in chronic pancreatitis: development and clinical implications. In: Beger HG, Büchler M, Ditschuneit H, Malfertheiner P (eds) Chronic pancreatitis. Berlin, Springer, pp 260-268
19. Anderson MC, Stroud WH (1981) Complications of chronic pancreatitis. In: Dent TL (ed) Pancreatic disease. New York, Grune & Stratton, pp 297-323
20. Aranha GV, Prinz RA, Freeark RJ, Greenlee HB (1984) The spectrum of biliary tract obstruction from chronic pancreatitis. Arch Surg 119: 595-600
21. Gregg JA, Carr-Locke DL, Gallagher MM (1981) Importance of common bile duct stricture associated with chronic pancreatitis; Diagnosis by ERCP. Am J Surg 141: 199-203
22. Petrozza JA, Dutta SK, Latham PS, Iber FL, Gadacz TR (1984) Prevalence and natural history of distal common bile duct stenosis in alcoholic pancreatitis. Dig Dis Sci 29: 890-895
23. Stabile BE, Calabria R, Wilson SE, Passaro E (1987) Stricture of the common bile duct from chronic pancreatitis. Surg Gynaecol Obstet 165: 121-126
24. Lankisch PG (1990) The spleen in inflammatory pancreatic disease. Gastroenterology 98: 509-516
25. Stabile BE, Wilson SE, Debas HT (1983) Reduced mortality from bleeding pseudocysts and pseudoaneurysms caused by pancreatitis. Arch Surg 118: 45-51
26. Reber HA (1990) Complications in chronic pancreatitis. In: Beger HG, Büchler M, Ditschuneit H, Malfertheiner P (eds) Chronic pancreatitis. Berlin, Springer, pp 253-255
27. Neoptolemos JP, Winslet MC (1990) Pancreatic ascites. In: Beger HG, Büchler M, Ditschuneit H, Malfertheiner P (eds) Chronic pancreatitis. Berlin, Springer, pp 269-279
28. Lowenfels AB, Maisonneuve P, Cavalllini G, Amman RW, Lankisch PG, Andersen JR, et al (1993) Pancreatitis and the risk of pancreatic cancer. N Engl J Med 328: 1433-1437

29. DiMagno EP, Go VLW, Summerskill WHJ (1973) Relations between pancreatic enzyme outputs and malabsorption in severe pancreatic insufficiency. N Engl J Med 288: 813–815
30. Andersen BN, Pedersen NT, Scheel J, Worning H (1982) Incidence of alcoholic chronic pancreatitis in Copenhagen. Scand J Gastroenterol 17: 747–752
31. Dominguez-Muñoz JE, Manes G, Pieramico O, Buechler M, Malfertheiner P (1995) Effect of pancreatic ductal and parenchymal changes on exocrine function in chronic pancreatitis. Pancreas 10: 31–35
32. Lankisch PG, Otto J, Erkelenz I, Lembke B (1986) Pancreatic calcifications: no indicator of severe exocrine pancreatic insufficiency. Gastroenterology 90: 617–621
33. Bank S, Marks IN, Vinik AI (1975) Clinical and hormonal aspects of pancreatic diabetes. Am J Gastroenterol 64: 13–22
34. Lankisch PG, Löhr-Happe A, Otto J, Creutzfeldt W (1993) Natural course in chronic pancreatitis. Pain exocrine and endocrine pancreatic insufficiency and prognosis of the disease. Digestion 54: 148–155

Painless Versus Painful Chronic Pancreatitis

C. Morán

Introduction

Chronic pancreatitis is an infrequent disease in Argentina. However, the abscence of adequate epidemiological data hinders our knowledge about its true prevalence and incidence.

Abdominal pain is the predominant symptom of presentation in the early phases of the disease. However, several studies have reported painless forms in 10%–20% of well-diagnosed series [1–3].

From January 1990 to December 1995, 57 patients were diagnosed of chronic pancreatitis in our unit and 30% of them were considered primary painless forms of the disease.

Our aim in the present study is to analyze the clinical aspects at the time of presentation and the outcome of the disease comparing primary painless patients with those with classic painful forms.

Material and Methods

Patients

During a period of 6 years, 57 patients (44 men, 13 women; mean age, 51.8 years; range, 17–79 years) were diagnosed with chronic pancreatitis (CP) at the Hospital de Gastroenterology in Buenos Aires. Diagnosis was based on the following major criteria: (a) pancreatic calcifications and (b) typical histological changes, which, with their presence alone are sufficient to establish diagnosis. Minor included criteria: (a) typical history of abdominal pain in alcoholic patient; (b) ultrasound (US)/computed tomography (CT)-compatible findings; (c) endoscopic retrograde cholangiopancreatography (ERCP)-compatible findings; (d) exocrine insufficiency, steatorrhea by abnormal Van de Kamer test ($>$ 7 g/day) or abnormal secretin-cholecystokinin (CCK) test; (e) endocrine insufficiency (overt diabetes or disturbed glucose tolerance); and (f) enzyme replacement response. Twenty-eight patients presented with one of the major criteria, and the remaining 29 presented with at least three of the minor criteria.

The patients were divided in two groups according to the presentation form of the (CP: (1) primary painless CP and (2) painful CP.

Statistical Analysis

Data are presented as mean ± SD. Comparisons were performed using chi-squared and Fisher exact tests, Student's (*t*-test), and Mann-Whitney rank sum test when appropiate.

Results

Presentation Form: Painless Versus Painful

In our series, pain was not present as the initial symptom in 17 patients (30%), while in the remaining 40 (70%), the disease started with a typical, painful presentation (Fig. 1).

Etiology

Forty-one patients (72%) out of 57 had alcohol intake histories (> 50 g/day). The etiology in the remaining patients was considered idiopathic after excluding other causes, such as hypertrigliceridemia, hypercalcemia, and hereditary and traumatic pancreatitis. In relation to the form of presentation, alcoholic etiology prevailed in both groups (average daily intake of 162 g for 23 years in the painless group and 240 g for 18 years in the painful group). Although this predominance was observed more clearly in the painful group, the differences between the two groups were not statistically significant (Fig. 2).

Epidemiological Data

The epidemiological characteristics of our population are summarized in Table 1.

Fig. 1. Percent age of patients (*n*=57) with painless (*light shading*) and painful (*dark shading*) chronic pancreatitis

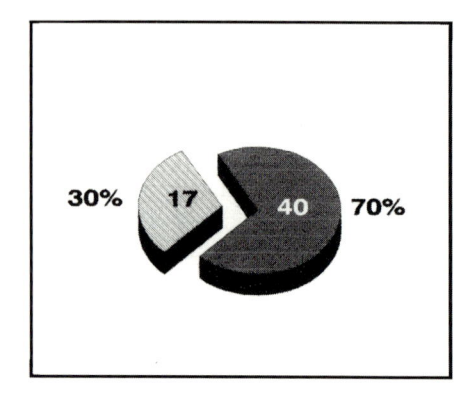

Fig. 2. Distribution of etiologies in relation to painless chronic pancreatitis *Black bars,* alcoholic; *shaded bars,* idiopathic. * NS, not significant (Fisher's exact test)

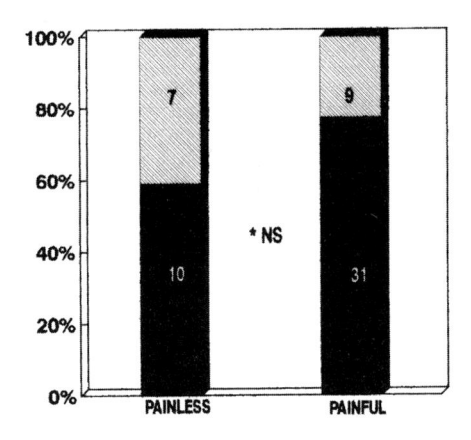

Sex. Globally, men prevailed over women in both groups. As regards the etiology, we also found a male predominance in the alcoholic patients, whereas sex distribution was more homogenous among patients with idiopathic CP.

Age at Onset of Symptoms. The age at which symptoms started was 57 years in the painless group versus 48 in the painful one. This statistically significant difference could be explained through the distribution of etiologies. Although the alcoholic prevailed in both groups, the percentage of alcoholic and idiopathic in the painless form was quite similar (59% vs. 41%). In this group all the idiopathic CP were of late-onset, which could have contributed to increase the average age at the moment of diagnosis. Only two of our patients presented with an early-onset idiopathic chronic pancreatitis (younger than 35 years), and both suffered pain from the beginning.

Prediagnostic Period. The time comprised between the beginning of the symptoms and the moment of diagnosis showed significant differences between both groups: 18 months in the painless group and 35 months in the painful one.

Table 1. Epidemiological features in patients with painless and painful chronic pancreatitis

	Painless (n=17) Men Women	Painful (n=40) Men Women	p value	Test
Sex	13 4	31 9	NS	Fisher's exact test
Alcoholic	9 1	27 4	NS	Fisher's exact test
Idiopathic	4 3	4 5	NS	Fisher's ecact test
Mean age at diagnosis (years) ± SD	56.6 ± 11.7	48.2 ± 12.0	$p < 0.03$	Student's t test
Prediagnostic period (months) ± SD	17.3 ± 18.8	35.5 ± 36.5	$p < 0.05$	Mann-Whitney U test

Ns, not significant.

Ns, not significant.

Clinical Features

Presentation Form. As regards the differences considered between the two groups, clinical presentation was one of the most prominent points. In this aspect, diarrhea with steatorrhea was the predominant sign in the primarily painless CP group, present in 13 out of 17 patients (76%). Jaundice caused by extrahepatic cholestasis was the initial symptom in two of the patients and diabetes and functional disorders were the first manifestations in the rest.

In the painful group most of the patients consulted for moderate pain. The weight loss was an accompanying symptom that appeared with a similar frequency in both groups (Table 2).

Exocrine and Endocrine Insufficiency. Among the patients in which fecal fat excretion was studied, 93% of the patients in the painless group presented an increased loss (mean, 39.6 ± 27.6 g/day).

In the painful group, the Van de Kamer test was done in 22 out of 40 patients, with 68% presenting a fat loss higher than 7 g/24 h (mean, 23.3 ± 20.9 g/24 h). These differences were not significant. The same statistical considerations were given to the endocrine insufficiency. Overt diabetes was detected in the initial consultation in six out of 17 patients group (32%) and in nine out of 40 in the painful group (22.5%) (Fig. 3).

Calcifications and Duct Abnormalities. Overall, pancreatic calcifications were present at the diagnosis time in 42% of patients. This figure showed a similar distribution when they were considered in each one of the groups (41% in painless group vs. 42% in painful group) (Fig. 4).

Related Diseases, Malignant Neoplasms and Surgery. There were three concomitant diseases that appeared more frequently in our patients with chronic pancreatitis: hepatic cirrhosis, gastroduodenal ulcer and gallstone disease. The distribution of these in both groups can be observed in Table 3. Four malignant neoplasms complicated our patients evolution: two in the painless group (pancreatic and colonic localizations) and two in the painful group (breast and esophagus localizations) (Table 3).

Table 2. Symptoms and signs at presentation

Clinical Features	Painless ($n = 17$) (n)	(%)	Painful ($n = 40$) (n)	(%)
Diarrhea	13	76	–	–
Extra-hepatic cholestasis	2	12	–	–
Diabetes	1	6	–	–
Functional disorders	1	6	–	–
Acute pancreatitis	–	–	8	20
Pain (moderate)	–	–	26	65
Pain (severe)	–	–	6	15
Weight loss	11	65	20	50

Fig. 3. Exocrine and endocrine insufficiency in patients with painless (*light shading*) and painful (*dark shading*) chronic pancreatitis. *NS*, not significant (Fisher's exact text)

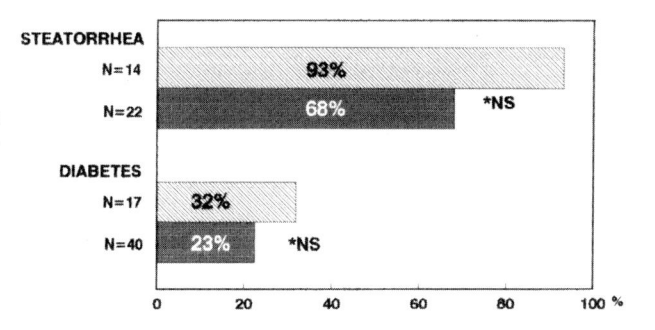

STEATORRHEA
N=14 93%
N=22 68% *NS

DIABETES
N=17 32%
N=40 23% *NS

There were no statistical differences in relation to the number of patients subjected to surgery. In the painless group, two were operated for obstructive jaundice, the sign that had marked the presentation of the disease. A pseudocyst in this group was successfully treated through percutaneous drainage. In the painful group, five out of 14 patients were operated on for pseudocysts and five out of five for jaundice, and three out of six patients required surgery for intractable pain (Table 4).

Discussion

It is a common observation that the abdominal pain constitutes the main symptom in the early stages of CP and it has been reported in more than 75 % of the patients in the different series [4, 5, 6].

When some authors considered the etiologies of CP separately, they found a higher incidence of idiopathic than alcoholic forms, among the primary painless patients [1, 4, 7]. In this sense, our data are not coincident, as the alcoholic etiology was slightly superior (59 % vs. 41 %) than the idiopathic one in the primary painless form. However, our limited number of patients may explain this difference.

While the clinical presentation form showed a clear distinction between both groups, there was an appreciable coincidence, as most of the patients consulted when the disease stage was already advanced: 13 patients in the painless group

Fig. 4. Calcifications and pancreatic duct abnormalities in patients with painless (*light shading*) and painful (*dark shading*) chronic pancreatitis. *NS*, not significant (chi-squared test, Yates corrected)

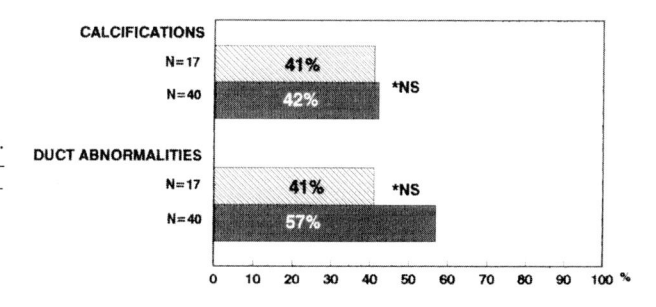

CALCIFICATIONS
N=17 41%
N=40 42% *NS

DUCT ABNORMALITIES
N=17 41% *NS
N=40 57%

Table 3. Related diseases and malignant neoplasms

	Painless (n = 17) (n)	Painful (n = 40) (n)
Related diseases		
Cirrhosis	2	2
Gastroduodenal ulcer	1	5
Gallstones	4	17
Malignant neoplasms		
Pancreas	1	
Colon	1	
Breast		1
Esophagus		1

Table 4. Specific complications and surgical treatment

	Painless (n = 17) (n)	(%)	Painful (n = 40) (n)	(%)
Pseudocyst				
Total	1	6	14	35
surgery	–	–	5	–
Jaundice				
Total	2	12	5	12.5
surgery	2	–	5	–
Intractable pain				
Total	–	–	6	15
surgery	–	–	3	–
Total surgery*	2	12	13	32.5

* Not significant (Fisher's exact test).

had steatorrhea, which implies extensive damage in the functional status of the pancreas and 17 patients (42.5 %) in the painful group (even when the pain was moderate in the majority of them) presented calcifications at diagnosis, with more than half in the same group having detectable duct abnormalities.

Several mechanisms have been involved in the production of pancreatic pain [8–10]. A question about the natural history of the disease is why, in some patients, minimal changes produce such an intense pain [11], making surgery necessary and others- like in our series-either have no pain or when they present it, it is moderate despite their advanced stage of the disease.

Our findings are in agreement with other Argentinian series which described 27.3 % of patients with painless chronic pancreatitis, although unlike our results, they had an even greater number of alcoholic patients (97 %) [12].

Our clinical comparison of the patients with CP with and without pain as a presentation form of disease did not show evidence or significant differences that could justify such a dissimilar evolution. It might be possible that a greater number of patients under stricter follow-up and research into immunological or genetic aspects of the disease could provide us with some answers in the near future. For the time being, we agree with Steer that chronic pancreatitis constitutes an enigmatic process with uncertain pathogenesis, unpredictable clinical course and unclear treatment [13].

References

1. Layer P, Yamamoto H, Kalthoff L, Clain JE, Bakken LJ, Di Magno EP (1994) The different courses of early- and late-onset idiopathic and alcoholic pancreatitis. Gastroenterology 86: 987-989
2. Ammann RW, Hammer B, Fumagalli I (1973) Chronic pancreatitis in Zurich, 1963-1972: clinical findings and follow-up studies of 102 cases. Digestion 9: 404-415
3. Domínguez-Muñoz JE, Malfertheiner P (1993) Diagnóstico y estadiaje de la pancreatitis crónica (I). El papel de los métodos de imagen. Rev. Esp. Enf. Digest. 83, 5: 367-372
4. Lankisch PG, Löhr-Happe A, Otto J, Creutzfeldt W (1993) Natural course in chronic pancreatitis. Digestion 54: 148-155.
5. Gullo L, Costa PL, Labo G (1977) Chronic pancreatitis in Italy; aetiological, clinical and histological observations based on 253 cases. Rendiconti Gastroenterol. 6: 35-44
6. Creutzfeldt W, Fehr H, Schmidt H (1970) Verlaufsbeobachtungen und diagnostische Verfahren bei der chronisch-rezidivierenden und chronischen Pankreatitis. Schweiz Med Wochenschr. 100: 1180-1189
7. Ammann RW, Akovbiantz A, Largiader F, Schuler G (1984) Course and outcome of chronic pancreatitis. Gastroenterology 86: 820-828
8. Bockman DE, Buchler M, Malfertheiner P, Beger HG (1988) Analysis of nerves in chronic pancreatitis. Gastroenterology 94: 1459-1469
9. Malfertheiner P, Mayer D, Buchler M, D Domínguez-Muñoz JE, Schiefer B, Ditschuneit H (1995) Treatment of pain in chronic pancreatitis by inhibition of pancreatic secretion with octreotide. Gut 36: 450-454
10. Banks PA (1991) Management of pancreatic pain. Pancreas 6, Suppl. 1: S52-S59
11. Walsh TN, Rode J, Theis BA, Russell RCG (1992) Minimal change chronic pancreatitis. Gut 33: 1566-1571
12. Parodi HC, Colombato LO, Villafañe VA, Gutierrez SC (1984) Chronic calcified pancreatitis. Our experience. Acta-Gastroenterol-Latinoam. 14(1): 1-12
13. Steer ML, Waxman I, Freedman S (1995) Chronic pancreatitis. The New England Journal of Medicine. 332: 1482-1490

II
Imaging Procedures

Role of Ultrasonography in the Diagnosis, Staging and Detection of Complications of Chronic Pancreatitis

R. Laugier

Introduction

Ultrasonography (US) has become an essential tool for gastroenterologists in their clinical practice, and in particular, in chronic pancreatits (CP). It contributes to the diagnosis of CP and the staging of the disease, as well as the detection of complications. Although US is more "operator-dependent" than computed tomography (CT), it gives essentially the same kind of anatomical and pathological data. Moreover, being simple, non-invasive and cheap, it now appears to be an easy method for monitoring the evolution of the disease.

Diagnosis

According to the duration of CP, one has to consider the precise place of US in two different conditions: in the early stage, just after the first or second painful episode, and later on, when repeated painful episodes have made the diagnosis obvious.

US demonstrates, in the early stage of CP, alterations of both the morphology and the echogenicity of the pancreatic gland [1, 2]. The main pancreatic duct might already be slightly irregular in diameter with abnormally visible edges (Fig. 1). The echogenicity of the pancreas is altered, being more heterogeneous than normally with numerous tiny hyperechoic spots throughout the gland, some of them giving shadowing.

Fig. 1. Early stage of chronic pancreatitis (CP). Within the hyperechoic pattern of the pancreas, note the main pancreatic duct, which is not yet dilated, although it is well delineated

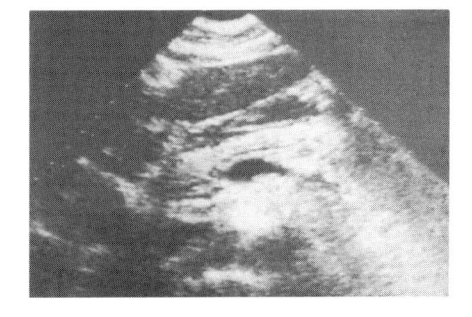

Fig. 2. Acute bout of acute pancreatitis on chronic pancreatitis (CP). The pancreas is swollen with periglandular oedematous reaction (*arrow*)

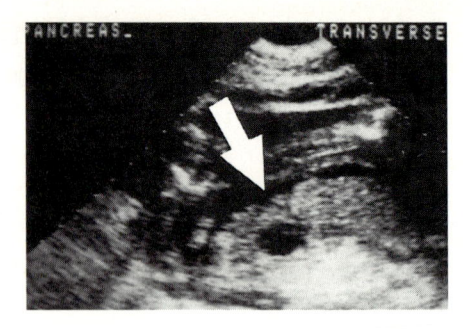

The injection of intravenous secretin has been utilized for enhancing the sensitivity of US at this early stage, but enlargement or lack of enlargement have been successively interpreted as signs of the disease [3, 4].

Immediately after an acute episode, the pancreas appears oedematous and swollen. Often periglandular hypoechoic oedema is noticeable (Fig. 2). In some cases, cystic formations are visible; at this stage, necrotic cysts might develop within the pancreas. They are usually heterogeneous and contain some solid material evocative of necrotic debris. Those cysts do not possess well delineated walls but rather very irregular limits which are difficult to define correctly [5]. Puncture or surgery usually confirms the presence of blood and necrotic material associated or not with pancreatic juice. Those cysts have a higher spontaneous tendency to heal than other retention cysts.

Endosonography allows a closer approach to the pancreatic tissue and thus a better imaging of its echogenicity [6, 7]. Hyperechoic spots are commonly found, the anatomic equivalent of which is not yet fully understood (fibrosis, microcalcifications). Multialveolar shape is usually associated. The main pancreatic duct has thickened walls and is irregular in diameter. Alterations of the parenchyma are very early in the disease: thus endosonography appears highly sensitive but with a poor specificity, the same alterations also being encountered in diabetic or alcoholic patients without CP, or during ageing.

As a consequence, endosonography is mostly useful in the differential diagnosis after an episode of pancreatic-type pain for demonstrating the absence of biliary disease (at the level of the gallbladder and the main bile duct).

Fig. 3. Atrophy of pancreas around a grossly dilated duct. Stones are visible within the dilated main pancreatic duct

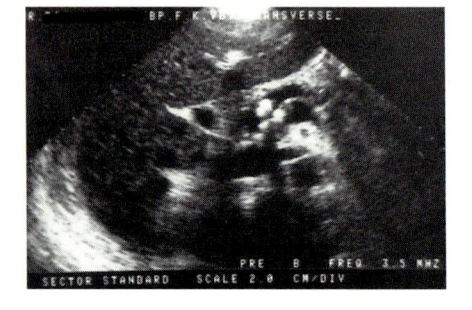

Later on, when the CP progresses, US is no longer useful for making a diagnosis but helps assess to the dimensions of both the gland and ducts. In most cases, the pancreatic gland appears atrophic with irregular edges. The echogenicity is markedly enhanced and stones are detected either within grossly dilated ducts as hyperechoic areas, giving rise to US shadowing, or as spots randomly dispersed throughout the parenchyma (Fig. 3). Ductal walls are thicker than normal and hyperechogenic due to the presence of fibrosis. At this stage, endosonography allows the detection of 88% of intraductal stones, but those structures prevent US propagation and a complete examination of the pancreatic gland [8].

Staging

US participates to the pretherapeutic staging of CP, but above all, one has to keep in mind that clinical and biological data are, at this stage, quite essential.

Echography easily enables the measurement of the pancreas which, in some cases, may be entirely reduced to a markedly dilated duct filled with stones. The diameter of the duct is accurately measured as well as the length of its dilation which is essential for assessing the possibility of a diversion surgery. Stones, either calcified or not, are searched for and usually found floating in the dilated duct or at the right part or the ductal dilation. Demonstrating a stenosis is difficult with transcutaneous echography but easy and reliable thanks to endosonography which enables one to follow the whole main duct from the papilla up to the tail [6, 7]. The existence of a pseudotumoral hypoechoic mass, raises the question of the reliability of US in differentiating CP and CP associated with a carcinoma. Although differential signs have been reported, clinical practice makes this association very difficult to analyze correctly.

Staging of CP Includes the Search for Complications

Main Bile Duct Involvement. This occurs as a form of regular stenosis throughout the pancreatic head associated with upstream dilatation. In some unusual cases, intrahepatic bile ducts may also be dilated as well as the gallbladder. In this situation, endosonography is helpful for eliminating the presence of any kind of other obstacle on the lower part of main bile tree (e.g. benign stricture of the sphincter of Oddi, carcinoma, stone).

Presence of Cysts. Cystic cavities appear as anechoic or very poorly echoic spheric areas due to the pressure of the pancreatic liquid within the cyst.

US is still the most efficient way to diagnose the development of cysts during CP [9]. It also allows one to analyze the size, localization and number of cysts.

Either entirely intrapancreatic, of small size and most often in the head, cysts may also develop outside the pancreatic gland. They may be unique or multiple, sometimes communicating. Later on, when cysts grow, they become intra- and also extrapancreatic: they are usually found at that stage of the disease, in the

Fig. 4. Typical retention cyst with well-delineated walls. A puncture needle and the corresponding "tip: effect" are visible near the centre of the cyst

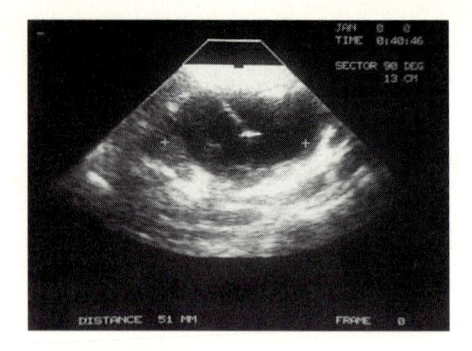

lesser sac cavity, or near the origin of mesenteric or hepatic vessels; they can also fuse towards colonic and pararenal spaces or communicate with the peritoneal cavity or the pleura, especially the left one. These two last cases represent an evolutive modality of a previously formed cyst, which may apparently disappear while communication with pleural or pertitoneal cavity develops (Fig. 4).

The pattern of the cystic content is of greatest interest: strictly anechoic cysts are filled only with pancreatic juice; they may be punctured transcutaneously or endoscopically without any special risk. By contrast, more echoic zones in the lower part of the cyst are evocative of a bleeding phenomenon [10]. When this pattern is associated with the recent, painful enlargement of the cyst, this represents signs of a recent intracystic bleeding. One has also to be very attentive to search for pericystic vascular development which represents detectable signs of portal segmental hypertension. Pulsed doppler, commonly available on new equipment, further analyzes the pericystic vascularization and its quantitative dynamic importance which, in any case, has to be taken into account in the therapeutic approach [4].

A cyst completely filled with rather echoic material is indicative of cystic infection. As it is observed and measured in CT scan, echogenicity is progressively growing as infection of the cystic content evolves towards pus transforming an infected cyst into an abscess [12].

Portal Hypertension. This may develop independently of the presence of the cyst in the tail of the pancreas. Lack of continuity of the sphenic vein is detectable thanks to US or endosonography. Abnormally visible vascularization should be systematically searched for in the splenic hilum as well as around the great curvature of the stomach.

Upstream Pancreatitis. Here, a stenosis of the main pancreatic duct is associated with dilation of the only ductal part that is localized left of the stenosis. Dilation of the duct appears more regular than that encountered in other cases of CP, and collateral branches are also regularly dilated. Stenosis may be replaced by an obstructing impacted stone.

Fig. 5. A transversal cut demonstrates the presence of a heteregeneous hyper-hypoechoic mass in the body of the pancreas representing an adenocarcinoma. The pancreatic head contains small calculi

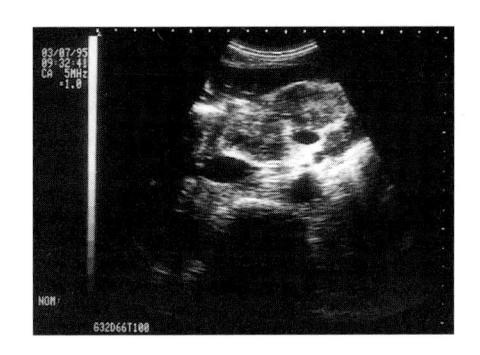

Association with a Carcinoma. This has already been envisaged. Lack of calcifications of an hypoechoic area within a gland which is entirely filled with typical spots might be alarming (Fig. 5). One should note that, in some cases, calfcifications may be surrounded by tumoral growth. Endosonography was considered some years ago as more efficient in the diagnosis of this association than US but this is no longer the opinion of most ultrasonographers. The differential diagnosis between carcinoma and CP is not difficult at all, the right part of the gland and consequently its duct being strictly normal; moreover, lesions located to the left of the tumor represent typical upstream pancreatitis (Fig. 5).

Cystic Dystrophy of the Duodenal Wall. This is arely detectable by US. Patients present with a typical pattern at endosonography [13]. It appears as cystic lesions strictly intraparietal within the duodenum and filled with anechoic material. They develop essentially in the submucosa, which is modified and always limited outside by the muscular layer which is normal.

Conclusion

In the early stage of CP, US fails sometimes because of a lack of sensitivity to the transparietal approach, while the endosonography lacks specificity. Nonetheless, typical alterations of the ductal system and early alterations of the parenchyma are almost always detected by this method.

In the later stages of the disease, US is the cheapest, simplest, and most efficient way of detecting all types of complications, including those of the main pancreatic duct. It is thus of infinite help in the staging, follow-up and therapeutical approach throughout the evolution of CP. It helps to avoid most endoscopic pancreatographies for diagnostic purposes only. Finally, US also participates in the therapeutic approach of guiding punctures and drainages either transcutaneously or endoscopically.

References

1. Foley WD, Stewart ME, Lawson TL et al (1980) CT, US and ERCP in the diagnosis of pancreatic disease: a comparative study. Gastrointest Radiol 5: 29–35
2. Grant JH, Efrasy ME (1981) Ultrasound in the evaluation of chronic pancreatitis. J.A.O.A. 81, 183–188
3. Bolondi L, Bassi S, Gaiani S et al (1989) Impaired response of main pancreatic duct to secretin stimulation in early chronic pancreatitis. Dig Dis Sci 34: 834–840
4. Glaser J, Hogemann B, Schneider J (1989) Significance of a sonographic secretin test in the diagnosis of pancreatic disease: result of a prospective study. Scand J Gastroenterol 24: 179–185
5. Segal I, Epstein B, Lawson HH, Solomon A, Patel V, Oettlé GJ (1984) The syndromes of pancreatic pseudocysts and fluid collections – Gastrointest Radiol 9: 115–122
6. Lee WR (1986) Endoscopic ultrasonography of chronic pancreatitis and pancreatic pseudocysts. Scand J Gastroenterol 21 (suppl 123): 123–129
7. Kaufman AR, Sivack MV (1989) Endoscopic ultrasonography in the differential diagnosis of pancreatic disease. Gastrointest Endosc 35: 214–219
8. Noguchi T, Aibe T, Amanoh et al (1986) The diagnosis of chronic pancreatitis and pancreatic cancer by endoscopic ultrasonography. Dig Dis Sci 31: 62 S
9. Williford ME, Foster WL, Halvorsen RA, Thompson WM (1983) Pancreatic pseudocyst: Comparative evaluation by sonography and computed tomography. Am J Roentgenol 140: 53–57
10. Frank B, Bolich P, Reichert J (1975) Sonographic appearance of organized blood within a cyst: 2 cases report. J Clin Ultrasound 3: 233–237
11. Gerolami R, Giovannini M, Laugier R (1997) Endosonographic guidance for cysts treatment. Endoscopy – in press
12. Laing FC, Gooding GA, Brown T, Leopold GR (1979) Atypical pseudocysts of the pancreas: and ultrasonographic evaluation. J Clin Ultrasound 7: 27–33
13. Andrieu J, Palazzo F, Chikli et al (1989) Dystrophie kystique sur pancréas aberrant. Apport de l'écho-endoscopie. Gastroenterol Clin Biol 3: 630–633

Diagnosis and Staging of Chronic Pancreatitis by Computed Tomography

W. Döhring

Introduction

Computed tomography (CT) belongs to the most important imaging procedures in the diagnosis and staging of chronic pancreatitis, alongside ultrasound (US) and endoscopic retrograde cholangiopancreatography (ERCP); other imaging techniques should be restricted to special diagnostic problems.

CT enables the detection of morphological alterations which cause sufficient changes of X-ray absorption within a sufficiently large tissue volume. Thus early parenchymal changes in chronic pancreatitis and effects on small pancreatic ducts cannot be detected by CT, but later stages, as well as pancreatic and extrapancreatic complications of the disease, can be evaluated with high reliability.

Two different CT techniques are available: the original single-slice technique and the newer spiral technique.

Spiral CT offers scanning of a complete body volume by continuous rotation of the X-ray tube/detector unit and constant table movement during a short scanning time of up to about 20 s. Vessels can be well delineated during the total scanning procedure because of the short scanning time, and transverse sections can be reconstructed in any requested axial plane due to the registration of the whole volume.

The CT examination of chronic pancreatitis demands, like examinations of other diseases, an optimized scanning technique. The slice thickness should be reduced at the level of the pancreas to 5 mm at the most, and in the use of spiral CT postcontrast scans should be performed during the arterial and the venous or parenchymal phase.

CT permits imaging of the various pancreatic structures with different reliability. For the detection of parenchyma it is comparable with ultrasound; however, for the detection of the pancreatic duct and the pancreatic and peripancreatic vessels it is less suitable than ERCP and angiography, respectively.

CT findings in chronic pancreatitis include

- Alterations in pancreatic size
- Irregularities in pancreatic margin
- Inhomogeneities of pancreatic parenchyma
- Dilatation and irregularities of the main pancreatic duct
- Ductal and "parenchymal" calcifications

- Cystic fluid collections
- Densification and obliteration of peripancreatic fatty tissue
- Thickening of peripancreatic fasciae and peritoneum
- Pancreatic and extrapancreatic complications

The *size* of the pancreas can vary during the course of disase. Ferrucci et al. found normal size in 16 % of cases, focal enlagement in 23 %, diffuse enlargement in 50 % and atrophy in 11 % [2]. Focal and diffuse enlargement can be caused by acute exacerbations of chronic pancreatitis, but also by pancreatic carcinoma. In such cases CT density measurements in precontrast and postcontrast scans, as suggested by Miura et al. [7], are not very helpful in differential diagnosis; fine-needle aspiration biopsies should be performed in uncertain cases. Pancreatic atrophy due to chronic pancreatitis is similar to atrophy as a result of senile involution or ductal obstruction caused by pancreatic cancer [5].

The *pancreatic margin* can be shaped normally or irrgularly. A generalized lobularity must be distinguished from intralobular fatty infiltration.

Irregular, beaded and smooth *dilatation of the main pancreatic duct* (Fig. 1a) are found in up to two thirds of cases of chronic pancreatitis [4]. The normal ductal caliber varies from 2 to 3 mm, in the elderly up to 4 mm. In contrast with ERCP, CT can show dilatations distal to total duct obstructions (Fig. 1b). CT, however, is not able to detect ectatic side branches.

Inhomogeneities of pancreatic parenchyma are mainly caused by necrosis, fat, hemorrhage and calcifications, whereas edema and fibrosis do not obviously influence CT density. Necrotic areas can be detected with increased sensitivity by contrast scans.

Calcifications are found in 30–50 % of cases [1, 4]. Usually they become detectable 1–3 years after the onset of clinical symtoms (Fig. 2a, b). In detection of calculi CT is more sensitive than film/screen radiography and in particular ultrasound. Pancreatic calcifications vary widely in size and distribution. In general they are tiny or coarse; anular configurations are rare and caused by calcified cystic walls or aneurysms. Mostly the calcifications are multiple; they are equally distributed over the gland in about 75 % and are limited to the head or tail in about 25 % of cases. Solitary calcifications are rare. Calculi can be

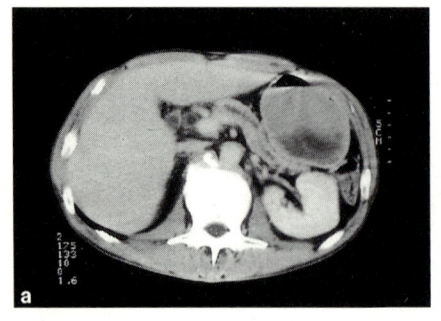

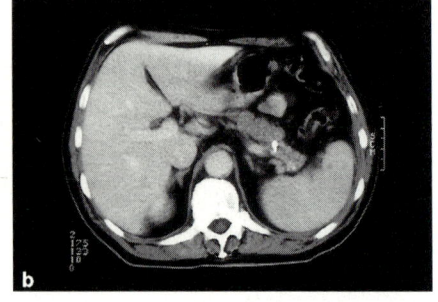

Fig. 1a, b. Dilatation of the main pancreatic duct in chronic pancreatitis. **a** Normally sized and smoothly marginated pancreas with a generally dilated main pancreatic duct. **b** Localized dilatation of the main pancreatic duct caused by an obstructing ductal calculus

Diagnosis and Staging of Chronic Pancreatitis by Computed Tomography

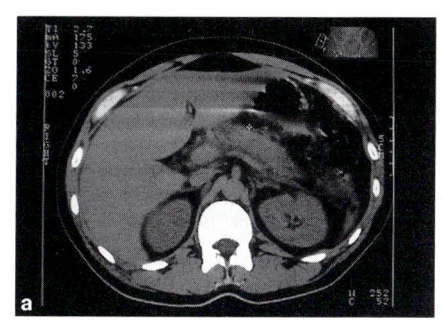

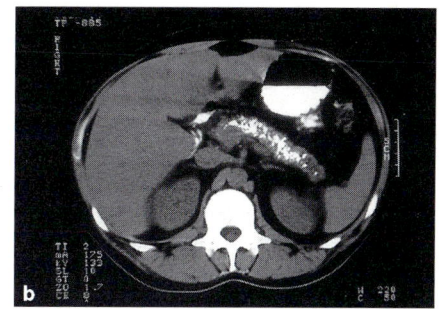

Fig. 2a, b. Appearance of pancreatic calcifications in chronic pancreatitis. **a** Acute onset of pancreatitis with a moderate enlargement and indistinct margination of the pancreas, exudation in front of the left-sided Gerota fascia. **b** Diffusely distributed pancreatic calcifications, detected 2 years later in the same patient

identified as ductal calcifications when they follow the course of the main pancreatic duct. Calculi within the ductal branches, however, appear as "parenchymal" calcifications. Usually the number and size of calculi increase during the progress of disease. Occasionally they can disappear (e.g. be engulfed by a growing carcinoma) or be displaced (e.g. by pseudocysts). Calcifications in chronic pancreatitis can be simulated by calcified splenic artery, by tumor calcifications or calcified lymph nodes, by calculi with the common bile duct, by calcified hematomas or infarctions, or by calcified hydatic cysts.

Cystic fluid collections are reported in 10-40% of cases of severe chronic pancreatitis [1, 3]. These are pseudocysts or retention cysts. In general they cannot be differentiated by CT, when they are localized within the pancreas and the pancreatic duct is not enhanced by contrast medium. Pseudocysts vary widely in size, shape and localization. They can be located intrapancreatically (Fig. 3a) or extrapencreatically and involve adjacent structures such as the spleen (Fig. 3b), liver, stomach, intestine, kidneys or mediastinum. Furthermore, they can be encapsulated or unencapsulated; sometimes they are septate, and occasionally their walls show calcifications. Pancreatic fluid collections have to be differentiated from cystic tumors (especially when septate) from ne-

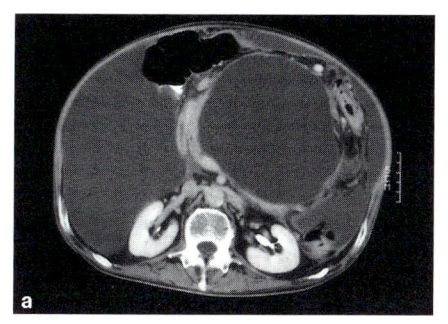

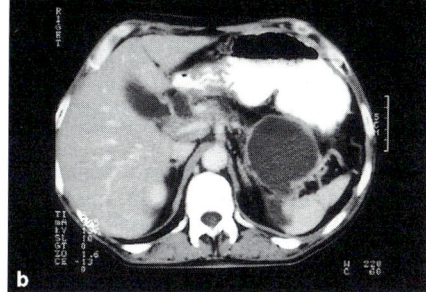

Fig. 3a, b. Cystic fluid collections in chronic pancreatitis. **a** Large pancreatic pseudocyst and extended ascites. **b** Pancreatic pseudocyst with involvement of the spleen

Diagnosis and Staging of Chronic Pancreatitis by Endoscopic Retrograde Cholangiopancreatography[*]

H. Bosseckert

The diagnosis of chronic pancreatitis in its early stages and the differential diagnosis of chronic focal pancreatitis versus pancreatic carcinoma present a great challenges.

Endoscopic retrograde cholangiopancreatography (ERCP) is one of various imaging modalities which are helpful in the diagnosis of chronic pancreatitis.

Other imaging modalities in the diagnosis of pancreatic diseases are the following:

- Aimed native X-ray pictures of the pancreas
- Ultrasonography
- Computed tomography (CT)
- Magnetic resonance imaging (MRI)
- Endoscopic ultrasonography
- Angiography
- Positron emission tomography (PET)
- Magnetic resonance cholangiopancreatography (MRCP)

Among these different imaging procedures MRI, PET, and MRCP are still at the experimental stage. Angiography is of no particular importance in the diagnosis and differential diagnosis of chronic pancreatitis. Ultrasonography and radiographic findings (calcifications; Fig. 1), shadows of soft parts (with and without displacement of organs in the vicinity) are the standard imaging methods in the diagnostic procedure of chronic pancreatitis. Computed tomography (CT) is sometimes helpful, but rarely provides new essential information.

Endoscopic ultrasonography (EUS) has the advantage of providing high-resolution images of the pancreas and the surrounding vessels. The method allows delineation of even small lesions of pancreatic parenchyma as well as pathological changes of the pancreatic duct. EUS is of great importance in diagnosis and staging of pancreatic cancer, but it is of much less value in differentiation between chronic pancreatitis and pancreatic carcinoma (Rösch 1994).

The benefits of ERCP include the following:
- High sensitivity and specificity
- Possibility of discovering additional findings (stomach, duodenum, papilla)
- Simultaneous evaluation of the bile ducts

---

[*] Dedicated to Professor Dr. D. Jorke on his 70th birthday.

Fig. 1. Calcification of the pancreatic head

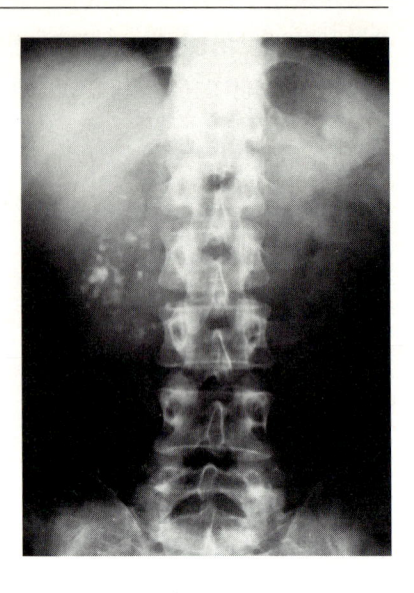

- Extension of diagnosis by biopsies, collection of pure pancreatic juice, manometry and pancreatoscopy

Possible findings during the passage to the papilla are protrusions of the stomach wall caused by pancreatic pseudocysts and varices of the fornix region. In the duodenum signs of obstruction and inflammation (edematous swelling of duodenal folds) and, additionally, adenomas and carcinomas of the papilla of Vater can be discovered. As a rare complication of chronic pancreatitis haemosuccus pancreatitis is sometimes observed.

A further advantage of ERCP is the possibility of recognizing changes of the common bile duct, which can give additional indications concerning the diagnosis of chronic pancreatitis (Fig. 2). A smooth narrowing of the intrapancreatic part of the common bile duct as well as a smooth symmetrical short-distance narrowing in the middle part of the common bile duct are typical signs

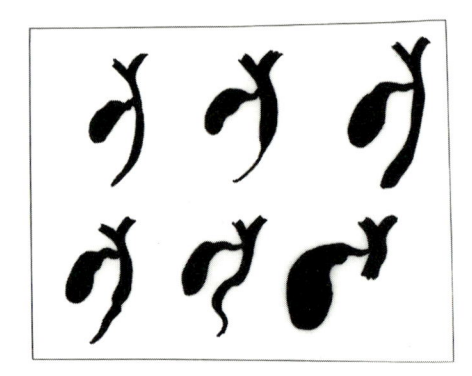

Fig. 2. Changes of the common bile duct in chronic pancreatitis or pancreatic cancer

of chronic pancreatitis, whereas other changes of the duct can be observed in both chronic pancreatitis and pancreatic carcinoma.

Furthermore, ERCP allows a classification of chronic pancreatitis in low, moderate, and high grades (Table 1, Figs. 3-5). Kasugai (1972) and the working group from Cambridge (Axon et al. 1984) classified chronic pancreatitis by means of ERCP, ultrasound, and CT. The findings are questionable if there are less than three altered side branches of the pancreatic duct. More than three changed side branches indicate a mild form of chronic pancreatitis. If there is an additional dilation and an irregular expansion of the main duct, a moderate stage of chronic pancreatitis can be postulated. All these findings, together with pseudocysts, intraductal or parenchymental calcifications, distinct strictures and involvement of the neighborhood (ultrasound or CT) present a severe form of the disease. Occasionally, ERCP gives some evidence for the etiology of chronic pancreatitis, e.g. if there are anomalies of the pancreatic and/or bile duct, e.g., pancreas divisum, choledochal cysts (Fig. 6, see page 199), adenomas of the papilla.

Via ERCP, further diagnostic procedures such as biopsies or brush cytology, collection of pure pancreatic juice, manometry, and at least pancreatoscopy can be done to support the diagnosis of chronic pancreatitis. In spite of the improvement of noninvasive imaging methods such as ultrasound, CT and MRT, there is no doubt about the importance of ERCP. The indications for ERCP in chronic pancreatitis are as follows:

- Differential diagnosis (pancreatic carcinoma)
- Exclusion of a mechanical outflow obstruction
- Suspicion of chronic pancreatitis without findings by common diagnostic procedures
- Preoperatively in pancreatic surgery
- Postoperatively if there are new complaints

An outflow obstruction has some importance in connection with recurring pain attacks in chronic pancreatitis. However, if the obstruction is abolished an uneventful recovery of the pancreas is possible in a patient with obstructive pancreatitis (retention pancreatitis).

In some cases of an early stage of chronic pancreatitis, only ERCP allows a diagnosis to be made, whereas all other procedures are negative. This it also the case in 10% of patients with a normal pancreozymin-secretin test; conversely, however, in about 15% of patients with a normal pancreatic duct, the stimulation test gives pathological results (own results).

Table 1. Classification of chronic pancreatitis by endoscopic retrograde cholangioancreatography

Grade	Features
Low	Dilatation with strictures and obstructions of the side branches
Moderate	Additional dilatations and stenoses of the main duct
High	Additional obstructions, cysts, and stones in the main duct and side branches

Fig. 3. Stage 1 chronic pancreatitis

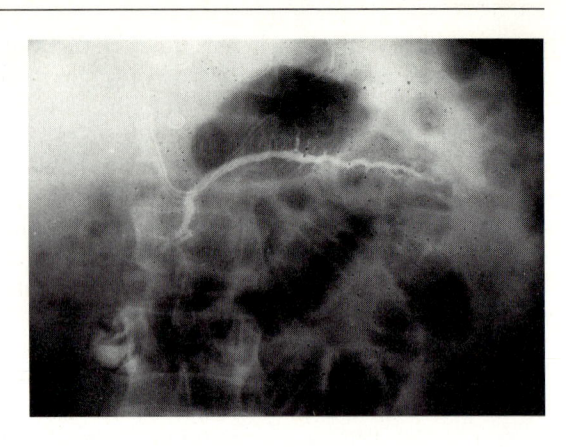

However, minimal changes of the pancreatic duct and its side branches have to be evaluated with caution, especially in the elderly, because of age-related changes. If an operation is being considered in chronic pancreatitis, ERCP may help to select the adequate surgical procedure, for example, a drainage or a resection approach. Differentiating between chronic pancreatitis and pancreatic carcinoma is still at present often very difficult. A pancreatic carcinoma may develop out of a preexisting chronic pancreatitis (Lowenfels et al. 1993), while on the other hand a pancreatic carcinoma is often accompanied by pancreatitis. Additionally, the alterations of the pancreatic duct are similar in both diseases. Some differences between chronic pancreatitis and pancreatic carcinoma are listed in Table 2.

If there is a stricture with dilation of the duct behind it, and there are also some signs of chronic pancreatitis in front of the stricture, then these findings are highly suspicious for chronic pancreatitis. In pancreatic carcinoma, changes which look like an obstructive pancreatitis are limited to the part of the duct which is located behind the tumor. In general the side branches of the main duct show only mild changes and often vanish in the region of the tumor.

Fig. 4. Stage 2 chronic pancreatitis

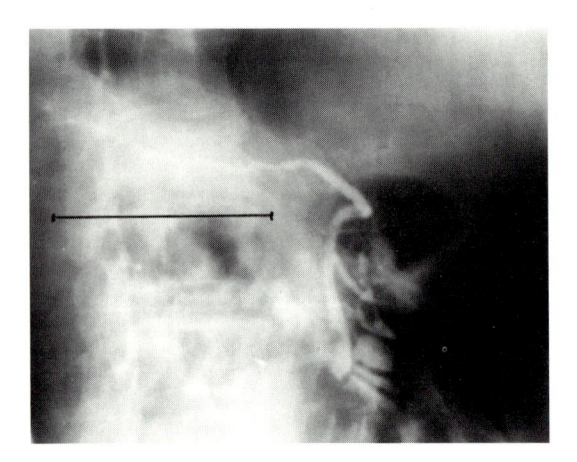

Fig. 5. Stage 3 chronic pancreatitis (a carcinoma of the head of the pancreas was excluded by a Whipple operation)

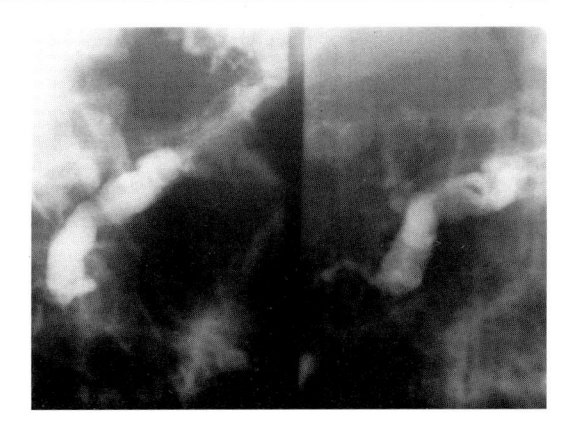

The sign of tapering of the main duct or the double duct sign can be found much more often in pancreatic carcinoma than in chronic pancreatitis.

However, calcifications are much more common in chronic pancreatitis, but do not exclude pancreatic carcinoma. A cavity in the pancreatic region without change of the pancreatic duct is highly suspicious for a pancreatic carcinoma.

Shemesh et al. (1990) suggested that a pancreatic duct stricture longer than 10 mm indicates pancreatic carcinoma instead of chronic pancreatitis, especially if the borders of the stricture are irregular. The ERCP of a patient who suffered from moderate pains in the upper abdomen showed a low-grade narrowing of the pancreatic duct (Fig. 7). Two and a half years later, the patient died of pancreatic carcinoma.

By cytological examination of pancreatic juice obtained during ERCP in connection with secretin stimulation, a better differentiation between chronic pancreatitis and pancreatic carcinoma may be possible (Endo et al. 1974). It may be that brush cytology from the pancreatic duct with or without the aid of pancreatoscopy will improve the diagnostic yield.

Fig. 6. Choledochal cyst and fusion anomaly of the pancreatic ducts

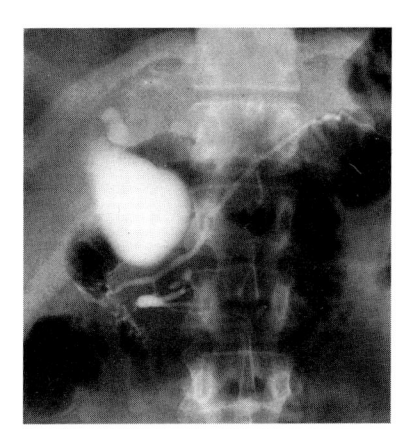

Table 2. Endoscopic retrograde cholangiopancreatography (ERCP) findings in chronic pancreatitis and pancreatic carcinoma

Sign	Chronic pancreatitis	Pancreatic carcinoma
Stricture	In front of and behind the stricture there are signs of chronic pancreatitis (only a short distance)	Duct is changed only behind the stricture
Side branches	Significantly changed	Minimally changed; in the region of the tumor they have vanished
Tapering	Seldom	More frequent
Double duct	Very rare	Frequent
Calcification	Frequent	Possible
Cavities	In relation to changes in the main duct	Often without changes in the main duct

Moreover, there are varying results concerning the determination of CA 19-9 in pancreatic juice obtained by ERCP. Whereas Malesci et al. (1987) report asthonishing by good results which would allow an early diagnosis of pancreatic carcinoma, Wakabayashi et al. (1993) could not reproduce these data. We will have to wait for further studies investigating the value of Ki-ras estimation in pancreatic juice (Tada et al. 1993).

Conclusion

ERCP is an important method in the diagnosis of chronic pancreatitis. It can be an aid to the surgeon in planning the operating procedure. The limitations of ERCP have to be kept in mind, e.g., the diagnosis of early stages of chronic pancreatitis and the difficulties in differentiating it from pancreatic cancer.

Fig. 7. Minimal changes of the pancreatic duct (the patient died 3 years later of pancreatic cancer)

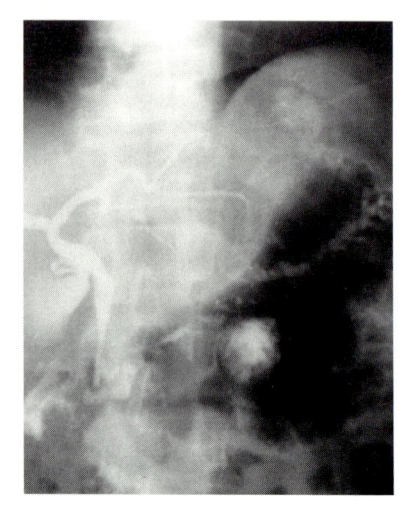

References

1. Rösch T (1994) Endoscopic Ultrasonography in Pancreatic Cancer. Endoscopy 26: 806–807
2. Kasugai T, Kizu M, Kabayashi S, Hattori K (1972) Endoscopic pancreatocholangiography. Gastroenterology 63: 227–234
3. Axon ATR, Classen M, Cotton PB, Cremer M, Freeny PC, Lees WR (1984) Pancreatography in chronic pancreatiits: international definitions. Gut 25: 1107–1112
4. Lowenfels AB, Maisonneuve P, Cavallini G, Ammann RW, Lankisch PG, Andersen JR, Dimagno EP, Andren-Sandberg A, Domellöf L (1993) Pancreatitis and the risk of pancreatic cancer. New England J of Med 328: 1433–1437
5. Shemesh E, Czerniak A, Nass S, Klein E (1990) Role of endoscopic retrograde cholangiopancreatography in differentiating pancreatic cancer coexisting with chronic pancreatitis. Cancer 65: 893–6
6. Endo Y, Morii J, Tamura N, Okuda S (1974) Cytodiagnosis of pancreatic malignant tumors by aspiration, under direct vision, using a duodenal fiberscope. Gastroenterology 67: 944–51
7. Malesci A, Evangelista A, Mariani A, Bersani M, Bonato C, Basilico M, Montorsi M, Beretta E (1988) CA 19-9 in serum and pancreatic juice: its role in the differential diagnosis of resectable pancreatic cancer from chronic pancreatitis. Int J Pancreatol. 3 Suppl. 1: 119–23
8. Wakabayashi T, Sawabu N, Takemori Y, Satomura Y, Kidani H, Ohta H, Watanabe H, Yamakawa O, Takahashi H, Watanabe K (1993) Pancreas 8 (2): 151–159
9. Tada M, Omata M, Kawai S, Saisho H, Ohto M, Saiki RK, Sninsky JJ (1993) Detection of ras gene mutations in pancreatic juice and peripheral blood of patients with adenocarcinoma. Cancer Res 53: 2472–2474

Radiologic Imaging of Chronic Pancreatitis

P. C. Freeny

Chronic pancreatitis comprises a broad spectrum of pathologic changes in the gland caused by a wide variety of etiologies. Our understanding of the morphologic changes produced by the chronic inflammatory process has expanded in the last decade as more sophisticated imaging modalities have been utilized for evaluation. This lecture will discuss the current concepts of diagnosis and the relationship between morphology and function of the pancreas.

Classification Systems

Two international symposia were held to evaluate the current status of the understanding of pancreatitis, to correlate new information now available regarding function and morphology, and to offer an improved classification system. The first was in Cambridge in 1983 [2], and the second in Marseille in 1984 [1].

Cambridge Classification

Chronic pancreatitis was defined as a continuing inflammatory disease of the pancreas, characterized by irreversible morphological change, and typically causing pain and/or permanent loss of function. Many patients with chronic pancreatitis may also have acute exacerbations, but the condition may be painless and the only evidence of an inflammatory process may be fibrosis indicating previous inflammation.

The sections on imaging and function at the Cambridge meeting recognized that there may be major discrepancies between the clinical severity of the inflammatory process, the degree of functional exocrine and endocrine impairment of the gland, and the morphological changes depicted by ultrasound (US), computed tomography (CT), and endoscopic retrograde cholangiopancreatography (ERCP). Moreover, it was apparent that diagnosis of chronic pancreatitis of mild to moderate severity often requires a combination of modalities, including clinical evaluation, laboratory studies and function testing, and one or more imaging procedures. Accordingly, a classification of the "severity" of the morphologic changes in chronic pancreatitis was proposed (Table 1) [3].

Table 1. Cambridge classification of pancreatic morphology in chronic pancreatitis

CHANGES	ERCP	CT and US
	No abnormal LSB	Normal gland size, shape Homogeneous parenchyma
Equivocal	MPD normal	One of the following: < 3 abnormal LSB MPD 2–4 mm gland enlarged < 2 × normal Heterogeneous parenchyma
Mild	MPD normal	Two or more signs for diagnosis: > 3 abnormal LSB MPD 2–4 mm Slight gland enlargement Heterogeneous parenchyma
Moderate	MPD changes LSB changes	Small cysts < 10 mm MPD irregularity Focal acute pancreatitis Increased echogenicity of MPD walls Gland contour irregularity
Severe	Any of the above changes plus one or more of the following: Cyst > 10 mm Intraductal filling defects Calculi MPD obstruction, stricture Severe MPD irregularity Contiguous organ invasion	

Focal change: less than one third of gland involved.
ERCP, endoscopic retrograde cholangiopancreatography; CT, computed tomography; US, ultrasonography; MPD main pancreatic duct; LSB lateral side branch ducts.

Marseille Classification

The Marseille and Cambridge clinical definitions of chronic pancreatitis agreed. The Marseille group emphasized morphology by defining chronic pancreatitis as characterized by irregular sclerosis with destruction and permanent loss of exocrine parenchyma. All types of inflammatory cells can be present in varying degrees, as well as edema and focal necrosis. Cysts and pseudocysts, with or without infection, which may or may nor communicate with ducts, are not uncommon. The morphological changes seen in chronic pancreatitis are progressive and eventually result in permanently diminished exocrine and endocrine function.

Acinar destruction may be either focal, segmental, or diffuse, and they may be associated with varying degrees of dilatation of the pancreatic duct. Duct dilatation is usually associated with strictures or intraductal protein plugs and calculi, although occasionally no apparent cause of dilatation may be seen. Compared to the degree of acinar destruction, the islets of Langerhans are relatively well preserved.

Based predominately on structural features, the following descriptive terms can be used:

(a) chronic pancreatitis with focal necrosis;
(b) chronic pancreatitis with focal, segmental or diffuse fibrosis;
(c) chronic pancreatitis with or without calculi.

Subtypes of Chronic Pancreatitis

A distinctive morphological form of chronic pancreatitis is *obstructive chronic pancreatitis*. It is characterized by dilatation of the ductal system proximal to an occlusion (e.g., by tumor or scar tissue from acute or traumatic pancreatitis), diffuse atrophy of the acinar parenchyma, and uniform diffuse fibrosis. Calculi and intraductal protein plugs are uncommon in obstructive chronic pancreatitis. This is the usual type of chronic pancreatitis which evolves from acute pancreatitis. In obstructive chronic pancreatitis, both structural and functional changes tend to improve if the obstruction is corrected.

Another distinctive form of chronic pancreatitis is *groove pancreatitis*. Groove pancreatitis describes a special form of pancreatitis that results in scarring that extends into the "groove" between the C-loop of the duodenum and the head of the pancreas [4, 5]. It has been described as occurring in up to 20 % of cases of chronic pancreatitis. The scarring leads to compression of the blood vessels and lymphatics, tubular stenosis of the common bile duct, and unilateral or concentric narrowing of the duodenum. The main pancreatic duct in the head of the gland may or may not be narrowed. The scarring produces a mass in the head of the pancreas which often is associated with cysts in the adjacent wall of the duodenum or within the groove. The mass can mimic pancreatic carcinoma.

Clinical Diagnosis

The clinical diagnosis of chronic pancreatitis is based upon the combination of one or more of the following symptoms and findings: abdominal pain, steatorrhea, jaundice, and diabetes mellitus. During exacerbations of symptoms, serum amylase and lipase levels may be elevated, but with advanced destruction of exocrine tissue, these enzymes may be normal or decreased. Unfortunately, these findings are quite nonspecific and can also be due to other diseases, particularly pancreatic carcinoma. In addition, chronic pancreatitis can be clinically silent owing to the fact that 80 % – 90 % of exocrine and endocrine function can be lost without manifesting steatorrhea or diabetes. Thus, considerable effort has been directed towards finding laboratory tests and imaging studies which will aid in diagnosis.

Pancreatic Function Tests

A variety of direct and indirect tests of pancreatic exocrine function can be used to help establish the clinical diagnosis of chronic pancreatitis. Two problems are inherent in each of the tests. First, in early or minimal disease, the degree of exocrine dysfunction may be too small to measure reliably. Secondly, pancreatic tumors, which cause obstruction of the main pancreatic duct, also produce exocrine dysfunction. Thus, these tests cannot discriminate between the exocrine dysfunction caused by chronic pancreatitis and that caused by pancreatic carcinoma.

Direct Tests. The secretin-cholecystokinin (SEC-CCK) and the secretin-caerulein (SEC-C) tests require intubation of the duodenum and collection of pancreatic juice during stimulation with secretin or cerulein. The amount of trypsin, amylase, lipase, and bicarbonate secreted is quantified. The sensitivity of the tests depends upon the severity of the disease and ranges from 74% to > 90% [6]. There are also a variety of other diseases, such as celiac sprue, primary diabetes mellitus, Billroth II gastrectomy, and hepatic cirrhosis, that can produce false positive SEC-CCK or SEC-C test results.

Indirect Tests. Considerable interest has been focused on indirect measurements of pancreatic function which do not require duodenal intubation. The most commonly used tests are the *N*-benzoyl-l-tyrosyl-*p*-aminobenzoic acid test, known as the bentiromide or NBT-PABA test, and the pancreolauryl (PLT). These tests invole oral administration of substrates for pancreatic digestive enzymes and then measurement of their products of digestion. The sensitivity of both of these tests also depends on the degree of exocrine dysfunction. Studies comparing NBT-PABA and PLT with SEC-CCK have shown that in patients with chronic pancreatitis and mild to moderate exocrine dysfunction, average senstivities are 46% and 39%, respectively, while in patients with severe exocrine dysfunction, average sensitivities are 71% and 79%, respectively [6].

Imaging Chronic Pancreatitis

Radiologic imaging has four primary roles in the evaluation of patients with chronic pancreatitis:

(1) diagnosis;
(2) staging the severity of the disease;
(3) detection of complications; and
(4) assistance in choosing treatment alternatives.

Diagnosis

Diagnosis of chronic pancreatitis is based upon clinical findings, assessment of endocrine and exocrine pancreatic function, and identification of morphologic changes in the gland as depicted by imaging studies. Evaluation of all three areas is essential, since many patients with chronic pancreatitis will have abnormalities of only one or two.

A morphologic diagnosis of chronic pancreatitis can be made with US, CT, and ERCP. ERCP continues to be the gold standard for diagnosis, but cross-sectional techniques are important for their ability to display changes in the parenchyma, as well as to detect complications of the inflammatory process.

Sonography (US). The overall sensitivity of US in the diagnosis of chronic pancreatitis shows considerable variation from a low of 48 % to a high of 96 % [7]. An average range in most studies is about 60 %-70 %. These figures reflect the morphologic spectrum of chronic pancreatitis, ranging from normal in early or mild disease to grossly abnormal in moderate to severe disease [8].

The most sensitive and specific US findings include pancreatic duct dilatation and intraductal calcifications (Fig. 1). However, these changes are usually found only in more advanced stages of the disease. In early or minimal chronic pancreatitis, the pancreatic duct may be normal and no calcifications are evident. Bolondi has shown that secretin-stimulated pancreatic duct sonography can be helpful in evaluating patients with suspected chronic pancreatitis and no demonstratable US morphologic abnormalities [8]. Following secretin stimulation, two responses are seen in patients with chronic pancreatitis: absent or decreased pancreatic duct dilatation (<50 % caliber change) or pancreatic duct dilatation (>100 % caliber change) with persistent dilatation at 15 min. Bolondi reports the sensitivity of secretin-stimulated pancreatic duct sonography as 86.6 % [8].

Endosonography. Endoscopic ultrasonography is a technique that produces very high-resolution images of the pancreatic parenchyma and pancreatic duct. Although it has been applied to the evaluation of patients with chronic pancreatitis, the exact role of the procedure vis-a-vis ERCP and CT has not as yet been defined [9, 10].

Computed Tomography. The CT findings of chronic pancreatitis consist of a broad spectrum of changes which depend on the severity of the chronic inflammatory process. These include alterations in size and shape of the gland,

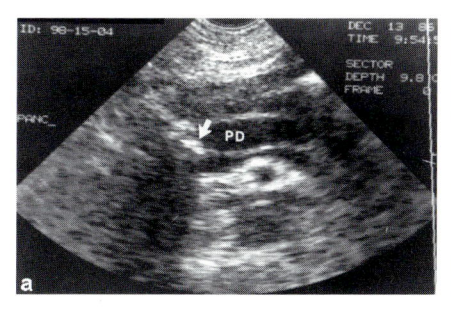

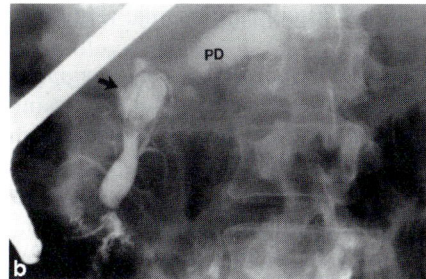

Fig. 1 a, b. Chronic calcific pancreatitis. **a** Transverse real time ultrasonogram shows a dilated main pancreatic duct (*PD*) owing to obstruction by a stone (*arrow*). **b** Endoscopic, retrograde cholangiopancreatography (ERCP) shows marked dilatation of the main PD upstream from the large, obstructing stone (*arrow*)

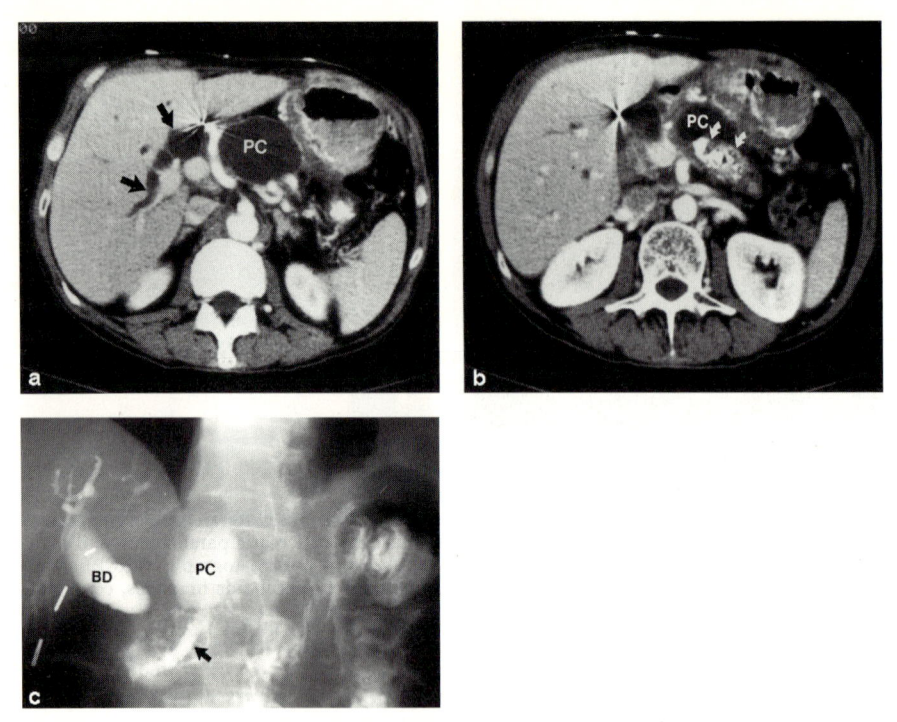

Fig. 4a–c. Chronic calcific pancreatitis, pseudocyst, and biliary obstruction. **a** Contrast-enhanced computed tomography (CT) scan shows dilated intrahepatic biliary ducts (*arrows*) owing to a pseudocyst (*PC*) in the region of the pancreatic head. **b** Scan in lower level shows continuation of the PC and calcifications in the tail of the gland (*arrows*). **c** Endoscopic retrograde cholangiopancreatography (ERCP) shows dilatation of the biliary duct (*BC*) with no filling of the intrapancreatic segment of the common bile duct. There are gross changes of chronic pancreatitis involving the main pancreatic duct (*arrow*) and there iscommunication of the PC with the pancreatic duct

overall assessment of the individual patient is correlation of morphology and endocrine-exocrine function with the clinical status of the patient.

The imaging section of the 1983 Cambridge Symposium attempted to develop a consistent set of definitions of morphological changes [2, 3]. Subsequently, several reports have been published which have correlated morphology, function, and clinical status of patients chronic pancreatitis [16–20].

Morphology and Function. We recently compared the Cambridge classification with clinical and functional information and showed that CT and clinical staging agreed in only 46% of patients. In the 54% where there was disagreement between CT and clinical staging, CT upstaged virtually all of these patients. Overall correlation of CT and clinical staging in patients with mild to moderate disease was only 29%, while in severe disease it was 100%.

The published reports [16–20] thus can be summarized by saying that in mild or early chronic pancreatitis, the most accurate diagnosis and assessment of the patient is achieved by the use of both function tests and imaging modalities, primarily CT and ERCP. The correlation was excellent in most cases, but there were a few patients with minimal morphological changes and marked functional abnormalities, and a few with marked morphologic changes and minimal functional alteration. Thus, although structure and function could not always be directly related, they showed the best correlation in patients with more advanced disease.

Pancreatic Duct Calcifications. An important recent observation concerns the relationship of pancreatic ductal calculi and exocrine function. In the past, duct calculi were believed to indicate advanced disease with severe exocrine dysfunction. In Lankisch's recent series, however, it was shown that 50% of patients with calculi had only mild to moderate exocrine dysfunction, while the other half had severe impairment [21]. In our experience, there is a definite trend toward increasing clinical severity of chronic pancreatitis and the presence of focal or diffuse calcifications: 89% of patients with severe chronic pancreatitis had calcifications. However, calcifications also were present in 55% of patients with only mild to moderate disease. Severe abdominal pain was present in 74% of patients with calcifications, but also was present in 44% of patients with no calcifications. Thus, calcification per se was a poor predictor of disease severity.

Morphology, Function, and Clinical Course. If all clinical stages of chronic pancreatitis are considered, the severity of the patient's clinical course (i.e., amount of pain, presence of diabetes mellitus, malabsorption, and complications, such as pseudocysts and vascular involvement) could not be predicted directly from the morphologic changes and vice versa. There was also no significant correlation between the degree of exocrine gland dysfunction and severity of clinical symptoms [18]. However, if only patients with advanced stages of chronic pancreatitis (defined as >75% reduction of enzyme and/or bicarbonate secretion in the SEC-C test), are considered, a significant correlation was found between the clinical and morphological severity of the disease in 80% of patients. However, patients with mild to moderate stages (<50%–75% reduction of enzymes and/or bicarbonate) showed poor correlation. Advanced morphologic changes (ERCP, CT) were found in 65% of these patients. The poor morphologic – clinical correlation raises the question of whether the morphologic grading of ERCP and CT is ill-defined, or whether the morphologic changes might precede the clinical course. Additional studies need to be performed to evaluate these questions.

Approach to Diagnosis and Staging of Chronic Pancreatitis

The clinical diagnosis of chronic pancreatitis is best confirmed with a combination of the imaging modalities of CT and ERCP. Although some investigators recommend US because of its lower cost, CT clearly is superior in the broad spectrum of information it provides and in the rarity of a technically unsatisfactory examination. In particular, CT is more useful for differentiating pancreatic cancer from chronic pancreatitis and for detecting the complications of chronic pancreatitis.

ERCP is more sensitive than CT in detecting chronic pancreatitis, particularly in the mild to moderate forms of the disease, and often provides valuable information if a surgical drainage procedure is contemplated (see Fig. 3). It also may be useful for differentiation of chronic pancreatitis and pancreatic carcinoma. The pancreatogram can be analyzed and brush cytology can be obtained from the pancreatic duct [22]. While MRCP does not allow for obtaining cytology, it can serve as an alternative procedure for defining ductal anatomy.

The role of pancreatic function tests remains controversial. While the tests are more widely used in Europe than in the United States, it seems clear from

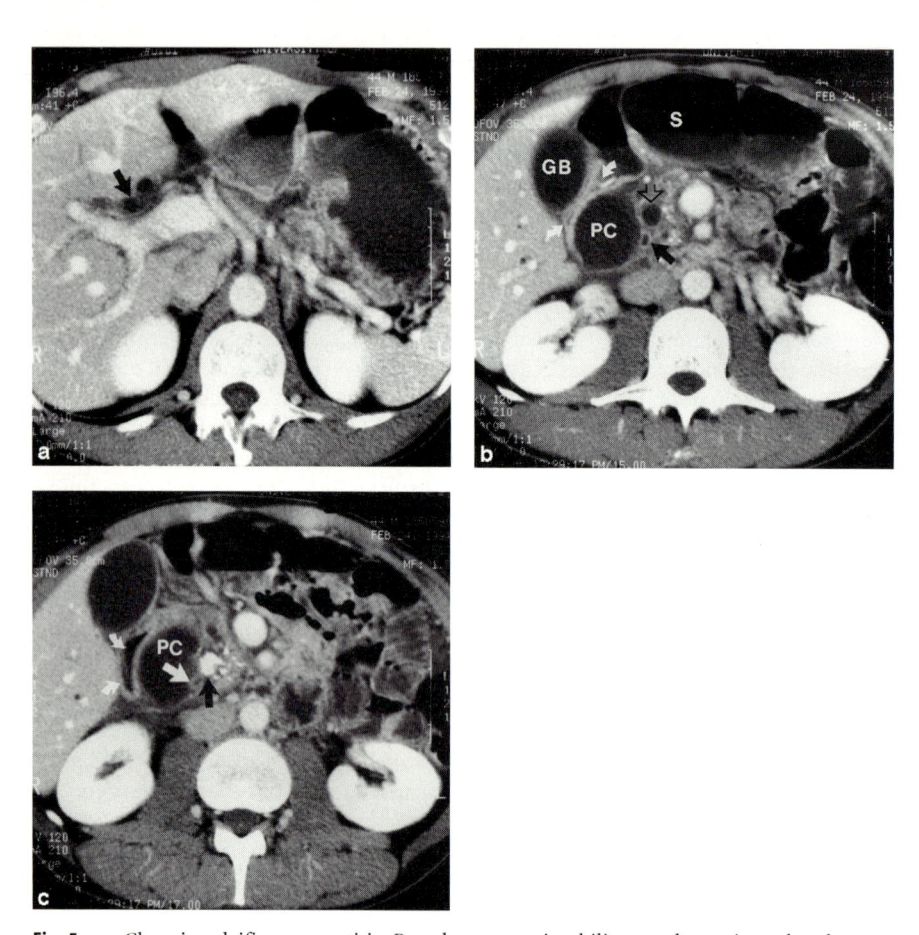

Fig. 5 a–c. Chronic calcific pancreatitis. Pseudocyst causing biliary and gastric outlet obstruction. **a** Contrast-enhanced computed tomography (CT) scan shows dilatation of the common hepatic duct (*arrow*). **b** Scan through the region of the pancreatic head shows a pseudocyst (*PC*) adjacent to the contiguous dilated main pancreatic duct (*open arrow*) and the common bile duct (*closed arrow*). The duodenum (*small white arrows*) is compressed by the PC, causing gastric outlet obstruction. Small calcifications are noted within the head of the gland. *GB*, gallbladder; *S*, dilated stomach. **c** Scan at a slightly lower level shows the PC compressing the duodenum (*small white arrows*) and adjacent common bile duct (*large white arrow*) and a large calculus obstructing the main pancreatic duct (*black arrow*)

the European data that function tests combined with imaging procedures provide the best diagnosis and the most accurate means of staging the severity of chronic pancreatitis. However, if diabetes and steatorrhea (malabsorption) are present, function tests are probably superfluous.

Complications of Chronic Pancreatitis

The primary complications of chronic pancreatitis are similar to those of acute pancreatitis: formation of fluid collections (including pseudocysts and abscesses), spread of the inflammatory reaction to involve the gastrointestinal tract, bile ducts, and vascular system, and pancreatic ascites (see Figs. 4, 5).

The association of chronic pancreatitis and pancreatic carcinoma continues to be debated [23, 24]. It is currently accepted that there is an increased incidence of pancreatic cancer, but it is very small. Gold estimated that in the US, only about 24 cases per year could be explained on the basis of chronic pancreatitis [23].

Treatment Alternatives

Patients with chronic pancreatitis can be treated with conservative medical therapy, surgery, or interventional endoscopic or radiologic techniques. Imaging procedures play a crucial role in selection of the appropriate therapeutic approach.

The primary indications for surgery are persistent pain and treatment of complications of chronic pancreatitis, such as biliary or duodenal obstruction or pseudocysts. Imaging studies are used to detect these complications and possible causes for pain, such as a pseudocyst or obstruction of the pancreatic or bile duct and to select the appropriate operation for treatment of a complication or for pain control, such as partial or total pancreatectomy versus a Puestow drainage procedure (longitudinal pancreatico-jejunostomy).

Some complications of chronic pancreatitis, such as fluid collections, biliary obstruction, pancreatic duct calculi and strictures, and acute arterial hemorrhage, can be treated with nonoperative endoscopic or radiologic techniques. These procedures include percutaneous or endoscopic drainage of fluid collections, endoscopic removal of pancreatic duct calculi, endoscopic or transhepatic dilatation of bile duct strictures and placement of stents for decompression, endoscopic pancreatic duct stricture dilatation or stent placement, sclerotherapy for control of variceal hemorrhage, and transcatheter embolotherapy for control of arterial hemorrhage or pseudoaneurysm formation [25–29]. Radiologic guidance and monitoring are crucial for safe and efficacious performance of most of these techniques.

References

1. Gyr K, Singer M, Sarles H (1984) Pancreatitis: Concepts and Classification. In: Gyr K, Sincer M, Sarles H, ed. Second International Symposium on the Classification of Pancreatitis. Amsterdam: Excerpta Medica, xxiii-xxvi
2. Sarner M, Cotton P (1984) Definitions of acute and chronic pancreatitis. Clin Gastroenterol 13: 865-870
3. Axon A, Classen M, Cotton P, et al (1984) Pancreatography in chronic pancreatitis: international definitions. Gut 25: 1107-1112
4. Itoh S, Yamakawa K, Shimamoto K, et al (1994) Groove pancreatitis. J Computr Assist Tomogr 18: 911-915
5. Becker V, Mischke U (1991) Groove pancreatitis. Internatl J Pancreatol 10: 173-182
6. Niederau C, Grendell J (1985) Diagnosis of chronic pancreatitis. Gastroenterology 88: 1973-1995
7. Freeny P, Lawson T (1982) Radiology of the Pancreas. New York: Springer-Verlag
8. Bolondi L (1989) Sonography of chronic pancreatitis. Radiologic Clinics of North Am 27: 815-833
9. Rosch T, Classen M (1992) Clinical relevance of endosonography in diagnosis of pancreatobiliary diseases. Z Gastroenterol 30: 878-884
10. Nattermann C, Goldschmidt A, Dancygier H (1993) Endosonography in chronic pancreatitis- a comparison between endoscopic retrograde pancreatography and endoscopic ultrasonography. Endoscopy 23: 565-570
11. Luetmer P, Stephens D, Ward E (1989) Chronic pancreatitis: reassessment with current CT. Radiology 171: 353-357
12. Axon A (1989) Endoscopic retrograde cholangiopancreatography in chronic pancreatitis (1989) The Cambridge classification. Radiologic Clinics of North Am 27: 39-50
13. Semelka R, Shoenut J, Kroeker M, et al (1993) Chronic pancreatitis: MR imaging features before and after administration of gadopentetate dimeglumine. J Mag Res Imag 3: 79-82
14. Takehara Y, Ichijo K, Tooyama N et al (1994) Breath-hold MR cholangiopancreatography with a long echo-train fast spin-echo sequence and a surface coil in chronic pancreatitis. Radiology 192: 19-21
15. Soto J, Barish M, Yucel E, et al (1995) Pancreatic duct: MR cholangiopancreatography with a three-dimensional fast spin-echo technique. Radiology 196: 459-464
16. Malfertheiner P (1986) Combined functional and morphological diagnostic approach in chronic pancreatitis. In: Malfertheiner P, Ditschuneit H, ed. Diagnostic Procedures in Pancreatic Disease. Berlin: Springer-Verlag, 262-267
17. Malfertheiner P, Büchler M, Stanescu A et al (1986) Correlation of morphological lesions, functional changes, and clinical stages in chronic pancreatitis. In: Malfertheiner P, Ditschuneit H, ed. Diagnostic Procedures in Pancreatic Disease. Berlin: Springer-Verlag, 268-273
18. Malfertheiner P, Büchler M (1989) Correlation of imaging and function in chronic pancreatitis. Radiologic Clinics of North Am 27: 51-64
19. Braganza J, Hunt L, Warwick F (1982) Relationship between pancreatic exocrine function and ductal morphology. Gastroenterology 82: 1341-1347
20. Girdwood A, Hatfield A, Bornman P, et al (1984) Structure and function in noncalcific pancreatitis. Dig Dis and Sci 29: 721-726
21. Lankisch P, Otto J, Erkelenz I, et al (1986) Pancreatic calcifications: no indicator of severe exocrine pancreatic insufficiency. Gastroenterology 90: 617-621
22. Steer M, Waxman I, Freedman S (1995) Chronic pancreatitis. New Engl J Med 332: 1482-1490
23. Gold E, Cameron J (1993) Chronic pancreatitis and pancreatic cancer. New Engl J Med 328: 1485-1486
24. Lowenfels A, Maisonneuve P, Calvallini G, et al (1993) Pancreatitis and the risk of pancreatic cancer. New Engl J Med 328: 1433-1437
25. Deviere J, Cremer M, Baize M, et al (1994) Management of common bile duct stricture caused by chronic pancreatitis with metal mesh self expandable stents. Gut 35: 122-126
26. Kozarek R, Ball T, Patterson D, et al (1991) Endoscopic transpapillary therapy for disrupted pancreatic duct and peripancreatic fluid collections. Gastroenterology 100: 1362-1370
27. Freeny P, Lewis G, Traverso L, et al (1988) Infected pancreatic fluid collections: percutaneous catheter drainage. Radiology 167: 435-441
28. Vujic I (1989) Vascular complications of pancreatitis. Radiologic Clinics of North Am 27: 81-91
29. vanSonnenberg E, Wittich G, Casola G, et al (1989) Percutaneous drainage of infected and noninfected pancreatic pseudocysts: experience in 101 cases. Radiology 170: 757-761

Role of Pancreatic Duct Drainage for Evaluation of Pancreatic Pain

M. Delhaye · M. Cremer

Introduction

Severe chronic pancreatitis (CP) is characterized by the formation of intraductal stones that may or may not be associated with stricture [1]. The resultant outflow obstruction can lead to pain via a mechanism of increased pancreatic ductal pressure [2] and to secondary obstructive CP if the duct obstruction remains for a long time. The consequences of parenchymal atrophy are steatorrhea and diabetes. Malnutrition is the result of decreased eating due to pain combined with exocrine and endocrine insufficiency.

The aims of management in severe CP are to relieve the pain which is present in about 80 % of patients with CP in Western countries and to prevent the development of glandular insufficiency.

Surgery has been the classic approach, with various drainage procedures being used for patients with a dilated pancreatic duct. However, surgical drainage procedures have a perioperative morbidity of 20 %–40 % and a mortality rate of about 2 %–5 % [3, 4]. Additionally, pancreaticojejunal anastomoses tend to become obstructed over time, and as a consequence the long-term success rate for these procedures is only 60 %–80 % [3–5]. Endoscopic pancreatic drainage is an appealing alternative associated with lesser morbidity and mortality and does not preclude future surgery, should that become necessary. Moreover, the success of temporarily lowering the pancreatic duct pressure by endoscopic drainage procedures might also be a predictor of the success of surgical drainage.

Diagnosis and staging of CP have now been dramatically improved by using magnetic resonance cholangiopancreatography (MRCP), a noninvasive technique not requiring endoscopy or injection of contrast medium. This imaging procedure is currently being evaluated [6, 7], and it can be predicted that in the near future endoscopic retrograde cholangiopancreatography (ERCP) will be used exclusively for therapeutic procedures.

Indications for endoscopic drainage of the pancreatic duct are the presence of outflow obstruction (ductal strictures, pancreatic stones) associated with chronic pain or recurrent attacks of pancreatitis.

The different procedures aimed at restoring pancreatic flow through the duodenum include endoscopic sphincterotomy [8], pancreatic stone disintegration [9], and pancreatic stenting [10]. Other endoscopic procedures such as bile duct drainage using stents or cyst and pseudocyst drainage are beyond the subject of this paper but can be performed to treat or to prevent the classical complications of CP.

Endoscopic Pancreatic Sphincterotomy

Indications

Endoscopic pancreatic sphincterotomy (EPS) is the first step to gain access to the main pancreatic duct (MPD); it is indicated for single or multiple stones in the MPD and may be the sole procedure when there is no stricture of the duct.

Methods

Endoscopic sphincterotomy is usually performed in two steps: first, biliary sphincterotomy, and then pancreatic sphincterotomy. Biliary sphincterotomy is mandatory to clear the opening of the MPD for better access and to avoid possible ascending cholangitis due to edema post-sphincterotomy, especially in patients with biliary stricture. After incision of the biliary sphincter, the pancreatic orifice is usually found at 5 o'clock on the sphincterotomy wall. An incision of 5–8 mm (pure cutting) of the pancreatic sphincter is then performed at the 12 o'clock position.

Stone extraction is attempted with a mini-Dormia basket (Medizin-Technische-Werkstätte, Wesel, Germany) or less efficiently with a Fogarty balloon catheter (Medizin-Technische-Werkstätte, Wesel, Germany, or Microvasive Wilson-Cook Medical Inc., Winston-Salem, NC, USA).

Results

The technical results of EPS were recorded in a series of 70 patients treated by EPS with or without extracorporeal shock wave lithotripsy (ESWL) for obstructive intraductal stones but without stenting of the MPD [8]. Partial or complete clearance of the MPD was obtained in 79 % of the cases (Table 1) and the availability of ESWL (since October 1987) is the best independent predictitve factor for the MPD clearance after EPS in a multivariate analysis.

Endoscopic drainage procedures are followed by immediate pain relief (complete or partial) in 95 % of the cases. A significant association was found between immediate disappearance of pain and complete or partial MPD clearance.

Long-term pain relief was associated with earlier treatment after onset of the disease, a low frequency of pain attacks before EPS and absence of MPD substenosis. Pain recurrences were often caused by migration of small fragments into the MPD and blockage at the level of substenosis. Such attacks of pain can be easily treated again by endoscopy.

No treatment-related deaths were observed. The overall complication rate was 13 %, including endoscopically controlled bleeding (three cases), clinical

Table 1. Results of pancreatic duct drainage procedures in chronic pancreatitis

Procedure	Total patients (n)	Technical success (%)	MPD clearance (%)	Pain relief Immediate	Pain relief Late	Essential conditions for pain relief	Morbidity rate (%)	Mortality rate (%) Early	Mortality rate (%) Late	Reference
EPS[a]	70	100	79	95	74	MPD stone clearance Early treatment Few pain attacks before EPS Absence of MPD substenosis	13	0	9	[8]
ESWL[b]	123	99	59	90	85	Decrease in MPD diameter	27	0	1.7	[9]
Pancreatic stenting[c]	76	99	n.d.	94	Permanent stenting: 75 Surgery: 15 Stent removed: 9	Decrease in MPD diameter	5	0	1.3	[10]

EPS, endoscopic pancreatic sphincterotomy; ESWL, extracorporeal shock wave lithotripsy; MPD, main pancreatic duct; n.d., not determined.
[a] Mean follow-up, 5 years.
[b] Mean follow-up, 14 months.
[c] Mean follow-up, 37 months.

post-ERCP acute pancreatitis (two cases), and sepsis controlled by antibiotics (four cases). Late mortality was recorded in five out of 58 patients (9%) from unrelated causes except one case of hypoglycemia.

Extracorporeal Shock Wave Lithotripsy

Indications

ESWL is indicated whenever calculi located in the MPD cannot be removed by endoscopic procedures and are responsible for upward ductal obstruction and dilatation.

Methods

ESWL is performed using the electromagnetic lithotriptor, the LITHOSTAR (Siemens, Erlangen, Germany) which delivers 100 shock waves (SW) per min with a power ranging from 0.08 to 0.54 mJ/mm^2. The pancreatic stones are located in the shock-wave focus by a bidimensional X-ray-focusing system. Sedation (midazolam 2-5 mg, pethidine 50-100 mg) is sufficient to reduce the pain. Most patients are treated in the prone position with slight left lateral decubitus to focus the stone clear of the spinal column. The first SW are targeted on the most distal stone located in the MPD and then on the other calculi from the head to the tail, allowing drainage of the fragments downwards through the papilla. EPS can be performed as the first step or more frequently after disintegration of the distal obstructive stone by SW, making deep cannulation of the MPD easier. Further endoscopic managements aimed at restoring pancreatic drainage through the duodenum: nasopancreatic catheter insertion followed by perfusion and flushing with saline, endoscopic extraction of stone fragments and pancreatic stenting if needed.

Results

Pancreatic stones can be disintegrated successfully and without major adverse effects in the majority of patients (99%) (Table 1).

Although complete clearance of the MPD is achieved in only 59% of patients, a decrease in MPD diameter is obtained in 90%, suggesting relief of ductal obstruction even if residual fragments remain in the duct. Failure of ductal drainage occurred in 10% in our series after successful ESWL mainly because of impassable ductal anatomy.

Spontaneous disappearance of the cysts and pseudocysts following endoscopic ductal decompression has been observed in 74% of the cases, mainly for small cavities (size, < 5 cm) and for distal cysts in the head of the pancreas.

Immediate pain relief was obtained for all patients with continuous pain. During a mean follow-up time of 14 months, complete or partial pain relief could be recorded for 85% of the patients. Recurrent pain resulted from stone migration, progressive stricture of the MPD or pancreatic stent obstruction or dislodgement. Each of these patients underwent another endoscopic treatment. In our series [9], pain relief was dependent on decrease in MPD diameter, while in Sauerbruch's series [11] it was dependent on MPD stone clearance, meaning that pain relief occurred in these patients after relief of ductal obstruction.

We observed no side effects after ESWL, but some minor complications were noted for about one third of the patients because of endoscopic procedures. These were easily controlled through medical treatment. No operative or hospital mortality was observed. Late mortality occurred in two patients (1.7%) 3 and 14 months after treatment of CP.

Pancreatic Stenting

Indications

Patients with persistent and significant stricture of the MPD in the head of the pancreas and a homogeneous upward dilatation of the MPD are considered good candidates for stenting.

Methods

Stent placement always follows EPS of the "dominant" duct (at the major or minor papilla) and clearance of MPD stones by ESWL and/or extraction. A guide wire is first passed across the stricture. Dilatation of the stricture is performed by bougienage (up to 11 F). Sometimes it is not possible to obtain such a dilatation on the first attempt. In these cases, a nasopancreatic catheter of 5, 6, or 7 F is left in place for 2 days allowing drainage of the MPD above the stricture. After this, it is usually easier to achieve dilatation up to 11 F and to place a 10-F pancreatic stent. The stent is threaded over a 6-F catheter (and a 0.035-in. guide wire) and introduced with a pusher tube.

Self-expanding metallic stents (Wallstent, Schneider, Switzerland) with open mesh or covered with silicone or polyurethane have been inserted in the MPD since 1989. These stents are actually easier to introduce in the MPD than the 10-F plastic stents. The Wallstent is constrained by an invaginated membrane over an introducing catheter which has an outer diameter of 9 F. The stent is deployed by progressive withdrawal of the membrane. The stent expands to a diameter of 6 mm and to a length of 23 mm.

Results

In a series of 76 patients presenting a MPD stricture with upstream ductal dilatation and persistent pain, a 10-F plastic stent could be inserted in the MPD with a high success rate (98.6%) [10].

Immediate decrease in pain or complete pain relief was noted in 71 of 75 (94%) patients successfully treated (see Table 1). A relationship between duct size reduction and pain disappearance was observed after stenting.

After a mean follow-up of 37 months ranging from 18 to 72 months, 11 patients underwent pancreaticojejunostomy after confirmation of pain resolution due to MPD decompression, seven patients had disappearance of the stricture after 13 (2–30) months of stenting, 22 patients received an 18-F self-expanding Wallstent after plastic stenting failed to have a significant effect on the ductal stenosis and 34 patients still had a stent in place which had to be changed systematically once a year – more frequently if pain recurred or MPD dilatation on abdominal ultrasonography occurred.

Pancreatic stent dysfunction, including clogging and migration of the stent, appears to be a major long-term problem in 15%–30% of patients.

Moreover a true calibration of the stricture and maintenance of the patient free of symptoms after removal of plastic stent succeeded in only 9% of the patients. This is why self-expanding metallic stents have been used in the pancreatic duct with excellent immediate results, but once again, the long-term patency of these stents has been disappointing because of inflammatory ingrowth through the meshes of the stent, because of spontaneous migration of covered stents, or because of resorption of the coating material in a few cases leading to relapsing stricture inside the stent. New developments in this area of pancreatic stents are awaited for the near future in order to provide a definitive "pancreaticoduodenostomy" for strictures located in the head of the pancreas.

Immediate and early complications related to EPS included three cases of cholangitis and one case of hemobilia following endoscopically controlled bleeding during EPS. The complications encountered during follow-up involved eight cases of sepsis due to stent clogging and three migrations of the stent into the MPD.

One patient died 1 year after implantation of a stent in the dorsal pancreatic duct from cholangitis associated with liver abscesses.

Conclusions

The indications for the endoscopic management of CP are specific and are based on complete imaging and functional assessment.

The endoscopic procedures are complex and difficult and require high-definition fluoroscopy, multiple sophisticated accessories and a skilled radio-endoscopic team.

The results are excellent for immediate pain relief and are comparable to those of surgical series after mid- to long-term follow-up.

Our results on pain relief support the etiologic role of ductal hypertension: multivariate analysis showed that the MPD clearance was the best independent predictive factor for disappearance of pain. Moreover, pain relief was significantly associated with the decrease in the MPD caliber. Pain relapses in CP seem to result most often from recurrent pancreatic duct obstruction usually caused by migration of stone fragments from the secondary ducts to the MPD.

These situations, leading to a subsequent increase in intraductal pressure, can again be managed endoscopically in some cases.

The complication rate is very low and can be medically controlled. The mortality rate is zero, which is definitely better than in a selection of surgical series in which resection was not performed.

To summarize, endoscopic management of CP associated with ESWL of intraductal calculi is generally safe, often effective for years, does not hinder further surgery, and can be repeated.

These advantages, along with the observation that the best results are obtained if endoscopic treatment is performed early, lead us to propose endoscopic management early in the course of calcifying CP. Finally, assessment of the clinical effect of ductal decompression is important before considering any further surgical treatment and could avoid inappropriate surgery. Moreover, endoscopic treatment represents the last possibility to treat the patients with relapsing pain after surgery, while any operation remains possible after failure of endoscopic management.

References

1. Ammann RW, Akovbiantz A, Largiader F, Schueler G (1984) Course and outcome of chronic pancreatitis. Longitudinal study of a mixed medical-surgical series of 245 patients. Gastroenterology 86: 820–828
2. Okazaki K, Yamamoto Y, Kagiyama S, Tamura S, Sakamoto Y, Nakazawa Y, Morita M, Yamamoto Y (1988) Pressure of papillary sphincter zone and pancreatic main duct in patients with chronic pancreatitis in the early stage. Scand J Gastroenterol 23: 501–507
3. Warshaw AL, Popp Jr JW, Schapiro RH (1980) Long-term patency, pancreatic function, and pain relief after lateral pancreaticojejunostomy for chronic pancreatitis. Gastroenterology 79: 289–293
4. Bradley EL III (1987) Long-term results of pancreaticojejunostomy in patients with chronic pancreatitis. Am J Surg 153: 207–213
5. Adams DB, Ford MC, Anderson MC (1994) Outcome after lateral pancreaticojejunostomy for chronic pancreatitis. Ann Surg 5: 481–489
6. Takehara Y, Ichijo K, Tooyama N, Kodaira N, Yamamoto H, Tatami M, Saito M, Watahiki H, Takahashi M (1994) Breath-hold MR cholangiopancreatography with a long-echo-train fast spin-echo sequence and a surface coil in chronic pancreatitis. Radiology 192: 73–78
7. Reinhold C, Bret PM, Guibaud L, Barkun ANG, Genin G, Atri M (1996) MR cholangiopancreatography: Potential clinical applications. Radiographics 16: 309–320
8. Dumonceau JM, Devière J, Le Moine O, Delhaye M, Vandermeeren A, Baize M, Van Gansbeke D, Cremer M (1996) Endoscopic pancreatic drainage in chronic pancreatitis associated with ductal stones: long-term results. Gastrointest Endosc 43: 547–555
9. Delhaye M, Vandermeeren A, Baize M, Cremer M (1992) Extracorporeal shock-wave lithotripsy of pancreatic calculi. Gastroenterology 102: 610–620
10. Cremer M, Devière J, Delhaye M, Baize M, Vandermeeren A (1991) Stenting in severe chronic pancreatitis: results of medium-term follow-up in seventy-six patients. Endoscopy 23: 171–176
11. Sauerbruch T, Holl J, Sackmann M, Paumgartner G (1992) Extracorporeal lithotripsy of pancreatic stones in patients with chronic pancreatitis and pain: a prospective follow-up study. Gut 33: 969–972

What Does the Surgeon Need in the Preoperative Evaluation of Chronic Pancreatitis?

H. Lippert · H.-U. Schulz

Introduction

Chronic pancreatitis is primarily not a surgical disease. In most cases this illness can be managed medically. Operative treatment remains a major challenge. The aims of surgical treatment are to relieve pain, treat complications and preserve pancreatic function. There is no operative procedure which is curative, and even following technically successful surgery symptoms such as pain may persist. Thus, the major issues are selection of the patient for operation, selection of the surgeon, the timing of operation, and the choice of the appropriate surgical procedure [1]. In general, resection of pancreatic parenchyma, drainage of the main pancreatic duct, or a combination of both methods can be performed. All the procedures have their individual indications and therefore cannot be evaluated in terms of relative merit.

The etiology of chronic pancreatitis is alcoholism in the vast majority of instances. However, it is essential to identify the occasional patient with an unusual cause who will gain most benefit from surgery [1]. So, for instance, pancreatic or periampullary cancer may give rise to chronic pancreatitis, especially in middleaged women who deny a history of alcoholism. Congenital anomalies of the duodenum (diverticula), bile duct (cysts) and pancreatic duct (Pancreas divisum) also may result in chronic pancreatitis.

The aims of surgical treatment are:
1. To treat complications of the disease
2. To relieve intractable pain
3. To eliminate causative conditions

Independent of the indication for operation, a fourth aim is to preserve functioning pancreatic parenchyma. The information the surgeon needs preoperatively depends mainly on the indication for operation. Following a brief introduction to the imaging procedures available, the surgeon's needs and wishes in the preoperative evaluation of a patient suffering from chronic pancreatitis will be outlined.

Imaging Procedures

Imaging procedures contribute to diagnosis, to differential diagnosis and to detection of complications of chronic pancreatitis. A broad spectrum of methods is available.

Plain Films

About 30% of patients with chronic pancreatitis display pancreatic calcifications which can ce visualized by abdominal X-ray. Duodenal stenosis is easily detected by contrast roentgenography of the stomach and duodenum.

Ultrasonography

By means of US, the size and shape of the pancreas and the diameter of the main pancreatic duct can be estimated. In addition, US can detect calcifications and give information on the presence, size and thickness of the wall of pseudocysts. US's sensitivity to diagnose chronic pancreatitis is 60–70%, its specificity 80–90% [2–4]. US can be used to guide percutaneous drainage of pseudocysts. Endoscopic US (EUS) is a novel method which allows imaging of the pancreas through the duodenal or gastric wall. EUS allows precise estimation of the thickness of the wall of a pseudocyst, yields information about vessels within the wall of a pseudocyst, and helps to differentiate inflammatory from neoplastic tumors of the pancreas.

Computed Tomography

CT scanning yields the same information about the pancreas as US, in general. CT is more sensitive than US, however. It can detect pseudocysts and calculi which have been missed by US. CT's sensitivity for chronic pancreatitis is 75–90%, its specificity about 85% [2–4]. Pancreatic size, shape, density and homogeneity can be estimated correctly. In addition, information on the main pancreatic duct, calculi, and neighboring vessels and organs can be obtained by contrast-enhanced CT. By means of CT, acute pancreatitis can be clearly differentiated from chronic pancreatic disease. The differentiation between chronic pancreatitis and pancreatic cancer can be difficult, however.

Endoscopic Retrograde Cholangiopancreatography

ERCP is the gold standard for the diagnosis of chronic pancreatitis. This method does not only visualize the main pancreatic duct but also its side branches. Ductal anatomy and pathology (strictures, dilatations, calculi) can be evaluated precisely. This information may prove invaluable for the selection of a patient for operation. In addition, ERCP provides information about the biliary tree (stones, tumor, distal stenosis of the choledochal duct). ERCP contributes most to the differential diagnosis between chronic pancreatitis and pancreatic cancer. Its sensitivity in this respect can be enhanced by aspiration of pancreatic juice or brush biopsy of ductal epithelium for cytologic or molecular biological analysis. For planning of the surgical strategy, ERCP is the most important imaging procedure of the pancreas nowadays.

Magnetic Resonance Cholangiopancreatography

MRCP is, like EUS, a novel procedure which is available only scarcely as yet. In general, it provides all the information obtained by ERCP. The major advantage of MRCP is its non-invasiveness. This method requires neither endoscopy nor administration of contrast medium and does not expose the patient to radiation. A minor disadvantage of MRCP is its tendency to over-estimate ductal stenosis [5].

Esophago-gastro-duodenoscopy

EGD allows evaluation of the hollow organs neighboring the pancreas. Indirect signs of pseudocysts or of pancreatic neoplasia may become visible. EGD detects causes (duodenal diverticula, pancreas divisum), complications (duodenal stenosis), and concomitant disease (gastric or duodenal ulcer, esophageal varices due to liver cirrhosis) of chronic pancreatitis. For this reason, EGD is a major procedure for the differential diagnosis of pain. EGD offers the opportunity to take biopsy samples for differentiation of inflammatory from malignant disease. Every patient with chronic pancreatitis needs to undergo endoscopy prior to operation, therefore.

Duplex Sonography

Duplex sonography (duplex) allows non-invasive evaluation of the vessels surrounding the pancreas, namely the portal and splenic vein, the superior mesenteric artery and vein, and the branches of the celiac artery. Portal or splenic vein thrombosis complicating chronic pancreatitis can be detected, as well as an involvement of vessel structures in the walls of pseudocysts localized in the head of the pancreas. Under circumstances of bleeding into a pseudocyst, duplex can identify the bleeding artery.

Angiography

Angiography is equivalent to duplex but is invasive and requires administration of contrast medium and exposure of the patient to radiation. It is performed when duplex is not available or does not yield the information required. In cases of bleeding into pseudocysts, angiography can be superior to duplex since hemostasis can quickly be achieved by embolization of the bleeding artery.

Preoperative Evaluation

Complications of Chronic Pancreatitis

The most frequent complications of chronic pancreatitis, exocrine insufficiency and diabetes mellitus, are not indications for surgery. In contrast, local complications such as pseudocysts, bleeding or thrombosis, obstruction of neighboring organs (e.g., duodenum, choledochal duct or splanchnic vessels), fistulas, ascites and suspected malignancy often lead the patient to the surgeon.

Pseudocysts
Pseudocysts develop in up to 10 % of patients suffering from chronic pancreatitis [2]. They are not always an indication for surgery. Surgical measures may be advisable in the following situations:

1. Bleeding into, rupture or infection of a pseudocyst
2. Displacement or compression of duodenum, choledochal duct, or vessels
3. Pseudocyst as the sole cause of pain
4. Suspected malignancy in a cystic tumor of the pancreas

The surgical procedures that can be employed include:

- Drainage of a pseudocyst into the stomach or jejunum
- Suture of a bleeding vessel
- Resection of the pseudocyst-bearing part of the pancreas

For planning the operative stragegy, the surgeon needs to obtain (→) the following information:

- What are the symptoms?
  → medical history
- Which treatment has been performed?
  → medical history
- In the case of bleeding, which artery is responsible?
  → duplex or angiography
- What is the site and size of the pseudocyst?
  → US or CT or ERCP or MRCP
- When drainage is planned, how thick is the wall of the pseudocyst?
  → US or EUS or CT

- When resection is planned, will sufficient parenchyma remain?
  → US or CT
- When malignancy is suspected: How large is the tumor? Are vessels involved? Is there suspicion of extrapancreatic tumor manifestation?
  → CT and ERCP (duplex or angiography only, when CT does not give sufficient information about the relevant blood vessels)

Bleeding/Thrombosis

Bleeding is often an indication for urgent or even emergency surgery. Bleeding occurs mainly into pseudocysts, and its treatment has already been described above. Thrombosis of the portal or splenic vein occurs rarely. In general, it is due to compression of the vessels by pseudocysts or inflammatory enlargement of the head of the pancreas. Portal hypertension and (as an exception) spontaneous rupture of the spleen may result.

The surgical procedures that can be employed include:

- Suture of a bleeding vessel
- Resection of the pseudocyst-bearing part of the pancreas
- Revascularization (thrombectomy or bypass)
- Splenectomy
- Shunting

For planning the operative strategy, the surgeon needs answers to the following questions.

- What are the symptoms of the patient and how long have they been present?
  → medical history
- What is the cause of the thrombosis?
  → CT
- What is the extent of the thrombosis?
  → CT (duplex or angiography)
- Is the spleen enlarged or ruptured?
  → CT or US

Obstruction of neighboring organs

Pseudocysts or inflammatory enlargement of the pancreatic head can cause obstruction of the duodenum, choledochal duct or splanchnic vessels.

The surgical procedures that can be employed include:

- Drainage of the pseudocyst
- Duodenum-preserving resection of the pancreatic head

In cases of suspected malignancy, the pylorus-preserving partial pancreatoduodenectomy is the method of choice. In cases of proven malignancy, Whipple's procedure is indicated under circumstances of resectability. Biliodigestive anastomosis without resection for chronic pancreatitis should be performed only exceptionally, because of its high risk of recurrent cholangitis and secondary biliary cirrhosis.

For planning the operative strategy, the surgeon needs the following information:

- What are the symptoms?
  → medical history
- What is the cause of the obstruction?
  → CT and ERCP
- What is the extent of the obstruction?
  → ERCP or MRCP, EGD or contrast roentgenography of the duodenum, duplex or angiography

Fistulas/Ascites

Fistulas and ascites develop following ductal ruptures.

The surgical procedures that can be employed include:

- Selective closure of the ruptured duct
- Distal pancreatic resection
- Drainage of the ruptured duct into the stomach or jejunum

For planning the operative strategy, the following information is required.

- Where is the duct ruptured?
  → ERCP or MRCP plus CT

Intractable Pain

Intractable pain can be an indication for surgery in patients:

- In whom no complication of chronic pancreatitis as the cause of pain and no extrapancreatic cause of pain could be identified
- Who have not responded to medical therapy
- Who are at risk of drug abuse or addiction

The surgical procedures that can be employed include:

- Distal pancreatic resection or total pancreatectomy
- Drainage of the main pancreatic duct by longitudinal pancreaticojejunostomy
- Combinations of parenchymal resection with ductal drainage

For planning the operative stragegy, the surgeon needs to know:

- What is the diameter of the pancreatic duct?
  → ERCP or MRCP or CT or US

Elimination of Causative Conditions

Surgically correctable causes of chronic pancreatitis include pancreas divisum, choledochal cysts, duodenal diverticula and hyperparathyroidism. The surgical procedure to be performed depends on the individual situation and cause. The surgeon needs to know the causative factor so that he can employ the appropriate procedure (i.e., resection of choledochal cysts and duodenal diverticula, hyperparathyroidectomy, drainage of the accessory pancreatic duct).

Chronic Pancreatitis: General Remarks

In every patient referred to surgery for chronic pancreatitis the surgeon needs to know the following:

1. What are the symptoms?
2. Which kind of treatment has been performed, with what result?
3. Has the entire spectrum of conservative approaches been exhausted?
4. Has the patient been operated on previously for chronic pancreatitis?
5. Has the patient already had other abdominal operations?
6. Is there concomitant disease that could influence the surgeon's decision?

Conclusion

Surgical treatment of chronic pancreatitis is never the therapy of first choice. Chronic pancreatitis becomes surgically relevant mainly when symptomatic and surgically correctable complications develop. Each patient must be treated carefully on an individual basis, and the reasons for choosing a particular procedure must be well delineated. The surgeon must always understand his limitations. He must recognize that even after a technically successful operation the symptoms of the patient may persist [1, 6, 7]. The principal information the surgeon needs in the preoperative evaluation of a patient with chronic pancreatitis can be obtained from careful history-taking, CT and ERCP. Other imaging procedures such as EGD, US, duplex and angiography are employed depending on the patient's individual situation. EUS and MRCP are promising novel procedures possessing considerable diagnostic potential.

References

1. Moossa AR (1987) Surgical treatment of chronic pancreatitis: an overview. Br J Surg 74: 661–667
2. Steer ML, Waxman I, Freedman S (1995) Chronic pancreatitis. N Engl J Med 332: 1482–1490
3. DiMagno EP, Layer P, Clain JE (1993) Chronic pancreatitis. In: Go VLW, DiMagno EP, Gardner JD, Lebenthal E, Reber HA, Scheele GA (eds) The pancreas: biology, pathobiology, and disease, 2nd Edn Raven Press, New York, pp 665–706
4. Niederau C, Grendell JH (1985) Diagnosis of chronic pancreatitis. Gastroenterology 88: 1973–1995

5. Reinhold C, Bret PM (1996) MR cholangiopancreatography. Abdom Imaging 21: 105–116
6. Reber PU, Friess H, Büchler MW (1996) Operative Therapie der chronischen Pankreatitis: Technik und Langzeitergebnisse. Chir Gastroenterol 12: 214–220
7. Rossi RL, Heiss FW, Braasch JW (1985) Surgical management of chronic pancreatitis. Surg Clin N Am 65: 79–101

III
Function Tests

Neuroendocrine Abnormalities of Upper Gut Function in Chronic Pancreatitis: Lessons for Physiology and Pathophysiology

D. K. Nelson

Introduction

The pancreas plays a central role in the integrated digestive processes of the upper gastrointestinal tract. It might, therefore, be expected that exocrine pancreatic insufficiency, such as occurs in chronic pancreatitis, would be reflected in abnormalities of extrapancreatic function or other (non-exocrine) aspects of intrapancreatic function. Over the past decade, we and others have begun to examine parameters of upper gut function which might be altered with the progressive changes in exocrine function accompanying chronic pancreatitis. The goals of this chapter are: (a) to provide an overview of these studies, (b) to discuss continuing areas of controversy, and (c) to attempt to draw lessons from these studies which might illuminate the integrated physiology and pathophysiology of the upper gut.

Cholecystokinin in Exocrine Pancreatic Insufficiency: Up, Down, All Around?

Nearly 70 years ago, Ivy and Oldberg [40] isolated a factor from the duodenal mucosa which induced gallbladder contraction. This was followed by the description of Harper and Raper [33] of pancreozymin, a duodenal substance which induced pancreatic secretion. Subsequent purification and sequencing clarified that these dual stimulatory functions are accomplished through a single peptide [12, 43, 57], which we now know by the historical atencedent as cholecystokinin (CCK). A physiologic role for CCK as a primary mediator of the postprandial response in humans has recently been confirmed through the application of CCK receptor antagonists [1, 3, 4, 37, 53]. However, the effect of the pathophysiologic condition of chronic pancreatitis on CCK release is not as clearly defined. While it appears to have passed into common knowledge that CCK levels are elevated in patients with chronic pancreatitis [30, 32, 73, 75], which in turn has been used to support the existence of CCK-mediated enteropancreatic feedback regulation in humans, a careful review of the literature suggests otherwise (Table 1). Earlier studies did, indeed, report increased plasma CCK concentrations in pancreatic insufficiency [34–36, 73], but there is a striking discordance in findings between and within groups. For example, Funakoshi and colleagues [26, 27] reported decreased plasma CCK response fol-

Table 1. Cholecystokinin (CCK) release in pancreatic insufficiency

Direction of change	Reference	Authors	Year	Comments
Increased	34-36	Harvey et al.	1973	
			1976	
			1977	
	73	Slaff et al.	1985	Fasting only
	70	Schafmayer et al.	1985	↑ Basal and peak, normal AUC
	27	Funakoshi et al.	1986	Mild CP
	44	Koide et al.	1989	Mild CP: ↑ basal, ↑ AUC
Decreased	24	Elderle et al.	1977	
	11	Byrnes et al.	1980	↓ Basal and postprandial
	71	Schafmayer et al.	1983	Normal basel, ↓ postprandial
	26	Funakoshi et al.	1985	Severe CP
	44	Koide et al.	1989	Severe CP: normal basal, ↓ AUC
	52	Masclee et al.	1989	Normalized with enzymes
	61	Nustede et al.	1991	Normalized with enzymes
	29	Glasbrenner et al.	1994	Progressive reduction with severity of CP
Unchanged	2	Allen et al.	1983	Cystic fibrosis
	42	Jansen et al.	1984	Alcoholic CP and cystic fibrosis, multiple region-specific assays
	13	Cantor et al.	1986	Advanced CP
	58	Nealon et al.	1986	No correlation with severity of CP, no control group
	7	Bozkurt et al.	1988	
	55	Mössner et al.	1989	Bioassay

CP, chronic pancreatitis.
AUC, area under the response curve

lowing ingestion of a liquid test meal in patients with chronic pancreatitis in 1985, but also reported high basal and postprandial CCK responses in another group of patients 1 year later in the same journal. In 1989, Koide et al. [44] showed that basal and integrated (area under the curve) CCK levels were increased in mild chronic pancreatitis, but in the same paper found no change in basal concentrations coupled with decreased integrated response in patients with severe chronic pancreatitis. Schafmayer et al. [70] reported increased basal and peak CCK levels (although no change was found in area under the curve, perhaps a better index of the global response), but the same group later found significant reduction of CCK release in patients with chronic pancreatitis [61]. Enzyme substitution therapy tended to raise postprandial CCK concentrations (i.e, the opposite of what might be predicted if exocrine insufficiency invariably elevates CCK), but never to the levels observed in healthy volunteers. This finding of a decreased CCK response in pancreatic insufficiency which was partially normalized toward healthy control levels confirmed a similar report by Masclee et al. [52], who used intraduodenal fat to stimulate CCK release. The authors from Göttingen [61] were forthright in addressing the discrepancy with their earlier report, noting several possible explanations for divergent observations. Among these must be considered differences in methods for CCK determination, in study design or in patient groups. CCK has proved to be a notoriously difficult molecule to assay, owing to cross-reactivity with other substances such as gastrin and a substantial molecular heterogeneity among forms of CCK [12].

Accordingly, the validity of assays used to measure CCK in earlier studies has been questioned [69]. Moreover, some investigators have used bioassays while others employed radioimmunoassays, and study designs have also differed with regard to stimuli used to induce CCK release. Finally, chronic pancreatitis is a progressive disease which, combined with the lack of any broadly accepted criteria for staging, results in heterogeneity among study populations. We [29] recently examined postprandial release of CCK and found that, while integrated response tended to be lower in a subgroup of chronic pancreatitis patients without steatorrhea as compared to healthy controls, statistical significance was not achieved until a subgroup of patients with severe exocrine insufficiency and steatorrhea was considered. In fact, close examination of several studies reporting normal postprandial responses reveals that CCK release tended to be reduced in these as well, but the reduction failed to reach statistical significance [7, 13, 42]. Whatever the explanation for discrepancies among studies, the majority of recent investigations suggest that *CCK release is either decreased or not altered in patients with exocrine pancreatic insufficiency* (Table 1). Recognition of the problems discussed above has resulted in methodologic improvements which would tend to favor conclusions drawn from later studies. However, the lack of consistency in findings should cause any reader or author to exercise some degree of caution in deriving declarative conclusions.

Lessons for Physiology

The studies reviewed above lead naturally to a discussion of negative feedback regulation of exocrine pancreatic secretion. If we accept the existence of such a mechanism, and there are those who do not [50], several questions arise: Is feedback regulation protease specific? Is it species specific? What is the role of CCK? It has been consistently shown in rat models that diversion of juice from the duodenum or inhibition of proteolytic activity is accompanied by an increase in the volume of pancreatic juice secreted [31, 48, 49, 62]. Conversely, intraluminal protease activity suppresses endogenous pancreatic secretory output. In rats, this feedback regulation is mediated via CCK [25, 48, 49]; the same manipulations which stimulate pancreatic enzyme secretion induce a concomitant rise in plasma CCK, and those which inhibit pancreatic secretion also suppress CCK release. Two peptides have been identified (CCK-releasing factor and monitor peptide, secreted by the duodenal mucosa and pancreas, respectively) which stimulate CCK release but are hydrolyzed by proteolytic enzymes, providing a mechanism for protease-dependent feedback in rats [41, 49]. In other animals, however, this mechanism has been more difficult to demonstrate unequivocally. In dogs this effect may be mediated via secretin or neurotensin, rather than CCK [15, 19]. Ihse et al. [39] first proposed the existence of negative feedback in man after studying a patient with a tumor of the papilla of Vater in whom pancreaticobiliary secretion was completely obstructed. Pancreatic secretion collected via percutaneous drainage of the common bile duct was shown to decrease when active enzymes (either mixed pancreaticobiliary juice or trypsin) were infused into the duodenum. This concept was subsequently supported by other human studies which showed stimulation of pancreatic secretion after duodenal perfusion with selective protease inhibitors and inhibition of secretion by perfusion of trypsin [1, 65, 72, 73]. Others, however, could not replicate these findings, concluding that negative feedback mechanisms were not operative in humans [22, 38, 45] or that, if present, CCK was not a major mediator [1]. At the least, the supraphysiologic quantities of intraluminal proteases required to elicit moderate inhibition of pancreatic enzyme output raises the question of relevance under physiologic conditions [19, 20, 47].

Lessons for Pathophysiology

Bearing in the mind the inconsistencies cited above, the feedback hypothesis provides a putative basis for understanding the pathophysiology of chronic pancreatitis, whereby the enteropancreatic response to intraluminal stimuli is altered. Following this line of reasoning, chronic pancreatitis involves a cascade of events in which low levels of intraluminal proteolytic enzymes in patients with exocrine insufficiency are inadequate to appropriately deactivate CCK-releasing factor, leading to hypersecretion of CCK and chronic stimulation of the exocrine pancreas. This in turn would result in ductal hypertension and consequently pain, particularly if accompanied by morphologic changes of chronic pancreatitis including ductal obstruction. As noted, however, the evidence documenting hypercholecystokinemia as a consistent feature of chronic pancreatitis is far from unequivocal (Table 1). Nevertheless, this hypothetical sequence of events has provided a basis for treatment of painful chronic pancreatitis with exogenous enzymes [20, 47, 72, 73, 75]. Once again, the clinical data in support of this approach are less than complete and therapeutic efficacy is variable [56, 72, 74]. As recently reviewed by DiMagno and colleagues [18-20], alternate explanations exist for mechanisms of pain relief and the underlying link to feedback regulation. It remains to be clearly demonstrated that CCK-mediated feedback mechanisms are operative under physiologic conditions in man, are altered under pathophysiologic conditions, or that a reduction in pancreatic enzyme output leads to pain relief.

Gallbladder Function in Pancreatic Insufficiency

The preceding discussion focused on the role of CCK in mediating pancreatic function and its potential involvement in related pathophysiologic processes. The role of CCK in mediating the intestinal phase of gallbladder contraction is, if anything, even more primary [4, 37, 53]. It follows that investigators, in their search for clarification on the role of CCK in pancreatic insufficiency, would also seek to determine if abnormal CCK release was reflected by abnormal gallbladder response. Masclee et al. [52] determined that the integrated plasma CCK response to intraduodenal fat was significantly impaired in patients with pancreatic insufficiency. This impaired CCK response was significantly enhanced by concomitant administration of pancreatic enzymes, so that values

Fig. 1. Gallbladder emptying in response to duodenal fat in patients with pancreatic insufficiency before (*open squares*) and after addition of pancreatic enzymes (*closed squares*), as compared to healthy controls (*open circles*). Gallbladder emptying was impaired in patients with pancreatic insufficiency, as was cholecystokinin (CCK) release, but both parameters were normalized by exogenous enzymes. (Reproduced with permission from [52])

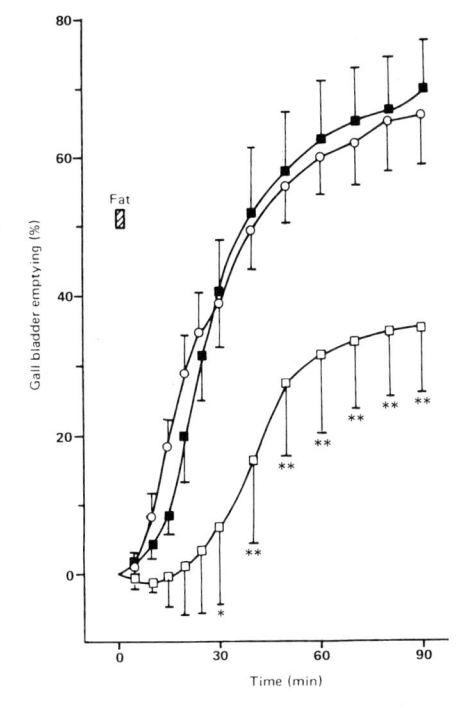

were no longer significantly different from healthy controls. Gallbladder emptying curves followed an identical pattern; gallbladder contraction was significantly impaired in patients with exocrine insufficiency before the addition of enzymes, but gallbladder emptying curves were superimposable with healthy controls after the addition of enzymes (Fig. 1). Masclee et al. [52] could demonstrate no effect on CCK secretion or gallbladder emptying in two patients administered pancreatic extracts in which enzyme activity was deactivated by boiling, suggesting enzyme-specific effects. Conversely, administration of pancreatic enzymes in the absence of intraduodenal fat had no effect on CCK release in two healthy subjects. Thus, patients with severe pancreatic insufficiency were shown to have impaired gallbladder emptying after duodenal fat, and this defect could be normalized by the addition of exogenous pancreatic enzymes. The authors attributed this impairment to a reduced plasma CCK response. In an earlier report [8], gallbladder contraction in response to exogenous CCK (intravenous cerulein) was also found to be impaired in patients with chronic pancreatitis, suggesting a decreased sensitivity of the gallbladder to CCK. While Masclee et al. [52] interpreted this finding as contradictory to their own, namely that impaired gallbladder emptying is a result of reduced endogenous CCK secretion, I see less conflict between these two sets of findings. It would not appear to be mutually exclusive that the putative impairment of gallbladder response in pancreatic insufficiency could be due to decreased sensitivity to CCK, or decreased CCK release, or a combination thereof. In a more recent study examining a similar question, Glasbrenner et al. [28] also found a significant reduction in postprandial CCK response in 14 patients with chronic pancreatitis. Although they found an increased fasting gallbladder volume in patients as compared to controls, there were no differences between these groups in gallbladder contraction curves following either ceruletide infusion or oral testmeal. These authors speculated that the alteration of gallbladder emptying detected by Masclee et al. [52] may have been compensated by multiple redundant regulatory systems, which were activated in their study by oral administration of food. While not entirely contradictory, these two later studies differed in terms of disease severity, stimuli used, and methods for quantitating gallbladder response (cholescintigraphy vs. ultrasonography).

Lessons for Physiology and Pathophysiology

Any lessons to be drawn would be much the same as those discussed in the preceding section, and hinge on consistent demonstration of abnormal CCK release in patients with exocrine pancreatic insufficiency. Many of the same pitfalls in interpretation (differences in methods, heterogeneous patient collectives) apply here as well, and definitive conclusions must await confirmation of the very few studies that have addressed this question. Clearly, the central role of CCK in the normal postprandial response of both pancreas and gallbladder provides a sound hypothetical basis for concurrent abnormalities in both systems.

Interdigestive Cycling in Chronic Pancreatitis

During the interdigestive state, pancreatic exocrine secretion cycles in synchrony with motor activity of the upper gut and with plasma concentrations of pancreatic polypeptide and motilin, which may serve as hormonal regulators. Approximately once every 90–120 min in humans, motor and secretory activity cycle progressively through periods of motor quiescence and minimal secretion (phase I), intermittent motor activity with moderate secretory output (phase II), and a short interval of regular propagating motor activity and maximal secretion (phase III). This periodic coupling between motor and secretory activity was described at the turn of the century by Boldyreff [6], working in the laboratory of Pavlov, and then rediscovered in 1979 by DiMagno et al. [21] and Vantrappen et al. [77]. Despite this longstanding recognition, mechanisms that regulate the link between motor activity and secretion remain poorly understood, and human studies are notably lacking. A physiological role for pancreatic secretion in modulating interdigestive motor activity was proposed by Owyang et al. [63, 64], who found that duodenal perfusion with pancreatobiliary juice increased plasma concentrations of motilin and pancreatic polypeptide. The same group observed impaired release of motilin in patients with exocrine pancreatic insufficiency. Based on these findings, they hypothesized that phasic pancreatobiliary secretion may play an important modulatory role during the interdigestive period and that patients with chronic pancreatitis may, therefore, present with associated abnormalities of motility. However, it was shown in dogs that pancreatectomy (i.e., removal of exocrine and endocrine pancreatic influences) did not alter the cyclic patterns of interdigestive gastrointestinal motility [51]. In order to test these hypotheses in humans, we examined temporal cycling of motility, pancreatic secretion, and hormones during the interdigestive period, using patients with chronic pancreatitis as a model of impaired pancreatic function [66]. Moreover, these multiple components acting in synchrony have been proposed to serve as an "intestinal housekeeper," preparing the upper gut for the next meal while sweeping it free of luminal debris and preventing bacterial overgrowth [17, 21, 78]. In this context, examination of cyclic phenomena during the fasting state, in which the gut spends a large portion of the day, might also shed light on the pathophysiology of chronic pancreatitis.

Results

We found [66] that interdigestive enzyme output was severely impaired in patients with chronic pancreatitis ($>80\%$ decrease), as expected. Nevertheless, secretory cycling was still evident in most patients upon close examination. All parameters describing interdigestive motility were similar in controls and patients with chronic pancreatitis, including duration of total cycle and individual phase, amplitude, frequency, propagation velocity, and motility index (Table 2). However, the time between cyclic peaks of enzyme secretion and pancreatic polypeptide was shortened in patients with chronic pancreatitis, and peaks were no longer temporally related to the migrating motor complex; only 56% of phase III activity fronts were associated with a concomitant secretory peak in patients as compared with 92% in healthy subjects. Thus, the link between motility cycle and secretory cycles was interrupted in patients with pancreatic insufficiency (Fig. 2). In a separate group of patients stratified by disease severity, we observed [67] a progressive diminution of both interdigestive and postprandial pancreatic polypeptide release with increasing severity of disease (Fig. 3). In particular, interdigestive release parameters were tightly correlated with exocrine function, so that the percent increase in pancreatic polypeptide concentrations during phase III over those in phase I was progressively decreased from controls (112%) to mild-moderate pancreatitis (62%) to severe pancreatitis (19%).

Lessons for Physiology

To the extent that patients with chronic pancreatitis may serve as a model of impaired pancreatic function, it seems unlikely that pancreatic secretion exerts a major influence over interdigestive events. Specifically, motor activity continues to cycle normally in patients with chronic pancreatitis, despite marked reductions in secretion from the exocrine and endocrine pancreas. As described

Table 2. Interdigestive cycling in chronic pancreatitis

Parameter	Controls	Chronic pancreatitis
Phase I motor activity		
Duration (min)	49 ± 10	41 ± 4
Phase II motor activity		
Duration (min)	69 ± 13	71 ± 20
Mean antral amplitude (mmHg)	74 ± 12	72 ± 8
Antral contractions (per 15 min)	10 ± 2	9 ± 1
Antral motility index	9.1 ± 2	8.9 ± 2
Duodenal contractions (per 15 min)	32 ± 3	27 ± 4
Phase III motor activity		
Duration (min)	6 ± 1	5 ± 1
Propagation velocity (cm/min)	10.3 ± 1.0	9.5 ± 1.5
Frequency (per h)	0.5 ± 0.4	0.6 ± 0.1
Total duration of motility cycle (min)	114 ± 15	107 ± 19
Peak trypsin (kU/h)	22.3 ± 8.4	2.3 ± 0.6*
Peak chymotrypsin (kU/h)	14.2 ± 4.8	1.6 ± 0.5*
Peak amylase (kU/h)	41.4 ± 7.2	7.7 ± 2.5*
Secretory cycle (min)	101 ± 4	76 ± 4*
Peak PP (ng ml^{-1} h^{-1})	11.6 ± 2.5	4.9 ± 1.2*
Hormonal cycle (min)	106 ± 7	63 ± 4*

Adapted from [66], with permission.
*$p < 0.05$.

in detail elsewhere [51, 60, 66], our findings in several animal and human models refute the concept that pancreatic mechanisms exert a major regulatory influence on interdigestive motor activity. A more likely explanation, as recently discussed by Layer [46], is that physiologic phenomena during the fasting state are driven and coupled by common regulatory pathways. Prominent among these integrating neurohormonal mechanisms is cholinergic innervation, which we have shown exerts its influence via M1-muscarinic receptors [60].

Lessons for Pathophysiology

Interdigestive cyclic events have not been thoroughly studied in chronic pancreatitis. Previous studies have not been consistent in detecting abnormalities in fasting plasma concentrations of pancreatic polypeptide in patients with chronic pancreatitis. However, it must be noted that "fasting" values in these studies were derived from a small number of basal samples obtained as a prelude to subsequent stimulation [9, 66]. No previous study had adequately examined the status of interdigestive secretory, motor, and hormonal events in chronic pancreatitis, nor was it known if the temporal coordination of these cyclic phenomena is maintained. As might have been predicted, interdigestive enzyme output is severely impaired in patients with exocrine insufficiency, yet secretory cycling persists [66]. In our study, cycles of pancreatic enzymes and pancreatic polypeptide were detectable in all but two patients with severe chronic pancreatitis and steatorrhea, although motor activity continued to cycle normally in the same two patients. In a separate group of patients stratified

Fig. 2. Individual examples of interdigestive trypsin output and pancreatic polypeptide (*PP*) release in a single healthy control subject (*top*) and a single patient with chronic pancreatitis (*bottom*). Arrows indicate the onset of duodenal phase III motor activity. Note the difference in the scale of *vertical axes*, which were expanded in the chronic pancreatitis example to allow visualization of cycling, which continues despite reduced secretion. The tight link between motor and secretory activity in health is broken in chronic pancreatitis. (Fig. adapted from [66], by permission)

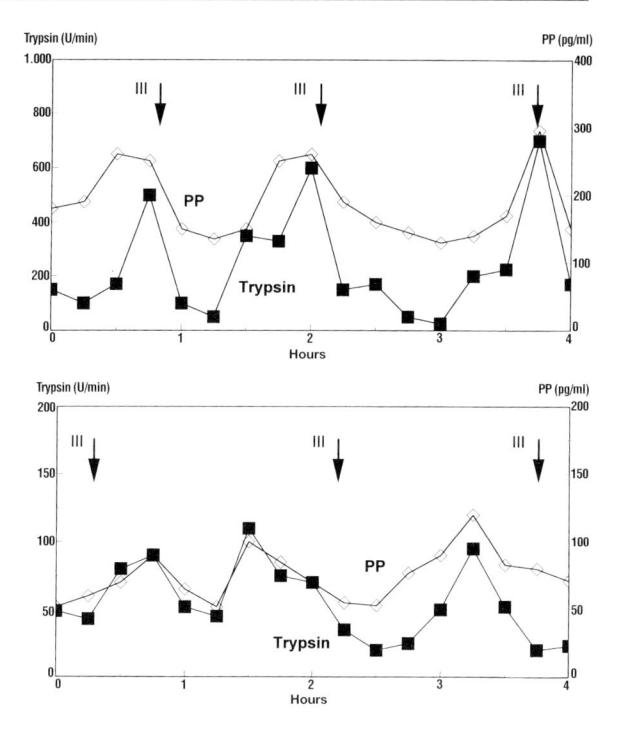

by severity of disease, we observed that changes in interdigestive release of pancreatic polypeptide are closely correlated to the stage of pancreatitis. The observation that these interdigestive abnormalities appeared in the early stages of disease, before postprandial impairment was evident, led us to hypothesize that impaired release of pancreatic polypeptide during phase III motor activity may represent an early hormonal disorder in chronic pancreatitis [67]. Interestingly, Dominguez-Muñoz et al. [23], discussed elsewhere in this volume, could find no alteration of interdigestive secretory output (enzymes or pancreatic polypeptide) in patients during the early phase of acute pancreatitis. Data describing motor activity in acute pancreatitis were, unfortunately, not reported, but this observation calls into question the therapeutic notion [23, 32] of "putting the gland at rest." While the clinical significance of our findings in patients with chronic pancreatitis [66, 67] remains to be determined, it is tempting to speculate that altered coordination among secretory and motor cycles may reduce the effectiveness of the "intestinal housekeeper" and/or other protective mechanisms [46]. According to this concept, secretions from the stomach, duodenum, and pancreas act in concert by digesting or inactivating substances before phase III motor activity sweeps luminal contents aborally [17, 21, 78]. Might the disrupted coordination between motor and secretory components contribute to bacterial overgrowth? If the normally tight coordination among upper gut phenomena serves to prevent duodenopancreatic reflux or pancreatic ductal hypertension, might the loss of this coordination promote

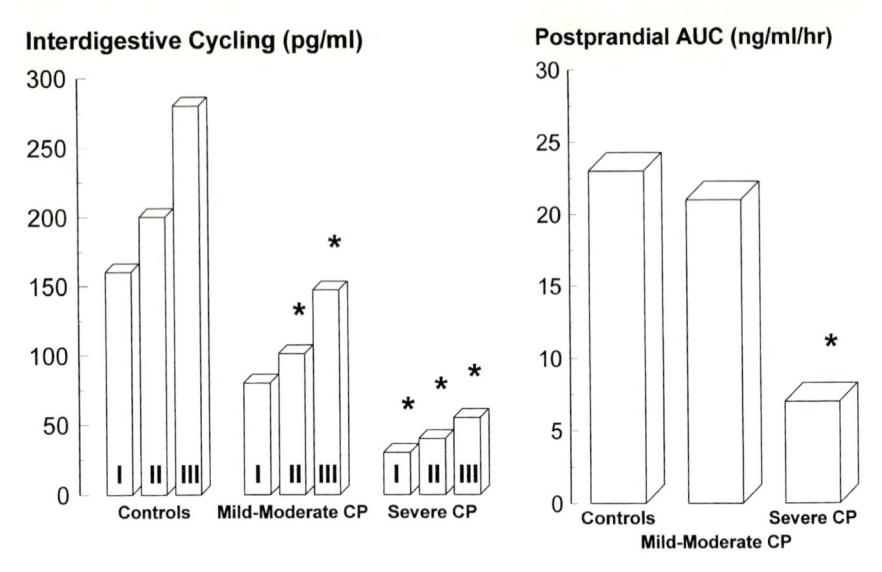

Fig. 3. Mean pancreatic polypeptide (PP) concentrations during phases of the interdigestive motor complex (*left*) in healthy controls and patients with mild-moderate and severe chronic pancreatitis (*CP*). Integrated postprandial release of PP is also shown for the same patients (*right*) (Fig. adapted from [67], by permission)

further pancreatic damage in patients with chronic pancreatitis? The clinical relevance of these findings must remain speculative for the time being, but these questions may provide theoretical underpinnings for future investigations.

Processing of Intrapancreatic Proenkephalin: A Link to Pain in Chronic Pancreatitis?

The endogenous opoids, including met-enkephalin (ENK), are involved as neurotransmitters throughout the central and peripheral nervous systems. In the pancreas, immunocytochemical studies have localized enkephalinergic nerve fibers which innervate acinar and islet cells, where ENK may serve to modulate exocrine and endocrine secretion via neural inhibition [14–16]. In a landmark paper of the last decade, Bockman et al. [5] demonstrated that the perineural elements of the pancreas are damaged in chronic pancreatitis, ultimately leading to alteration of the neural microenvironment. This has led to the hypothesis that alterations of neurotransmitter substances are involved in the pathophysiology of chronic pancreatitis [10]. Given the role(s) of ENK in mediating nociception, inflammation, and pancreatic function [14–16, 54, 68, 76], it was of interest to examine the status of ENK-containing elements in chronic pancreatitis [59]. Specifically, we investigated posttranslational processing of the proenkephalin A precursor, during which multiple encrypted copies of ENK are enzymatically cleaved from this large prohormone [54, 76, 79].

Methods

Tissue samples were obtained from the pancreatic head of 20 patients with alcohol-induced chronic pancreatitis who had been operated with the duodenum-preserving pancreatic head resection. Identical tissues were obtained from nine organ donors with no gastrointestinal disease. Tissues were extracted in boiling HCl, and concentrations of ENK in acid extracts (denoted as FREE-ENK) were determined by specific radioimmunoassay [79]. Additional aliquots of supernatant were assayed after treatment [76, 79] with trypsin and carboxypeptidase B to enzymatically expose ENK which remained encrypted within the precursor molecule (denoted as TOTAL-ENK). The ratio of TOTAL-ENK to FREE-ENK within each tissue sample provided an index of the degree of processing which had occurred.

Results

We found [59] that intrapancreatic concentrations of FREE-ENK were increased in chronic pancreatitis as compared to controls (2.9 ± 0.4 vs. 0.8 ± 0.3 ng/g; $p < 0.01$). Conversely, concentrations of TOTAL-ENK were significantly decreased (104.4 ± 8.0 vs. 159.8 ± 4.9 ng/g; $p < 0.001$). These changes resulted in a sixfold decrease in ratio of TOTAL-ENK:FREE-ENK in chronic pancreatitis. When these same data were viewed in relation to pain score, we observed that concentrations of FREE-ENK increased steadily with pain (assuming that organ donor controls were pain free, at least with regard to pain of pancreatic origin). TOTAL-ENK decreased as pain became more severe, resulting in an inverse relationship between the processing index and pain that was highly significant ($p < 0.0001$ ENK ratio vs. pain score). There was no correlation, however, between exocrine function (as tested by the pancreolauryl serum test [29]) and pain score, or between exocrine function and enkephalin processing parameters. Immunostaining against extended ENK fragments revealed primary localization in intrapancreatic ganglia and associated nerve fibers.

Lessons for Physiology

Our data suggest that there is normally a large reserve of unprocessed proenkephalin in the healthy pancreas. On the background of what is already known about posttranslational processing of endogenous opioids, we would speculate that proteolytic cleavage by trypsin and carboxypeptidase B-like enzymes can generate biologically active enkephalin to subserve a variety of neural mechanisms [54, 68, 76].

Lessons for Pathophysiology

It has previously been shown that processing of proenkephalin A precursor is altered in some disease states [79]. Our findings suggest that post-translational processing of intrapancreatic proenkephalin is enhanced in chronic pancreatitis [59]. In other words, there is a shift from TOTAL to FREE leaving encrypted enkephalin to release by subsequent enzymatic cleavage. Possible explanations include irregular activity of intrapancreatic enzymes in chronic pancreatitis, or changes in processing linked to perineural damage [5, 10]. We further speculate that aberrant processing in the endogenous opioid system may underlie, or respond to, the persistent pain associated with chronic pancreatitis.

Acknowledgements. The author thanks Susan Sullivan, The Genesee Hospital, Rochester, New York, for preparation of the manuscript, and the many colleagues who collaborated in the studies described herein.

References

1. Adler G, Reinshagen M, Koop I, Göke B, Schafmayer A, Rovati LC, Arnold R (1989) Differential effects of atropine and a cholecystokinin receptor antagonist on pancreatic secretion. Gastroenterology 96: 1158–1164
2. Allen JM, Penketh ARL, Adrian TE, Lee YC, Sarson DL, Hodson ME, Batten JC, Bloom SR (1983) Adult cystic fibrosis: postprandial response of gut regulatory peptides. Gastroenterology 85: 1379–1383
3. Beglinger C, Fried M, Whitehouse I, Jansen JB, Lamers CB, Gyr K (1985) Pancreatic enzyme response to a liquid meal and to hormonal stimulation: correlation with plasma secretin and cholecystokinin levels. J Clin Invest 75: 1471–1476
4. Beglinger C, Hildebrand P, Adler G, Werth B, Luo H, Delco F, Gyr K (1992) Postprandial control of gallbladder contraction and exocrine pancreatic secretion in man. Eur J Clin Invest 22: 827–834
5. Bockman DE, Büchler M, Malfertheiner P, Beger HG (1988) Analysis of nerves in chronic pancreatitis. Gastroenterology 94: 1459–1469
6. Boldyreff W (1911) Einige neue Seiten der Tätigkeit des Pankreas. Ergeb Physiol 11: 121–217
7. Bozkurt T, Adler G, Koop I, Koop H, Turmer W, Arnold R (1988) Plasma CCK levels in patients with pancreatic insufficiency. Dig Dis Sci 33: 276–281
8. Bradshaw MJ, Mauad EC, Richardson RB, et al (1983) Impaired gallbladder response to intravenous caerulein in patients with chronic pancreatitis. Digestion 28: 15–16
9. Brugge WR, Burke CA, Brand DL, Chey WY (1985) Increased interdigestive pancreatic trypsin secretion in alcoholic disease. Dig Dis Sci 30: 431–439
10. Büchler M, Weihe E, Friess H, Malfertheiner P, Bockman DE, Müller S, Nohr D, Beger HG (1992) Changes in peptidergic innervation in chronic pancreatitis. Pancreas 7: 183–192
11. Byrnes DJ, Borody T, Henderson L (1980) Plasma cholecystokinin. Regul Peptides Suppl 1: S15
12. Cantor P (1989) Cholecystokinin in plasma. Digestion 42: 181–201
13. Cantor P, Petronijevic L, Worning H (1986) Plasma cholecystokinin concentrations in patients with advanced chronic pancreatitis. Pancreas 1: 488–493
14. Cetin Y (1990) Immunohistochemistry of opioid peptides in the guinea pig endocrine pancreas. Cell Tissue Res 259: 313–319
15. Chey WY (1993) Hormonal control of pancreatic exocrine secretion. In: Go VLW et al (eds) The Pancreas: Biology, Pathobiology, and Diseases, 2nd edn. Raven, New York, pp 403–424
16. Chey WY, Coy DH, Konturek SJ, Schally AV, Trasler J (1980) Enkephalin inhibits the release and action of secretin on pancreatic secretion in the dog. J Physiol 298: 429–436
17. Code CF, Marlett JA (1975) The interdigestive myo-electrical complex of the stomach and small bowel of dogs. J Physiol 246: 289–309

18. DiMagno EP (1993) A short, eclectic history of exocrine pancreatic insufficiency and chronic pancreatitis. Gastroenterology 104: 1255-1262
19. DiMagno EP, Layer P (1993) Human exocrine pancreatic enzyme secretion. In: Go VLW et al (eds) The Pancreas: Biology, Pathobiology, and Diseases, 2nd edn. Raven, New York, pp 275-300
20. DiMagno EP, Clain JE, Layer P (1993) Chronic pancreatitis. In: Go VLW et al (eds) The Pancreas: Biology, Pathobiology, and Disease, 2nd edn. Raven, New York, pp 665-706
21. DiMagno EP, Hendricks JC, Go VLW, Dozois RR (1979) Relationships among canine fasting pancreatic and biliary secretions, pancreatic duct pressure and duodenal phase III motor activity-Boldyreff revisited. Dig Dis Sci 24: 689-693
22. Dlugosz J, Fölsch UR, Creutzfeldt W (1983) Inhibition of intraduodenal trypsin does not stimulate exocrine pancreatic secretion in man. Digestion 26: 197-204
23. Dominguez-Muñoz JE, Pieramico O, Büchler M, Malfertheiner P (1995) Exocrine pancreatic function in the early phase of human acute pancreatitis. Scand J Gastroenterol 30: 186-191
24. Elderle A, Vantini J, Harvey RF, et al (1977) Fasting serum cholecystokinin levels in chronic relapsing pancreatitis. Ir J Med Sci 146: 30
25. Fölsch UR, Cantor P, Wilms HM, Schafmayer A, Becker HD, Creutzfeldt W (1987) Role of cholecystokinin in the negative feedback control of pancreatic enzyme secretion in conscious rats. Gastroenterology 92: 449-458
26. Funakoshi A, Nakano I, Shinozaki H, Ibayashi H, Tateishi K, Hamaoka T (1985) Low plasma cholecystokinin response after ingestion of a test meal in patients with chronic pancreatitis. Amer J Gastroenterol 80: 937-940
27. Funakoshi A, Nakano I, Shinozaki H, Tateishi K, Hamaoka T, Ibayaski H (1986) High plasma cholecystokinin levels in patients with chronic pancreatitis having abdominal pain. Am J Gastroenterol 81: 1174-1178
28. Glasbrenner B, Malfertheiner P, Pieramico O, Klatt S, Riepl R, Friess H, Ditschuneit H (1993) Gallbladder dynamics in chronic pancreatitis: relationship to exocrine pancreatic function, CCK, and PP release. Digestive Diseases and Sciences 38: 482-489
29. Glasbrenner B, Dominguez-Muñoz JE, Nelson DK, Riepl RL, Büchler M, Malfertheiner P (1994) Relationship between postprandial release of CCK and PP in health and in chronic pancreatitis. Regulatory Peptides 50: 45-52
30. Go VLW (1990) Gastrointestinal hormones in chronic pancreatitis. In: Beger HG et al (eds) Chronic pancreatitis. Springer-Verlag, Berlin Heidelberg New York, pp 163-170
31. Green GM, Lyman RL (1972) Feedback regulation of pancreatic enzyme secretion as a mechanism for trypsin inhibitor-induced hypersecretion in rats. Proc Soc Exp Biol Med 140: 6-12
32. Greenberger NJ, Toskes PP, Isselbacher KJ (1994) Acute and chronic pancreatitis. In. Isselbacher KJ et al (eds) Harrison's principles of internal medicine. 13th edn. McGraw-Hill, New York, pp 1520-1532
33. Harper AA, Raper HS (1943) Pancreozymin: a stimulant of the secretion of pancreatic enzymes in extracts of the small intestine. J Physiol 102: 115-125
34. Harvey RF, Dowsett L, Hartog M, Read AE (1973) A radioimmunoassay for cholecystokinin-pancreozymin. Lancet ii: 826-828
35. Harvey RF, Rey JF, Howard JM, Read AE, Elderle A, Vantini I, Groarke JF, Fitzgerald JF (1977) Bioassay and radioimmunoassay of serum cholecystokinin in patients with pancreatic disease. Rend Gastroenterol 9: 15-16
36. Harvey RF, Rey JF, Howard JM, Read AE, Groarke JF, Fitzgerald O, Elderle A, Vantini I (1976) Serum cholecystokinin in pancreatic disease. Gut 17: 827
37. Hildebrand P, Beglinger C, Gyr K, Jansen JBMJ, Rovati LC, Zuercher M, Lamers CBHW, Setnikar I, Stalder GA (1990) Effects of a cholecystokinin receptor antagonist on intestinal phase of pancreatic and biliary responses in man. J Clin Inves 85: 640-646
38. Hotz J, Ho SB, Go VLW, DiMagno EP (1983) Short-term inhibition of duodenal tryptic activity does not affect human pancreatic, biliary or gastric function. J Lab Clin Med 101: 488-495
39. Ihse I, Lilja P, Lunquist I (1977) Feedback regulation of pancreatic enzyme secretion by intestinal trypsin in man. Digestion 15: 303-308
40. Ivy AC, Oldberg E (1928) A hormone mechanism of gallbladder contraction and evacuation. Am J Physiol 86: 599-613
41. Iwai K, Fukuoka Sl, Fushiki T, Tsujikawa M, Hirose M, Tsunasawa S, Sakiyama F (1987) Purification and sequencing of a typsin-sensitive cholecystokinin-releasing peptide from rat pancreatic juice. J. Biol Chem 262: 8956-8959

42. Jansen JBMJ, Hopman WPM, Lamers CBHW (1984) Plasma cholecystokinin concentrations in patients with pancreatic insufficiency measured by sequence-specific radioimmunoassays. Dig Dis Sci 29: 1109–1117
43. Jorpes E, Mutt VE (1966) Cholecystokinin and pancreozymin one single hormone? Acta Physiol Scand 66: 196–202
44. Koide M, Okabayashi Y, Hasegawa H, Fujisawa T, Okutani T, Kido Y, Otsuki M (1989) Plasma cholecystokinin bioactivity in patients with chronic pancreatitis. Pancreas 4: 624
45. Krawisz BR, Miller LJ, DiMagno EP, Go VLW (1980) In the absence of nutrient pancreatic-biliary secretions in the jejunum do not exert feedback control of human pancreatic or gastric function. J Lab Clin Med 95: 13–18
46. Layer PH (1995) Motor cycles and other cycles in chronic pancreatitis. Gastroenterology 109: 316–319
47. Layer PH, Holtmann G (1994) Pancreatic enzymes in chronic pancreatitis. International Journal of Pancreatology 15: 1–11
48. Louie DS, May D, Miller P, Owyang C (1986) Cholecystokinin mediates feedback regulation of pancreatic enzyme secretion in rats. Am J Physiol 250: G262–259
49. Lu L, Louie D, Owyang C (1989) A cholecystokinin releasing peptide mediates feedback regulation of pancreatic secretion. Am J Physiol 256: G430–G435
50. Magee DF (1991) Is there a duodenum-pancreas negative feedback? Int J Pancreatol 8: 367–377
51. Malfertheiner P, Sarr MG, DiMagno EP (1989) Role of pancreas in the control of interdigestive gastrointestinal motility. Gastroenterology 96: 200–205
52. Masclee AAM, Jansen JBMJ, Corstens FHM, Lamers CBHW (1989) Reversible gallbladder dysfunction in severe pancreatic insufficiency. Gut 30: 866–872
53. Meyer BM, Werth BA, Beglinger C, Hildebrand P, Jansen JBMJ, Zach D, Rovati LC, Stalder GA (1989) Role of cholecystokinin in regulation of gastrointestinal motor functions. The Lancet ii: 12–15
54. Morgan IG, Chubb IW (1991) How peptidergic neurons cope with variation in physiological stimulation. Neurochemical Research 16: 705–714
55. Mössner J, Back T, Regner U, Fischbach W (1989) Plasma-Cholezystokininspiegel bei chronischer Pankreatitis. Z Gastroenterol 27: 401–405
56. Mössner J, Secknus R, Meyer J, Niederau C, Adler G (1992) Treatment of pain with pancreatic extracts in chronic pancreatitis: results of a prospective placebo-controlled multicenter trial. Digestion 53: 54–66
57. Mutt V, Jorpes JE (1971) Hormonal polypeptides of the upper intestine. Biochem J 125: 57–58
58. Nealon WH, Beauchamp RD, Townsend CM jr, Boyd G, Shabot M, Thompson JC (1986) Diagnostic role of gastrointestinal hormones in patients with chronic pancreatitis. Ann Surg 204: 430–436
59. Nelson DK, Gress TM, Lucas DL, Muller-Pillasch F, DiSebastiano P, Friess H, Adler G, Buchler M and Malfertheiner P (1993) Gene expression and post-translational processing of intrapancreatic proenkephalin: a link to pain in chronic pancreatitis? Gastroenterol 104: A558
60. Nelson DK, Pieramico O, Dahmen G, Dominguez-Muñoz, Malfertheiner P, Adler G (1996) M1-muscarinic mechanisms regulate interdigestive cycling of motor and secretory activity in human upper gut. Dig Dis Sci 41: 2006–2015
61. Nustede R, Köhler H, Fölsch U, Schafmayer A (1991) Plasma concentrations of neurotensin and CCK in patients with chronic pancreatitis with and without enzyme substitution. Pancreas 6: 260–265
62. Owyang C (1994) Neurohormonal control of the exocrine pancreas. Current Opinion in Gastroenterology 10: 491–495
63. Owyang C, Achem-Karam SR, Vinik AI (1983) Pancreatic polypeptide and intestinal migrating motor complex in humans. Effect of pancreaticobiliary secretion. Gastroenterology 84: 10–17
64. Owyang C, Funakoshi A, Vinik AI (1983) Evidence for modulation of motilin secretion by pancreatico-biliary juice in health and in chronic pancreatitis. J Clin Endocrinol Metab 57: 1015–1020
65. Owyang C, Louie D, Tatum D (1986) Feedback regulation of pancreatic enzyme secretion: suppression of cholecystokinin release by trypsin. J Clin Invest 77: 2042–2047
66. Pieramico O, Dominguez-Muñoz JE, Nelson DK, Böck, W, Büchler M, Malfertheiner P (1995) Interdigestive cycling in chronic pancreatitis: altered coordination among pancreatic secretion, motility, and hormones. Gastroenterology 109: 224–230

67. Pieramico O, Nelson DK, Glasbrenner B, Malfertheiner P (1994) Impaired interdigestive pancreatic polypeptide release: early hormonal disorder in chronic pancreatitis? Dig Dis Sci 39: 69–74
68. Przewlocki R, Hassan AHS, Lason W, Epplen C, Herz A, Stein C (1992) Gene expression and localization of opioid peptides in immune cells of inflamed tissue: functional role in antinociception. Neuroscience 48: 491–500
69. Rehfeld JF (1984) How to measure cholecystokinin in plasma? Gastroenterology 87: 434–438
70. Schafmayer A, Becker HD, Werner M, Fölsch UR, Creutzfeld W (1985) Plasma cholecystokinin levels in patients with chronic pancreatitis. Digestion 32: 136–139
71. Schafmayer A, Werner M, Becker HD (1983) Radioimmunological determination of CKK in normal subjects and patients with chronic pancreatitis. Gastroenterology 84: 1299
72. Slaff J, Jacobson D, Tillmann CR, Curington C, Toskes PP (1984) Protease-specific suppression of pancreatic exocrine secretion. Gastroeneterology 87: 44–52
73. Slaff JI, Wolfe MM, Toskes PP (1985) Elevated fasting cholecystokinin levels in pancreatic exocrine impairment: evidence to support feedback regulation. J Lab Clin Med 105: 282–285
74. Steer ML, Waxman I, Freedman S (1995) Chronic pancreatitis. NEJM 332: 1482–1490
75. Toskes PP, Frey CF, Halsted CH, Steer ML (1995) The use of pancreatic enzymes in postpancreatectomy. Proceedings of a roundtable on diagnosis and management of chronic pancreatitis. December 3, 1994. Available from Scienta Healthcare Education, Durham, NC
76. Udenfriend S, Kilpatrick DL (1984) Proenkephalin and the products of its processing: chemistry and biology. In: Gross E, Meienhofer J (eds), Vol 1. The Peptides. Academic, New York, pp 25–68
77. Vantrappen GR, Peeters TL, Janssens J (1979) The secretory component of the interdigestive migrating motor complex in man. Scand J Gastroenterol 14: 663–667
78. Vantrappen G, Janssens J, Hellemans J, Ghoos Y (1977) The interdigestive motor complex of normal subjects and patients with bacterial overgrowth of the small intestine. J Clin Invest 59: 1158–1166
79. Yaksh TL, Carmichael SW, Stoddard SL, Tyce GM, Kelly PJ, Lucas D, VanHeerden JA, Ahlskog JE, Byer DE (1990) Measurement of lumbar CSF levels of met-enkephalin, encrypted met-enkephalin, and neuropeptide Y in normal patients and in patients with parkinson's disease before and after autologous transplantation of adrenal medulla into the caudate nucleus. J Lab Clin Med 115: 346–351

Direct Pancreatic Function Tests in the Diagnosis and Staging of Chronic Pancreatitis

L. Gullo

Ten years ago at the Symposium on Diagnostic Procedures in Pancreatic Diseases [1], I spoke in detail about direct pancreatic function tests and illustrated their diagnostic superiority over other methods. I then concluded by expressing the hope that a simple, noninvasive, and highly sensitive pancreatic function test would be developed in the near future, so that we could abandon duodenal intubation. Unfortunately, this has not occurred, and the direct tests are still the best means of evaluating pancreatic function. Because they are invasive and time-consuming, but also because several sophisticated imaging techniques have become available, they are performed infrequently. Nonetheless, these tests remain, without a doubt, the best means of defining the diagnosis and stage of chronic pancreatitis.

Direct tests of pancreatic function are based on duodenal intubation and the study of bicarbonate and enzyme secretion after pancreatic stimulation [2]. Stimulation may be direct, by administration of exogenous hormones, or indirect, by ingesting a standardized meal. Of the two means, direct stimulation is by far the most widespread; this is performed using secretin alone or, more commonly, secretin in combination with cholecystokinin or cerulein. As far as the doses are concerned, it is generally agreed that they should be maximal or near maximal. The hormones may be administered as a rapid IV injection or as a continuous IV infusion. In the first case, the maximum concentration of bicarbonate and enzymes is taken as an index of pancreatic function. In the case of continuous infusion, the pancreatic outputs during the last 30 min of stimulation are taken as an index of pancreatic function.

About 20 years ago, we proposed a method based on continuous IV infusion of secretin and cerulein [3]. In order to augment the sensitivity of the test, we used a combination of maximal doses of secretin and cerulein and prolonged stimulation by 90 min. In previous studies, continuous stimulation had been carried out for 45 or 60 min, and generally secretin alone had been used. We reasoned that if we stimulate the pancreas both maximally and for a long period of time, we would probably have a greater chance of assessing the whole mass of secretory cells and thus obtaining a more accurate measure of the reserve capacity of the gland. This should lead to better separation of normal from pathological functions and detection of milder degrees of pancreatic insufficiency. Indeed, we showed that in patients with chronic pancreatitis, the output of bicarbonate and enzymes, but mainly the latter, tended to decrease during stimulation, whereas in healthy subjects it remained stable or tended to increase (Fig. 1). An

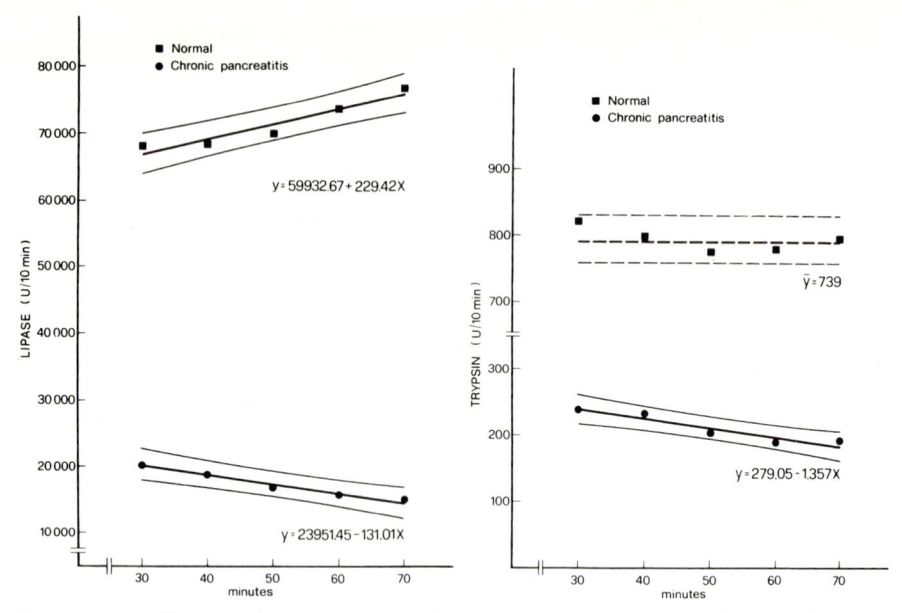

Fig. 1. Pattern of lipase and trypsin secretion during 90-min pancreatic stimulation with secretin (1 CU/kg per h) plus cerulein (100 ng/kg per h) in 30 healthy normal subjects and 32 patients with chronic pancreatitis. Analysis of variance

insufficient reserve capacity of the pancreas in patients with chronic pancreatitis is one possible explanation. From a diagnostic point of view, this method offered improved discrimination between normal and pathological responses [3].

We have shown that this method of continuous pancreatic stimulation has a greater sensitivity than that employing rapid injection of hormones [4].

In another study [5] we compared the sensitivity of this test of pancreatic function with that of endoscopic retrograde cholangiopancreatography (ERCP) and ultrasonography in a large series of patients with chronic pancreatitis who had various degrees of insufficiency. The sensitivity of duodenal intubation was clearly superior to that of the other techniques (Table 1).

In another study (not yet published) we examined some characteristics of exocrine pancreatic insufficiency in relation to the clinical duration of chronic pancreatitis. Table 2 shows the percentage of pathological results for bicarbonate and enzymes in 128 patients studied with the secretin-cerulein test, who were divided into five groups according to the clinical duration of the pancreatitis. It is of interest to note that among the 27 patients studied within one year of clinical onset (first attack of abdominal pain), seven (25.9%) had normal bicarbonate output, five (18.5%) had normal chymotrypsin output, but only one (3.7%) had normal lipase output. Among the patients studied more than 1 year after clinical onset of the disease (Table 2), the percentage of pathological results was similar for bicarbonate and enzymes. These results indicate that enzyme secretion, and especially secretion of lipase, is impaired sooner than

Table 1. Sensitivity of the secretin-cerulein test (S-C test), endoscopic retrograde cholangiopancreatography (ERCP), and ultrasonography (US) in the diagnosis of chronic pancreatitis (140 cases)

Test	Sensitivity
S-C test	97%
ERCP	90%
US	70%

From [5].

Table 2. Percentage of pathological results on the secretin-cerulein test in relation to clinical duration of chronic pancreatitis (128 cases)

Group	Patients (n)	Bicarbonate (%)	Chymotrypsin (%)	Lipase (%)
1	27	74.1	81.5	96.3
2	34	94.1	97.1	97.7
3	17	94.1	94.1	94.1
4	33	93.9	90.9	90.9
5	17	94.1	82.4	100.0

Group 1 patients were studied within 1 year of clinical onset, group 2, within 2-3 years, group 3, within 4-5 years, group 4 within 6-10 years, and group 5, more than 10 years clinical onset.

Table 3. Patterns and staging of exocrine pancreatic insufficiency in chronic pancreatitis

Insufficiency	Degree
Lipase alone	Usually mild[a]
Enzymes alone	Usually mild or moderate[b]
Enzymes and bicarbonate	Mild, moderate, or severe[c]
Bicarbonate alone	Usually mild

[a] Mild, loss of function of less than 30% of normal.
[b] Moderate, between 30% and 80%.
[c] Severe, more than 80%.

that of bicarbonate in chronic pancreatitis. A similar observation, i.e., that enzyme secretion is a more sensitive indicator of pancreatic pathology than bicarbonate secretion, had already been made by Burton et al. [6] in their pioneering work on the secretin-pancreozymin test. These data underline the importance of using cholecystokinin or cerulein in direct tests of pancreatic function and of studying enzyme secretion in the investigation of pancreatic function.

Our results contradict a diffuse belief that exocrine pancreatic insufficiency in patients with chronic pancreatitis develops several years after clinical onset of the disease [7]. It should be noted, however, that this belief was based on pancreatic function studies employing indirect tubeless tests [7], the sensitivity of which is considerably lower than that of the secretin-cerulein test we used [4].

Our studies have shown that, from a qualitative point of view, three types of pancreatic insufficiency may develop in patients with chronic pancreatitis (Table 3): one consisting of a selective deficit of lipase alone, another of a deficit of enzymes but not bicarbonate, and yet another in which both enzymes and bicarbonate are impaired. The insufficiency is usually mild in the first case, mild or moderate in the second, and mild, moderate, or severe in the third. Quantitatively, we define as mild a loss of function of less than 30 % of normal; as moderate a loss between 30 % and 80 %; and as severe when the loss of function is more than 80 % of normal. A selective deficit of only bicarbonate secretion is extremely rare.

Thus, despite its age (it was introduced in clinical practice more than 50 years ago), duodenal intubation and stimulation of the pancreas with exogenous hormones still represent a very important tool in the detection of pancreatic insufficiency as well as in the diagnosis and staging of chronic pancreatitis. Clearly, it is not a routine test, but one for selected patients only.

References

1. Gullo L (1986) Pancreatic function test by means of duodenal intubation. In: P. Malfertheiner and H. Ditschuneit, eds. Diagnostic procedures in pancreatic disease. Springer-Verlag, Berlin Heidelberg, 201–207
2. Wormsley KG (1972) Pancreatic function tests. Clin Gastroenterol 1: 27–51
3. Gullo L, Costa PL, Fontana G, Labò G (1976) Investigation of exocrine pancreatic function by continuous infusion of caerulein and secretin in normal subjects and in chronic pancreatitis. Digestion 14: 97–107
4. Gullo L, Costa PL, Labò G (1978) A comparison between injection and infusion of pancreatic stimulants in the diagnosis of exocrine pancreatic insufficiency. Digestion 18: 64–69
5. Gullo L (1986) Direct pancreatic function test (duodenal intubation) in the diagnosis of chronic pancreatitis. Gastroenterology 90: 799–800
6. Burton P, Evans DG, Harper AA, Howat HT, Oleesky S, Scott JE, Varley H (1960) A test of pancreatic function in man based on the analysis of duodenal contents after administration of secretin and pancreozymin. Gut 1: 111–118
7. Ammann RW, Akovbiantz A, Lardiader F, Schueler G (1984) Course and outcome of chronic pancreatitis. Longitudinal study of a mixed medical-surgical series of 245 patients. Gastroenterology 86: 820–828

Oral Pancreatic Function Tests in the Diagnosis and Staging of Chronic Pancreatitis

M. Rünzi · P. Layer

The diagnosis of chronic pancreatitis is based on assessment of morphological and functional alterations [1]. In contrast to direct tests of pancreatic secretory capacity involving collection of duodenal or pancreatic juice after pancreatic stimulation with exogenous hormones such as secretin and cholecystokinin [2, 3], indirect pancreatic function tests are frequently used in clinical routine as complementary measures for the diagnosis of chronic pancreatitis. The development of indirect pancreatic function tests has provided potential alternatives and diagnostic comfort because they are noninvasive and simple, less time-consuming, and inexpensive.

Two indirect pancreatic function tests are currently widely used: the *NBT-PABA (bentiromide)* and the *pancreolauryl test*. While the NBT-PABA test is preferably used in the USA (and no longer available in Germany), the pancreolauryl test is the major indirect test within Europe.

Principle of Oral Pancreatic Function Tests

Both the NBT-PABA and pancreolauryl test require the pharmacological combination of a special substrate and a marker substance in capsules ingested amidst a standard breakfast. The marker and the substrate are cleaved enzymatically by pancreas-specific enzymes within the gut lumen, and the marker is then absorbed by intestinal cells, thereby detectable in the serum, conjugated and/or metabolized in the liver, and finally excreted in urine (Fig. 1).

The *NBT-PABA test* (*N*-benzoyl-L-tyrosyl-*p*-aminobenzoic acid; bentiromide) uses a synthetic peptide that is specifically cleaved by the pancreatic enzyme chymotrypsin. The p-aminobenzoic acid (PABA) released is the measurable substance in the serum and/or urine, and the recovery rate of PABA indirectly reflects the amount of intraluminal chymotrypsin [4–8].

The *pancreolauryl test* (fluorescein dilaurate test) is basically similar to the NBT-PABA test. The synthetic, poorly water-soluble ester, fluorescein dilaurate, is specifically hydrolyzed by pancreatic cholesterolesterhydrolase (arylesterase). The fluorescein released is water-soluble, measurable in the serum after absorption, and serves as an indicator for exocrine pancreatic function after metabolization and conjugation with glucuronic acid followed by excretion into the urine.

Fig. 1. Principle of NBT-PABA (bentiromide) and pancreolauryl test as oral pancreatic function tests

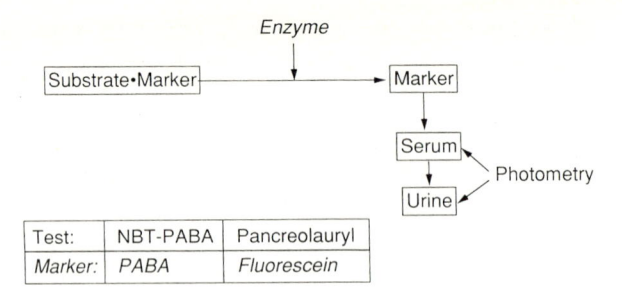

Test:	NBT-PABA	Pancreolauryl
Marker:	PABA	Fluorescein

Standard Methods

Briefly, the two-step procedure of the *pancreolauryl test* is as follows: on the first day, fluorescein dilaurate is given amidst a standard breakfast (50 g white bread, 20 g butter, a cup of tea) to stimulate the pancreas. To enhance diuresis, the patient is asked to drink 1.5 l tea (no milk or sugar) or mineral water. The test has to be repeated on the third day using only free fluorescein to correct the result for individual intestinal absorption, conjugation, and urinary excretion. The urinary fluorescein recovery over 10 h is measured photometrically on both days. Photometric reading is performed at 492 nm. Recovery of the fluorescein on the test (T) and control days (C) can then be calculated and expressed as a T/C ratio [=(T/C)×100]. A T/C ratio greater than 30 signifies normal pancreatic function, a ratio less than 20 indicates exocrine pancreatic insufficiency. If the T/C ratio is between 20 and 30, the test must be repeated [9].

Concentrations of fluorescein can be measured before and at various time points after administration of the test capsules in blood samples, which are then processed as described elsewhere [10]. The fluorescein concentration of each blood sample is analyzed in comparison with a fluorescein standard curve.

The *NBT-PABA test* runs a very similar test procedure: 1 g NBT-PABA is considered to be the optimum concentration and ingested with a test meal (i.e., mostly liquid formulation containing 3.6% fat, 4% protein, 14.7% carbohydrates). The urinary recovery of PABA is measured over 6 h. The lower limit of normal for 6-h PABA excretion is defined to be 50% of the dose given to healthy controls [11, 12]. PABA can be measured in the serum at the same time intervals as fluorescein, and the blood samples are processed as reported elsewhere [12]. Photometric reading is performed at 546 nm, and results are compared with the PABA standard curve.

Methodological Improvements

Two further improvements were reported recently: it could be shown that with a modified protocol running over 10 h overnight, the fluorescein concentration in the serum can be a helpful marker in the diagnostic work-up of exocrine pancreatic function in anuric patients on hemodialysis [13].

An interesting alternative to the conventional test procedure has been the introduction of a single-day test with fluorescein dilaurate plus mannitol, which has been validated in children with cystic fibrosis [14]. Mannitol resists metabolism within the gastrointestinal tract and also systemically. It is wholly and solely excreted in the urine with a clearance rate similar to that of creatinine. By combining fluorescein dilaurate and mannitol in the same test, the factors that affect absorption, distribution, and excretion of free fluorescein and mannitol apply equally to both, and changes in the urinary recovery of the former compared with the latter (F/M ratio) will be an indirect measure of pancreatic digestion. This test eliminates the second day of the classic protocol and shortens the duration of urine collection. However, this test awaits validation in chronic pancreatitis.

Current Status of Clinical Experience

NBT-PABA Test

In a meta-analysis of five European studies comprising $n = 1500$ patients, the clinical value of the NBT-PABA test was evaluated. Sensitivity ranged from 80 % to 100 %, and specificity was 85 %–94 % [15]. The North American experience showed similar data [16]; however, a dose of 500 mg instead of 1000 mg NBT-PABA was used.

Since one of the major problems of oral pancreatic function tests is the sampling of urine, several studies have put forward the idea of measuring the marker substance (PABA) in the serum. For the NBT-PABA test a sensitivity of 87 % and a specificity of 71 %, comparable to urine measurements, have been reported (Table 1) [12]. The optimal time point for the highest concentration of PABA detectable in the serum is about 3 h after ingestion of the test compound with the standard breakfast.

Several groups have tried to improve the PABA test. To this end, a single-day NBT-/^{14}C-PABA test has been proposed, showing better results in the serum than in the urine [17]. However, use of radioactive PABA has its limitations in pregnancy and children, and is expensive. Because of this, a combination with paraaminosalicylic acid (PAS) as a second marker substance ingested in combination with PABA has been suggested and has shown reasonable sensitivity and specificity values [18].

Table 1. Specificity and sensitivity of pancreolauryl and NBT-PABA (bentiromide) tests according to meta-analysis from the literature

OPFT	Urine method Specificity (%)	Sensitivity (%)	Serum method Specificity (%)	Sensitivity (%)
Pancreolauryl test	90 [10]	82 [10]	82 [12, 19]	85–90 [12, 19]
NBT-PABA test	85–94 [15]	80–100 [15]	71 [12]	87 [12]

OPFT, oral pancreatic function test.

Pancreolauryl Test

In a meta-analysis of 11 studies comprising $n = 975$ patients, sensitivity was 82% (range 39% to 100%) and specificity 90% (range 55% to 100%). The large discrepancy in the range numbers is probably due to different patient and criteria choices [10]. Similar to the PABA test, atempts have been made to improve the pancreolauryl test by introduction of serum measurement of the marker, resulting in a sensitivity of 97% and a specificity of 82% in one study [12]. However, results from other investigations suggest a lower sensitivity of 85%–90% [19] (Table 1).

To further improve the serum test, Malfertheiner et al. added metoclopramide and secretin to fluorescein dilaurate (to obtain a faster and greater pancreatic secretory response). This resulted in a shorter test protocol (peak fluorescein value in the serum after 180 min) and a specificity and sensitivity comparable to the urine method [19]. Although the serum measurement of the marker substance is a very attractive and less time-consuming procedure with similar sensitivities and specificities as the original urine test, it is somewhat more expensive. The serum test may have its main advantages in the elderly, the severely ill, and especially in outpatients. An important prerequisite is a good case history because the predictive value of the test increases considerably with the prevalence of the disease [20].

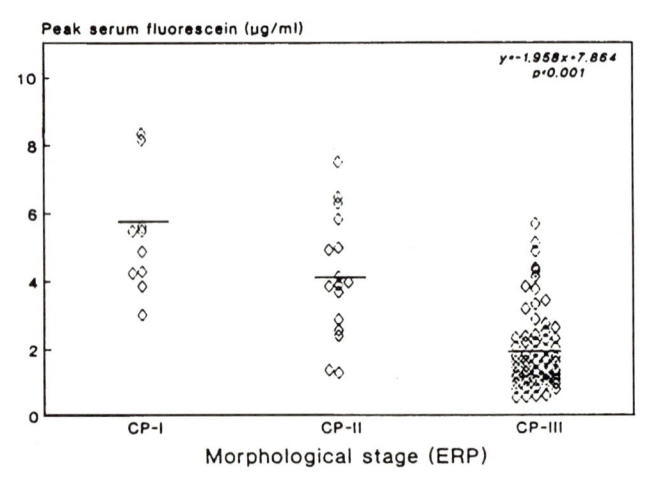

Fig. 2. Correlation of serum pancreolauryl test with ductal changes seen on endoscopic retrograde pancreatography (ERP) according to the Cambridge classification system (stage CP-I°–CP-II°). (Modified from [21])

Value of Indirect Tests for Staging of Pancreatic Disease

Recently, the results of the pancreolauryl test were correlated with the morphology seen on endoscopic retrograde pancreatography (ERP) and/or computed tomogaphy (CT scan in the same patients by using the improved serum test procedure with metoclopramide and secretin and discriminating two different cuttoff levels at 4.5 µg/ml and 2.5 µg/ml peak serum fluorescein [21], respectively. The results showed that the serum pancreolauryl test correlates with the degree of ductal abnormalities as assessed by ERP (according to the Cambridge classification). Furthermore, a level of ≤ 4.5 µg/ml probably suggests the presence of chronic pancreatitis. A level of ≤ 2.5 µg/ml indicates advanced disease; this cutoff might therefore be used to stage chronic pancreatitis (Fig. 2).

Although an over all correlation with ERP could be demonstrated, the pancreolauryl test could not be used to stage chronic pancreatitis I° and II° [21].

Limitations of Oral Pancreatic Function Tests

The major disadvantage of both the PABA and pancreolauryl tests is the low accuracy in mild or early insufficiency. Detection of chronic pancreatitis in early stages remains a difficult diagnostic problem. The efficacy of the pancreolauryl test in the early diagnosis of chronic pancreatitis is poor with a sensitivity of 52% and a specificity of less than 70% [21]. In addition, low accuracy is also reported for other or concomitant gastrointestinal diseases such as peptic ulcer disease, reflux esophagitis, extensive intestinal disease, or hepatobiliary disease associated with impaired bile acid secretion – all of which are known to result in an abnormal pancreolauryl test [21–24]. In addition, drug interferences (i.e., vitamin B_{12}, salazosulphapyridine) have also been reported [24, 25].

It is well known that in patients with partial or subtotal gastric resections (i.e., BI/BII resection, Roux-en-y anastomosis), the specificity of oral tests is decreased (PABA test 70% and pancreolauryl test 10% specificity) [26]. The clearly abnormal urine or serum concentrations in these postgastrectomy states are a result of pancreatic maldigestion secondary to abnormally rapid gastric

Fig. 3. Influence of previous surgical manipulation with pancreatico-biliochymous asynchrony on pancreolauryl and NBT-PABA (bentiromide) test results: limitation of the methods. (Modified from [26])

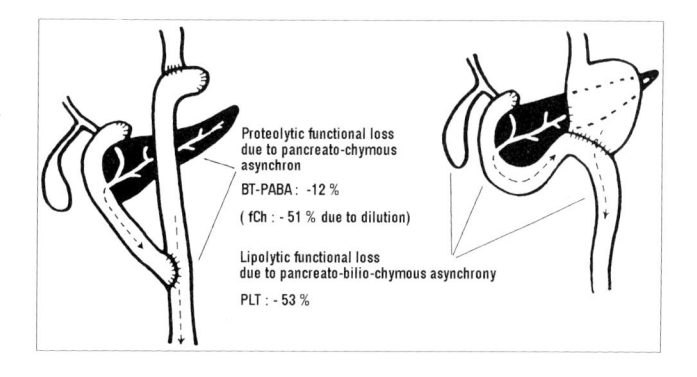

Proteolytic functional loss due to pancreato-chymous asynchron
BT-PABA: -12%
(fCh: -51% due to dilution)

Lipolytic functional loss due to pancreato-bilio-chymous asynchrony
PLT: -53%

emptying and delayed pancreatic secretion [27, 28]. This is caused by postsurgical anatomy resulting in an asynchrony of the intestinal deliveries of pancreaticobiliary secretions and chyme (Fig. 3). In these patients, oral tests are not applicable for the diagnosis of chronic pancreatitis. However, they may be used as an indicator of severe luminal maldigestion.

Conclusions

Oral pancreatic function tests are widely accepted as noninvasive diagnostic tools in chronic pancreatitis. However, their clinical value is only established for severe pancreatic insufficiency. Compared to the urinary test procedure, serum modification, especially for the pancreolauryl test, allows better control of the patient's compliance, is less time-consuming, and appears more sensitive. In contrast to this, the serum test is currently more expensive.

At present, the secretin-pancreozymin test remains the "gold standard" since oral pancreatic function tests have no clinical value for the detection and/or exclusion of mild pancreatic disease due to their inherent limitations (Fig. 4). In the landmark study of DiMagno et al., the major mechanism for this significant disadvantage of oral pancreatic function tests has been illustrated: only when the secretory capacity of the exocrine pancreas (i.e., lipase output) has decreased below 10% of normal, luminal digestion becomes significantly abnormal [29]. This, however, usually reflects advanced chronic pancreatic disease.

Fig. 4. Correlation of pancreolauryl test and fecal fat excretion. *T/C*, ratio of fluorescein recovery on test to control days. (Modified from [12])

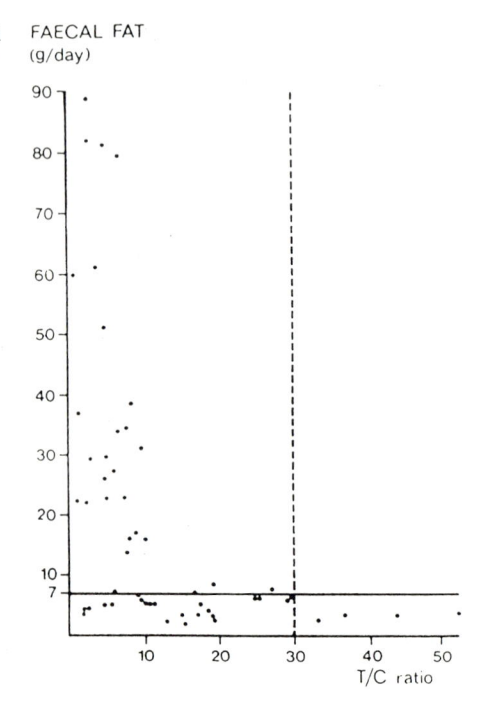

References

1. Gyr KE, Singer MV, Sarles H, eds (1984) Pancreatitis: Concepts and classification. Amsterdam: Excerpta Medica
2. Wormsley KG (1978) Tests of pancreatic secretion. Clin Gastroenterol 7: 529-544
3. Lankisch PG (1982) Exocrine pancreatic function test. 23: 777-798
4. Imondi AR, Wolgemuth RL (1979) Improved sensitivity of the BT-PABA pancreatic function test in animals with meals of raw egg white. Am J Dig Dis 24: 214-216
5. Gyr KE (1975) Tests of exocrine pancreatic function. Huber, Bern (Current problems in clinical biochemistry 5
6. Arvanitakis C, Greenberger N (1976) Diagnosis of pancreatic disease by a synthetic peptide: a new test of exocrine pancreatic function. Lancet I: 663-666
7. Bornschein W, Goldmann FL, Otte M (1976) Methodische und erste klinische Untersuchungsergebnisse mit einem neuen indirekten Pankreasfunktionstest. Clin Chim Acta 67: 21-27
8. Hosoda S, Kashima K, Bamba T, Kinugasa K, Nakaki T, Masuda M (1979) PFD, a new test of exocrine pancreatic function using BT-PABA (Bentiromide). In: Masuda M (ed) Pancreatic function diagnostic. Igaku-Shoin, Toyko; pp 27-37
9. Lankisch PG, Schreiber A, Otto J (1983) Pancreolauryl test: evaluation of a tubeless pancreatic function test in comparison with other indirect tests for exocrine pancreatic function. Dig Dis Sci 28: 490-493
10. Lankisch PG (1986) The indirect pancreatic function test "pancreolauryl" in chronic pancreatitis. Diagnostic Procedures in Pancreatic Disease. Ed. by P. Malfertheiner und H. Ditschuneit, Springer Verlag. Berlin Heidelberg
11. Lankisch PG, Ehrhardt-Schmelzer S, Koop H, Caspary WF (1980) Der NBT-PABA-Test in der Diagnostik der exokrinen Pankreasinsuffizienz. Dtsch Med Wochenschr 105: 1428-1423
12. Lankisch PG, Brauneis J, Otto J, Göke B (1986) Pancreolauryl and NBT-PABA Tests. Are serum tests more practicable alternatives to urine tests in the diagnosis of exocrine pancreatic insufficiency? Gastroenterology 90: 350-354
13. Lerch MM, Nolte I, Riehl J, Gladziwa U, Mann H, Sieberth HG, Matern S (1994) Diagnostic value of indirect pancreatic function test in serum of anuric patients with chronic renal failure. Scand J Clin Lab Invest 54: 247-250
14. Green MR, Austin S, Weaver LT (1993) Dual marker one day pancreolauryl test. Arch Dis Child 68: 649-652
15. Lang C, Gyr K (1986) Indirect pancreatic function test with NBT-PABA. Diagnostic Procedures in Pancreatic Disease. Ed. by P. Malfertheiner and H. Ditschuneit, Springer Verlag. Berlin Heidelberg
16. Toskes PP (1983) Bentiromide as a test of exocrine pancreatic function in adult patients with pancreatic exocrine insufficiency. Gastroenterology 85: 565-569
17. Tanner AR, Robinson DP (1988) Pancreatic function testing: serum PABA measurement is a reliable and accurate measurement of pancreatic function. Gut 29: 1736-1740
18. Hoek FJ, van den Bergh FAJTM, Klein Elhorst JT, Meijer JL, Timmer E, Tytgat GNJ (1987) Improved specificity of the PABA test with p-aminosalicylic acid (PAS). Gut 28: 468-473
19. Malfertheiner P, Büchler M, Müller A, Ditschuneit H (1987) Fluorescein dilaurate serum test: A rapid tubuless pancreatic function test. Pancreas 2: 53-60
20. Freise J, Ranft U, Fricke K, Schmidt FW (1984) Chronische Pankreatitis: Sensitivität, Spezifität und prädiktiver Wert des Pankreolauryltests. Z Gastroenterol 22: 705-712
21. Domínguez-Muñoz JE, Pieramico O, Büchler M, Malfertheiner P (1993) Clinical utility of the serum pancreolauryl test in diagnosis and staging of chronic pancreatitis. Am J Gastroenterol 8: 1237-1241
22. Malfertheiner P, Büchler M, Müller A, Ditschuneit H (1985) Influence of extra pancreatic digestive disorders on the indirect pancreatic function test with fluorescein dilaurate. Clin Physiol Biochem 3: 166-173
23. Kay G, Hine P, Braganza J (1982) The pancreolauryl test. A method of assessing the combined functional efficacy of pancreatic esterase and bile salts in vivo? Digestion 24: 241-245
24. Rosemeyer D, Brackmann P, de Boer H, Freitag J, Koblitz DK, Müller K (1986) 1000 Pancreolauryl-Tests: Beurteilung von Sensitivität, Spezifität und Verwendbarkeit in der klinischen Routine. Z Gastroenterol 24: 635-644
25. Scharpé S, Iliano L (1987) Two indirect tests of exocrine pancreatic function evaluated. Clin Chem 33: 5-12

26. Heptner G, Domschke S, Domschke W (1989) Exocrine pancreatic function after gastrectomy. Specificity of indirect tests. Gastroenterology 97: 147–153
27. Mac Gregor IL, Parent J, Meyer JH (1977) Gastric emptying of liquid meals and pancreatic and biliary secretion after subtotal gastrectomy or truncal vagotomy and pyloroplast in man. Gastroenterology 72: 195–205
28. Malfertheiner P, Junge U, Ditschuneit H (1984) Pancreatic digestive function after subtotal gastrectomy – evaluation of an indirect method. Hepatogastroenterology 31: 172–175
29. DiMagno EP, Go VLW, Summerkill WHJ (1973). Relations between pancreatic enzyme outputs and malabsorption in severe pancreatic insufficiency. N Engl J Med 288: 813–815

Present and Future of Breath Tests in the Diagnosis of Pancreatic Insufficiency

B. Lembcke

There is a gap between the application of breath tests for pancreatic insufficiency in clinical routine in some parts of the world and their role among scientific efforts, towards achieving a better characterization of impaired pancreatic function as a routinely applicable indicator of exocrine pancreatic disease in others. Currently, two facts need to be considered:

(1) at the end of 1995, except for research purposes, not a single institution in Germany ever used any type of breath tests for the diagnosis of pancreatic insufficiency or the malabsorption of fat;
(2) on the other hand, in 1993 the Editorial Office of the *Lancet* commented "that faecal fat estimations are probably not the gold standard method for assessing malabsorption" and that "labelled triglyceride (such as C 14 triolein) is more commonly used to diagnose pancreatic disease" and is a "more accurate measure of fat malabsorption."

This discrepancy leads to the question of how the current and future role of breath tests for exocrine pancreatic insufficiency can be defined.

Historical Perspective

Analyzing the breath in a pig in 1784, Lavoisier and LaPlace were the first to describe a relationship between ventilation and oxidation. Later, Charles Dodds applied breath analysis to gastrointestinal (GI) diseases. In 1920, he was able to demonstrate that postprandial increases in pCO_2 varied depending on the underlying GI tract disease (e.g., exocrine pancreatic insufficiency).

Thus breath tests for fat maldigestion and malabsorption have long tradition among GI function tests in general, and among breath tests in particular. While R. Schönheimer, the founder of stable isotope tracer techniques, was the first to adopt stable isotopes for the investigation of fatty acid metabolism as early as 1938, clinical fat balance studies in humans were performed with triglycerides labeled with radioactive isotopes (^{131}I) until radioactive (^{14}C) and stable (^{13}C) isotope breath tests became available.

Balance studies with ^{125}I- or ^{131}I-labeled substrates and equivalent techniques have been studied and reviewed in detail. As radioactive and time-consuming procedures (even using a double-marker technique) that still require the collection of stool, they cannot be considered to be suitable in current medical practice [1].

In addition to the study of fat maldigestion as a sequel to lipase deficiency, another approach was to investigate starch maldigestion as a consequence of diminished amylase secretion in patients with exocrine pancreatic insufficiency.

Rice Starch H$_2$ Breath Test and [^{13}C]Starch Breath Test

In 1984, Kerlin et al. [2] described a rise in breath hydrogen (H$_2$) concentrations after ingestion of 100 g rice starch in patients with exocrine pancreatic insufficiency, which indicates the maldigestion/malabsorption of the carbohydrate substrate in the case of impaired pancreatic amylase secretion. While this test was not sensitive enough to be helpful as a diagnostic test, the study clearly demonstrated that salivary amylase and intestinal glucosidase activities might not be sufficient to prevent carbohydrate malabsorption after starch ingestion and that this, subsequently may be a cause of symptoms of carbohydrate malabsorption in pancreatic insufficiency.

In an elegant report, Hiele and colleagues [3] used 50 g raw crystalline (naturally ^{13}C-enriched) corn starch as a substrate for their [^{13}C]starch breath test. This group again showed a significant malabsorption of (raw) starch in the case of rather severe exocrine pancreatic insufficiency, predominantly in patients with chronic calcifying pancreatitis. A substantial overlap of 6-h cumulative ^{13}CO$_2$ excretion in controls and patients with exocrine pancreatic insufficiency, however, prevents the use of this breath test as a diagnostic test.

In conclusion, there is no evidence that carbohydrate-based breath tests for exocrine pancreatic insufficiency might have similar diagnostic potential as breath tests for impaired lipolysis. Furthermore, breath tests assessing the maldigestion of fat can also be used to monitor the efficacy of pancreatic enzyme supplementation, which is in the first line a replacement of lipase activity.

[^{14}C]Triglyceride Breath Tests

Several ^{14}C breath tests were developed to diagnose fat maldigestion and fat malabsorption from 1960 to 1980, using [^{14}C]tripalmitin, [^{14}C]triolein, or [^{14}C]trioctanoate as the substrate [4-16].

The general principle behind these tests as a measure of exocrine pancreatic function is that LCT-hydrolysis by pancreatic enzymes (lipase) is the rate-limiting step after oral ingestion and gastric emptying. Accordingly, the resulting fatty acids must be absorbed and oxidized at excess capacities compared to lipolysis. Ideally, the generation of CO$_2$ from the substrate would be constant among different individuals (thereby allowing the calculation of CO$_2$ recoveries using discontinuous breath-sampling techniques) and unaffected by other diseases. However, this is apparently not the case, because cardiovascular and severe pulmonary disease, diabetes, disorders of lipid metabolism, obesity, fever, thyroid dysfunction, and severe liver disease have been demonstrated to interfere with the results [4]. Nevertheless, continuous analysis has been completely replaced by the discontinuous sampling technique.

[^{14}C]Triolein Breath Test

An important study addressing the question of which substrate is the most suitable was reported by Newcomer et al. [4]. The authors prospectively compared the analysis of serum β-carotene, qualitative fecal fat estimation, the [^{14}C]triolein test, the [^{14}C]tripalmitin test, and the [^{14}C]trioctanoate test in a carefully selected cohort of patients.

Time Course. Peak $^{14}CO_2$ exhalation after triolein predominantly occurred after 6 h.

Sensitivity. In this study, the [^{14}C]-triolein breath test was unequivocally superior to the other breath tests, with 100% sensitivity and 86% specificity of peak $^{14}CO_2$ exhalation for diagnosing pancreatic steatorrhea. Later, investigations both questioned and supported the clinical significance of the [^{14}C]triolein breath test [6, 12, 13]. At least within the British Empire, however, the method seems to have been established as a clinical test.

But why was this test – irrespective of another differential diagnostic modification [9] – supplanted by other breath tests at the end of the 1980s?
There are two main reasons:

1. The Mayo study by Newcomer et al. [4] predominantly included patients with moderate to severe steatorrhea, i.e., patients with late-stage pancreatic disease (pancreatic steatorrhea does not usually occur with a deficit in exocrine function of less than 90% [17, 18]). Therefore, a breath test suitable for detecting mild to moderate exocrine pancreatic insufficiency (without or with mild steatorrhea) was regarded a useful diagnosic test.
2. A major advantage of all breath tests (already mentioned by Dodds in 1921: "The analysis of alveolar air does not cause the subject any discomfort whatever") is their clinical feasibility. Relevant in this context are not only the unwillingness to work with malodorous feces and the invasiveness of intubation techniques, but also time requirements. The time course of fatty acid oxidation after the ingestion of the respective triglycerides, however, is strikingly different for octanoate, oleic acid, and palmitic acid [8].

Mixed Triglyceride Breath Test

The mixed triglyceride breath test was developed by the group of Vantrappen, Rutgeerts, and Ghoos in Leuven, Belgium, for the study of intraluminal lipase activity. The test molecule, i.e., either 1,3-dioleyl-2-(carboxyl-^{14}C)-octanoyl glycerol, the substrate initially used, or 1,3-distearyl-2-(carboxyl-^{13}C)-octanoyl glycerol, the stable isotope substrate (91% ^{13}C-enriched, purity > 98%), consists of a medium-chain fatty acid in the 2-position and long-chain fatty acids in the 1- and 3-positions [7, 16].

Fig. 1. Principle of the mixed triglyceride breath test

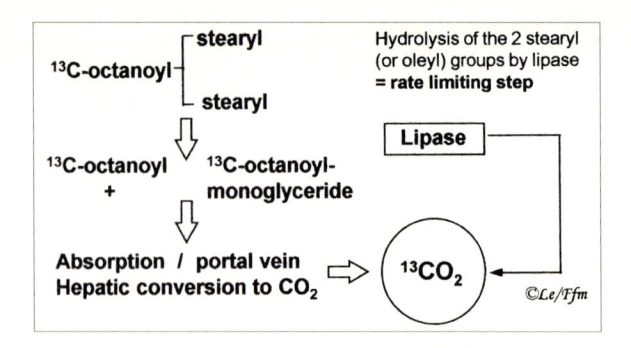

The rationale for both substrates is that the long-chain fatty acid groups have to be split off the glycerol by the action of lipase before [$^{13/14}$C]octanoyl monoglyceride or [$^{13/14}$C]octanoate is absorbed and transported to the liver (via the portal vein), where it is rapidly metabolized to $^{13/14}CO_2$ (Fig. 1).

Time Course. While with the ^{14}C-mixed triglyceride 1,3-dioleyl-2-(carboxyl-^{14}C)-octanoyl glycerol peak $^{14}CO_2$ exhalation was found at 4 h after the test meal, the $^{13}CO_2$ response after ingestion of 1,3-distearyl-2-(carboxyl-^{13}C]-octanoyl glycerol showed peak $^{13}CO_2/^{12}CO_2$ ratios at 4–6 h, and the 6-h cumulative recovery rate was used for correlation with the lipase output [7, 16].

Dosage Requirements. For the stable isotope test, the test meal consisted of 100 g toast with 0.25 g butter/kg body weight, to which 16 mg of the labeled substrate was added.

Sensitivity. Lipase output and cumulative $^{13}CO_2$ excretion (6 h) followed a hyperbolic correlation which allowed patients to be detected who had impaired lipase output without steatorrhea as well as those with severe exocrine insufficiency. As a test for exocrine pancreatic insufficiency, the ^{13}C-mixed triglyceride breath test had a sensitivity of 89%, with 81% specificity [16].

Similarly, in the ealier investigation with the ^{14}C-mixed triglyceride, a positive breath test was reported in patients with impaired lipase output but no steatorrhea. Thus the mixed triglyceride breath test appears to be more sensitive in detecting impaired pancreatic function than fecal fat determination. However, in a large proportion of patients, intestinal causes of malabsorption will also lead to a positive breath test.

Comments. The determinants for the $^{13}CO_2$ response of the mixed triglyceride $^{13}CO_2$ breath test, other than factors related to pancreatic insufficiency, are largely unexplored. Initial studies indicate that reproducibility might be limited, in particular with respect to $^{13}CO_2$ expiration rates. While the importance of prolonged fasting during the test might be overemphasized, standardisation of physical activity appears advisable (M. Kalivianakis et al. 1996, unpublished data).

Cholesteryl Octanoate Breath Test

Principle. The cholesteryl octanoate test is based on the fact that the ester bond of cholesteryl-1-^{13}C (or -^{14}C) octanoate is hydrolyzed by pancreatic carboxyl ester lipase (cholesterol lipase), and that this is the rate-limiting step, including intestinal absorption and hepatic oxidation of ^{13}C- (or ^{14}C-) octanoate (Fig. 2) [14, 15]. The test molecule is thought to be only slightly different from cholesterol esters naturally present in foods.

Fig. 2. Principle of the cholesteryl-octanoate breath test

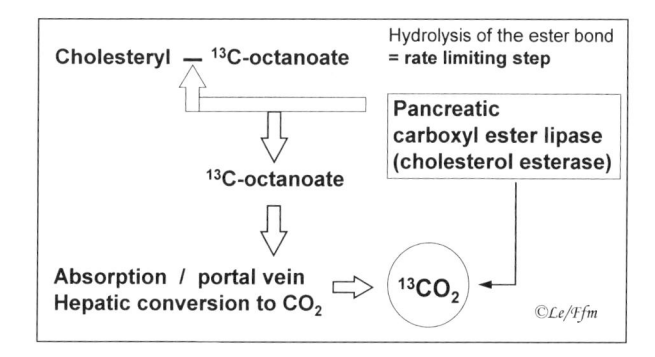

Time Course. CO_2 responses after oral administration peak at 60–120 min in healthy subjects and at 60–180 min in patients with pancreatic insufficiency. In patients with severe exocrine pancreatic insufficiency, responses may be further delayed [14].

Dosage Requirements. The tracer (dosage in humans not specified in the only published work) is administered together with 2 g cholesteryl octanoate and 18 g cholesterol-free vegetable oil (soya). While published data refer to the ^{14}C breath test, a ^{13}C breath test was only performed in a single subject.

Sensitivity. Regardless of experimental data in rats which suggested a test that is sensitive enough to detect mild degrees of pancreatic insufficiency, data in humans clearly demonstrate that the cholesteryl-^{14}C octanoate breath test does not differentiate between patients with exocrine insufficiency and pancreatic steatorrhea of 7.7–10.8 g fat excretion per day and normal controls. Four patients with pancreatic steatorrhea (55.7–123.2 g/day) were well recognized by the test, and one subject with steatorrhea (25 g/day) was slightly abnormal. No study in humans has assessed the cholesteryl octanoate breath test in correlation with direct pancreatic function tests (secretin pancreozymin test, Lundh test). Thus this test is fast, but currently it neither meets the criteria of a sufficiently validated breath test nor does it detect mild or moderate degrees of pancreatic insufficiency. Although allegedly not affected by gastric lipase and lingual lipase, even pancreatic steatorrhea is underdiagnosed by the cholesteryl octanoate test [14].

[^{13}C]Hiolein® Breath Test

Principle. Derived from algae living in an atmosphere with $^{13}CO_2$ as the sole source of carbons, hiolein® is a microalgal oil comprised of neutral triglycerides with a mixture of different long-chain fatty acids. The composition of these fatty acids is shown in Table 1. Unlike chemically synthesized 1-^{13}C-labeled triolein, in which only the carboxyl carbon of oleic acid is labeled, every carbon of hiolein, including the glycerol carbons, is labeled with ^{13}C.

Time Course. Comparing the time course of $^{13}CO_2$ exhalation following ingestion of either (1,1,1-^{13}C-triolein, 99%) at a dose of 20 mg/kg body weight, hiolein (U-^{13}C, 6.6%) at the same dose or hiolein (U-^{13}C, 66%) at a dose of 2 mg/kg body weight in seven healthy women, Peter Klein et al. from Houston confirmed that the oxidation kinetics of hiolein are indistinguishable from those of triolein. With both substrates, peak $^{13}CO_2$ exhalation occurred at 6 h [19]. The same profile was obtained in a study by Lembcke et al. [20] using 98% U-^{13}C-labeled hiolein in both healthy controls and in patients with exocrine pancreatic insufficiency.

Dosage Requirements. Using 98% U-^{13}C hiolein, 1 g rice snack/kg body weight was used as the test meal (21% fat), to which 2 mg hiolein/g rice snack was added [20].

Sensitivity. Although the nonlinear relation of lipase output and the $^{13}CO_2$ response could be described by a mathematical function (Fig. 3), an abnormal breath test was only observed in patients with severe pancreatic insufficiency, i.e., in those with pancreatic steatorrhea (Table 2). While the sensitivity of the test for the detection of pancreatic steatorrhea was 91.7% (specificity, 85.7%), the hiolein breath test had only 47% sensitivity as a test for exocrine pancreatic insufficiency (specificity, 90%). Subsequently, the Hiolein breath test it not an adequate test in patients with mild or moderate degrees of impaired pancreatic function, but a reliable indicator of pancreatic steatorrhea [20].

Table 1. Composition of hiolein® (lot no. # 0242, Martek Biosciences Corporation, Columbia, Maryland, USA) [20]

Common name	Fatty acid	Amount (%)
Oleic acid	18:1 ω-6	50.6
Linoleic acid	18:2 ω-6	19.6
Stearic acid	18:0 ω-6	2.3
Palmitic acid	16:0 ω-6	16.9
No common name	16:2 ω-6	1.4
α-Linolenic acid	18:3 ω-3	3.0
No common name	16:3 ω-3	1.2
Palmitoleic acid	16:1 ω-9	1.8

Fig. 3. 95 % confidence interval ($m = 0.01856 - 0.02266$) of the linear regression of lipase output$_{30\,min}$ versus lipase output$_{30\,min}$/DOB$_{max}$ (kU/30 min per δ‰). $r = 0.949$, $n = 46$; $p < 0.0001$ (data from ref. [20])

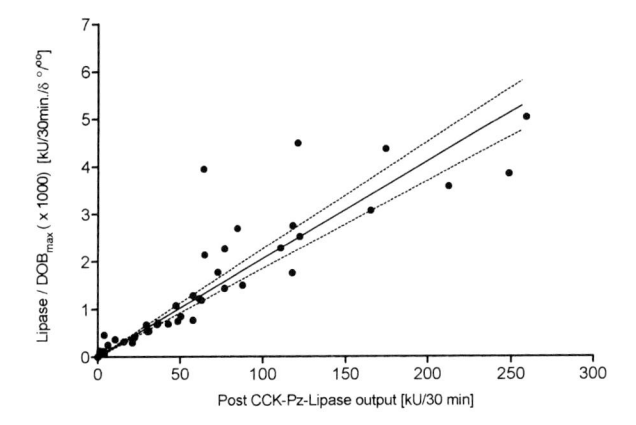

Comparative aspects

Although the pros and cons concerning breath tests for the diagnosis of exocrine pancreatic insufficiency might be weighed on the basis of objective criteria, the current discussion and judgement seem to be dominated by more general criteria.

General Importance

Breath tests neither support the differential diagnosis of pancreatic cancer and chronic pancreatitis, nor do they indicate malignant transformation in the course of chronic pancreatitis. Further, they are of no help in the management of pain in chronic pancreatitis. If these questions are more important than guiding and treating patients with chronic pancreatitis or cystic fibrosis sophisticatedly, breath tests in exocrine pancreatic insufficiency could be regarded as dispensible.

Accurate Targeting of Tests

Some authorities claim the need for a noninvasive and feasible test which allows detection of even minor degrees of exocrine pancreatic insufficiency. This view seems to be less widespread in countries where chronic pancreatitis is usually diagnosed on the basis of imaging methods (ultrasound; endoscopic retrograde cholangiopancreatography, ERCP) and where the potential role of breath tests is confined to replacing fecal fat analysis in the detection of pancreatic steatorrhea and to monitoring enzyme replacement therapy [21, 22].

With regard to an ultrasensitive indirect measure of pancreatic function, all the breath tests described above will probably fail, with the mixed triglyceride breath test being the *primus inter pares*. Furthermore, it is questionable

Table 2. Hiolein breath test in patients with and without exocrine pancreatic insufficiency of different severity as compared to healthy controls and patients with gastrointestinal disease without pancreatic involvement (peak increments, DOB, $\Delta \delta$‰)

Patient group	Number	Lower 95% CI	Mean ± SD	Upper 95% CI
Control	7	41.4	53.9 ± 13.6	66.5
+ EPI[a], + steatorrhea[c]	12	13.3	21.7 ± 13.2	30.1
+ EPI[a], − steatorrhea[d]	18	44.7	51.0 ± 12.7	57.3
− EPI[b], − steatorrhea[d]	10	43.5	50.2 ± 9.3	56.9
Disease Controls	6	29.1	44.9 ± 15.0	60.6

[a] Proven exocrine pancreatic insufficiency.
[b] Exocrine pancreatic insufficiency excluded by the secretin pancreozymin test.
[c] Fecal fat excretion ≥ 7 g/day.
[d] Fecal fat excretion < 7 g/day.

whether any breath test which relies on the maldigestion of fat will ever become an indicator of mild pancreatic insufficiency, because the functional reserve capacity of the pancreas allows 90% destruction before steatorrhea occurs [17, 18].

As far as the second scenario is concerned, the hiolein breath test and the ^{13}C-mixed triglyceride breath test will definitely be applicable [16, 20]. The same is true of the [^{14}C]triolein breath test, but at the end of this millenium ^{14}C substrates should be replaced in medicine by stable isotopes, and [^{13}C]triolein at the required amounts is a prohibitively expensive substrate.

The "Haves" and the "Have-Nots"

^{13}C breath tests are still hampered by both high substrate expenses and the low cooperation in gaining access to ^{13}CO$_2$ analysis facilities. While substrate expenses for breath tests with ^{13}C-labeled fats are generally too high for routine applications (e.g., $ 200–300 for a single hiolein breath test), prices will (hopefully) become increasingly subject to market forces.

Measurement facilities, however, formerly confined to isotope ratio mass spectrometry (IR-MS) in high-tech research laboratories, are gaining a broader application as a result of two developments:

1. In many European countries and the United States, there are now enough laboratories equipped with robust IR-MS facilities to provide an adequate number of analyses on a commercial and shipping basis. However, at least in Germany, a broad tendency towards significant overequipment both in hospitals and especially in private practice is currently seen.
2. Non-mass spectrometry methods have recently gained increasing acceptance. Nondispersive isotope-selective infrared spectrometry (NDIRS) as an affordable method (appr. $ 50 000) which allows the application of ^{13}C breath tests in the clinical routine has been validated versus IR-MS, and other similar developments will soon become available [23, 24].

Conclusion

It is likely that test kits for different breath tests will become availably commercially in the near future in several countries. In Germany, reimbursement has become possible for some breath tests only recently; the respective amounts, however, were obviously unsatisfactory. In view of this, the future of breath tests in the diagnosis of pancreatic insufficiency will still remain closely associated with research facilities. The search for pancreatic insufficiency in cystic fibrosis and the control of pancreatin therapy, however, are good candidates for a clinical application of the ^{13}C breath tests in pediatric patients.

Acknowledgement. This work was supported by a grant from the Else-Kröner-Fresenius Foundation.

References

1. Lembcke B, Lösler A, Caspary WF, Schürnbrand P, Emrich D, Creutzfeldt W (1986) Clinical value of a dual isotope fat absorption test system (FATS) using glycerol ^{125}I-trioleate and glycerol ^{75}Se-triether. Dig Dis Sci 31: 822–828
2. Kerlin P, Wong L, Harris B, Capra S (1984) Rice flour, breath hydrogen, and malabsorption. Gastroenterology 87: 578–585
3. Hiele M, Ghoos Y, Rutgeerts P, Vantrappen G (1989) Starch digestion in normal subjects and patients with pancreatic disease, using a ^{13}CO$_2$ breath test. Gastroenterology 96: 503–509
4. Newcomer AD, Hofmann AF, DiMagno EP, Thomas PJ, Carlson GL (1979) Triolein breath test: a sensitive and specific test for fat malabsorption. Gastroenterology 76: 6–13
5. Nasrallah S, Al-Khalidi UAS (1980) Clinical value of 14C-phenylacetic oil as a fat absorption test. Lancet i: 229–231
6. West PS, Levin GE, Griffin GE, Maxwell JD (1981) Comparison of simple screening tests for fat malabsorption. Br Med J 282: 1501–1504
7. Ghoos YF, Vantrappen GR, Rutgeerts PJ, Schurmans PC (1981) A mixed triglyceride breath test for intraluminal fat digestive capacity. Digestion 22: 239–247
8. Watkins JB, Klein PD, Schoeller DA, Kirschner BS, Park R, Perman JA (1982) Diagnosis and differantiation of fat malabsorption in children using 13C-labeled lipids: trioctanoin, triolein, and palmitic acid breath tests. Gastroenterology 82: 911–917
9. Goff JS (1982) Two-stage triolein breath test differentiates pancreatic insufficiency from other causes of malabsorption. Gastroenterology 83: 44–46
10. Einarsson K, Björkhem I, Eklöf R, Blomstrand R (1983) 14C-Triolein breath test as a rapid and convenient screening test for fat malabsorption. Scand J Gastroenterol 18: 9–12
11. Benini L, Scuro LA, Menini E, Manfrini C, Vantini I, Vaona B, Brocco G, Talamini G, Cavallini G (1984) Is the ^{14}C-triolein breath test useful in the assessment of malabsorption in clinical practice? Digestion 29: 91–97
12. Mylvaganam K, Hudson PR, Ross A, Williams CP (1986) 14C triolein breath test: A routine test in the gastroenterology clinic? Gut 27: 1347
13. Turner JM, Lawrence S, Fellows IW, Johnson I, Hill PG, Holmes GKT (1987) [14C]-triolein absorption: a useful test in the diagnosis of malabsorption. Gut 28: 694–700
14. Cole SG, Rossi S, Stern A, Hofmann AF (1987) Cholesteryl octanoate breath test. Gastroenterology 93: 1372–1380
15. Mundlos S, Rhodes JB, Hofmann AF (1987) The cholesteryl octanoate breath test: a new procedure for detection of pancreatic insufficiency in the rat. Ped. Res. 22: 257–261
16. Vantrappen GR, Rutgeerts PJ, Ghos YF, Hiele MI (1989) Mixed triglyceride breath test: a noninvasive test of pancreatic lipase activity in the duodenum. Gastroenterology 96: 1126–1134
17. DiMagno EP, Go VWL, Summerskill WHJ (1973) Relations between pancreatic enzyme outputs and malabsorption in severe pancreatic insufficiency. N Engl J Med 288: 813–815

18. Lankisch PG, Lembcke B, Wemken G, Creutzfeldt W (1986) Functional reserve capacity of the exocrine pancreas. Digestion 35: 175–181
19. Klein PD, Hachey DL, Opekun AR, Tacquard PE, Kyle D (1991) Oxidation studies of a biosynthetic randomly ^{13}C-labeled triglyceride. Gastroenterology 100: 528 A
20. Lembcke B, Braden B, Caspary WF (1996) Exocrine pancreatic insufficiency: accuracy and clinical value of the uniformly labeled ^{13}C-Hiolein breath test. Gut 39: 668–674
21. Mundlos S, Kühnelt P, Adler G (1990) Monitoring enzyme replacement treatment in exocrine pancreatic insufficiency using the cholesteryl octanoate breath test. Gut 31: 1324–1328
22. Braden B, Picard H, Caspary WF, Lembcke B (1997) Monitoring pancreatin supplementation in cystic fibrosis patients with the ^{13}C-Hiolein breath test: evidence for normalized fat assimilation with high dose pancreatin therapy. Z Gastroenterol 35
23. Braden B, Haisch M, Duan LP, Lembcke B, Caspary WF, Hering P (1994) Clinically feasible stable isotope technique at a reasonable price: analysis of $^{13}CO_2/^{12}$-CO_2-abundance in breath samples with a new isotope selective nondispersive infrared spectrometer. Z Gastroenterol 32: 675–678
24. Braden B, Schäfer F, Caspary WF, Lembcke B (1996) Nondispersive isotope-selective infrared spectroscopy: a new analytical method for ^{13}C-urea breath tests. Scand J Gastroenterol 31: 442–445

Value of Serum Pancreatic Enzymes in the Diagnosis of Chronic Pancreatitis

J. Mössner

What is the value of serum pancreatic enzymes in the diagnosis of chronic pancreatitis? This question includes several aspects

1. Can we detect pancreatic insufficiency by measuring serum pancreatic enzymes?
2. Can we detect acute inflammatory relapses?
3. Can we differentiate between acute pancreatitis and acute inflammatory relapses of chronic pancreatitis?
4. Can we differentiate between pancreatitis and pancreatic carcinoma?

Value of Serum Pancreatic Enzymes in Detecting Pancreatic Insufficiency

Benini et al. (1991) studied the variations in time of serum pancreatic enzyme levels in chronic pancreatitis and compared them with the clinical course of the disease. According to their study design, 34 patients with chronic pancreatitis were evaluated prospectively every 9 months for up to 3 years. Painful relapses were excluded. Serum elastase-1, trypsin, lipase, and amylase were determined. At study entry, high levels of elastase were found in 41.1 %, low levels in 11.7 %; high levels of lipase and trypsin only in 11.7 % and 5.8 %, low levels in 32.3 % and 47.8 %, respectively. There was a significant reduction of serum elastase-1 over time. This reduction was not seen for trypsin, lipase, or amylase. However, patients with severe exocrine impairment had low levels of elastase in only 20 % of cases in contrast to lipase which was decreased in 53.3 % and trypsin in 73.3 %. In an another study from Italy, Ventrucci et al. (1989) determined amylase, pancreatic isoamylase, trypsinogen, and elastase-1 in 145 patients with pancreatic disease and in 66 with pain of nonpancreatic origin. Fifty-two patients with chronic pancreatitis in clinical remission showed serum enzyme behavior with great variations Normal assays were found in 60 % even in severe pancreatic insufficiency. Steinberg et al. (1984) measured serum trypsinogen and found considerable variations in the same patient over time. They emphasized that a low trypsinogen level indicates pancreatic insufficiency with high specificity. However, a normal serum trypsinogen level does not exclude chronic pancreatitis. High specificity but rather low sensitivity of another pancreatic enzyme were also reported by Lankisch et al. (1986). They investigated the role of serum pancreatic isoamylase in the diagnosis of exocrine pancreatic insufficiency. Only 67.9% of 82 patients with pathological secretin-pancreozymin test had decreased serum levels of pancreatic isoamylase. Some better results were reported by Kitagawa et al. (1991) by measuring phospholipase A_2 using radioimmunoassay. They found an increase of this enzyme in most patients with acute pancreatitis and a decrease in patients with severe pancreatic insufficiency. The sensitivity of this enzyme seems to be greater than that of amylase; however, it is still too low at only 62%. Other groups tried to increase sensitivity in diagnosing pancreatic insufficiency by measuring the ratios of different serum pancreatic enzymes. Dominguez-Muñoz et al. (1993) investigated 296 patients with clinically suspected chronic pancreatitis. Of these, 167 patients had a final diagnosis of chronic pancreatitis. Serum values of pancreatic amylase, lipase, immunoreactive trypsin, and their ratios were measured. Abnormally low values of individual serum pancreatic enzymes were highly specific in the diagnosis of chronic pancreatitis (92%–98%), yet very insensitive (20%–32%). Thus, one can not improve sensitivity by calculating ratios of serum values of pancreatic enzymes.

More than 10 years ago, another attempt to differentiate between chronic pancreatiitis with slight impairment of pancreatic exocrine function, patients with severe insufficiency, and controls was the so-called evocation-test. It was assumed that in patients with chronic pancreatic inflammation, pancreatic serum enzyme activities increase after stimulation with either secretin or cholecystokinin due to disturbances in either directed secretion of the acinar cell or in barrier function of ducts. Malfertheiner et al. (1982) evaluated the diagnostic significance of pancreatic serum-enzyme patterns after stimulation with secretin in chronic pancreatitis. They determined immunoreactive trypsin and pancreatic isoamylase. A significant abnormal increase in serum trypsin was seen in 34 patients with proven chronic pancreatitis associated with mild to moderate dysfunction. However, no increase was seen in marked insufficiency. Vezzadini et al. (1984) confirmed these results by measuring serum immunoreactive trypsin response to secretin. They claim that a markedly elevated increase of serum immunoreactive trypsin in response to stimulation with secretin seems to differentiate between patients with mild pancreatic insufficiency, those with severe insufficiency, and controls. Despite these promising results, sensitivity of this test for differentiating between early and late stages of chronic pancreatitis is obviously too low. Thus this test is no longer performed in most centers.

Value of Serum Pancreatic Enzymes in Detecting Acute Inflammatory Relapse

It is common knowledge that acute pancreatitis and acute relapse of chronic pancreatitis are most often associated with marked elevations of serum amylase and lipase. In severe necrotizing pancreatitis, enzyme levels may already be normal when the patient enters hospital due to destruction of pancreatic tissue. Furthermore, there are numerous studies clearly demonstrating that serum levels of pancreatic enzymes do not correlate with severity of the disease. An acute relapse of chronic pancreatitis may not be accompanied by elevations of serum enzymes either when most of the pancreatic exocrine tissue has already been displaced by fibrotic tissue or when acute clinical relapse is not due to acute inflammation of the acinar tissue but due to other causes such as development of a pseudocyst. It is well known that one cannot differentiate between acute relapse of chronic pancreatitis and acute pancreatitis by measuring serum amylase or lipase. Thus, Kemmer et al. (1991) studied the potential diagnostic value of serum ribonuclease activity in various pancreatic diseases. In edematous pancreatitis, ribonuclease activity was similar to that of healthy controls. In necrotizing pancreatitis, serum ribonuclease was clearly elevated, suggesting that this enzyme may help to differentiate between edematous and necrotizing pancreatitis. However, in chronic pancreatitis, pancreatic carcinoma, and renal insufficiency, serum ribonuclease activity was also elevated. Thus, sensitivity and specificity of this enzyme seem to be rather low.

Ventrucci et al. (1992) studied the diagnostic sensitivity of various pancreatic enzymes in 100 patients with acute abdomen. 27 selected patients with proven acute pancreatitis served as controls. Amylase, pancreatic isoamylase, lipase, trypsinogen, and elastase-1 were determined. All enzymes were elevated in the 8 patients having acute pancreatitis as cause of acute abdomen. In the remaining 92 patients, serum amylase was abnormal in seven and at least one pancreatic enzyme abnormal in 16. Patients were correctly classified by isoamylase and lipase in 96% of cases, amylase in 93%, elastase-1 in 91%, and trypsinogen in 84%. The authors recommend a turbidometric assay of serum lipase as the most suitable test for emergency diagnosis. This test seems to be highly sensitive, specific, simple, and can be performed quickly.

Value of Serum Pancreatic Enzymes in Differentiating Between Acute Pancreatitis and Acute Inflammatory Relapse of Chronic Pancreatitis

Funakoshi et al. (1991) investigated the problem of whether serum pancreatic enzymes can help to differentiate between acute pancreatitis and a relapse of chronic pancreatitis. They determined phospholipase A_2 and prophospholipase A_2 by monoclonal antibodies. Phospholipase A_2 was elevated in acute pancreatitis. However, no differentiation was possible between a relapse of chronic pancreatitis and acute pancreatitis. Similar "negative" findings were reported by Basso et al. (1990). They measured serum phospholipase A_2 acitivity in addition to elastase-1, total, and pancreatic isoamylase activity in chronic pancreatitis, pancreatic cancer, and controls. Elastase-1, phospholipase A_2, and isoamylase were elevated in cancer (56%, 25%, 15%, respectively) and in chronic pancreatitis (40%, 31%, 41%, respectively). In addition, all four enzymes gave pathological values in a number of extrapancreatic diseases. The authors concluded that diagnostic efficacy of phospholipase A_2 is similar to other pancreatic enzymes and that its sensitivity and specificity are rather unsatisfactory. LeMoine et al. (1994) tested the hypothesis that trypsin activity may be a new marker of acute alcoholic pancreatitis. They studied 32 patients with acute pancreatitis, with 17 cases due to alcohol and 15 due to other causes (11 cases of gallstone pancreatitis). High trypsin activity was found in all patients with alcoholic pancreatitis, even when amylase was normal. However, trypsin activity did not differ among alcoholic controls and nonalcoholic causes of acute pancreatitis.

Value of Serum Pancreatic Enzymes in Differentiating Between Pancreatitis and Pancreatic Carcinoma

Fabris et al. (1986) measured serum elastase-1, imunoreactive trypsin, α_1-antitrypsin, and α_2-macroglobulin in controls and in patients with pancreatic cancer, chronic pancreatitis, and extrapancreatic diseases. Increases of all parameters apart from immunoreactive trypsin were found in all diseases tested. Multiple regression analyses revealed that the variations of proteases and antiproteases in chronic pancreatitis were independent of each other. Again, measurement of these parameters did not help to differentiate between chronic pancreatitis and pancreatic cancer.

Conclusion: Value of Serum Pancreatic Enzymes in the Diagnosis of Chronic Pancreatitis?

The following points can be made:

1. They have no value in detecting pancreatic insufficiency. Serum pancreatic enzymes may be decreased only in severe pancreatic insufficiency.
2. They have some value in detecting acute inflammatory relapse.
3. Determination of serum pancreatic digestive enzymes cannot differentiate between acute pancreatitis and acute inflammatory relapse of chronic pancreatitis.
4. Serum pancreatic enzymes can not reliably detect pancreatic carcinoma.

References

1. Basso D, Fabris C, Panozzo MP, Meggiato T, Del Favero G, Naccarato R (1990) Serum phospholipase A2 activity in chronic pancreatic diseases. Clin Biochem 23: 229–232
2. Benini L, Caliari S, Vaona B, Brocco G, Micciolo R, Rizzotti P, Fioretta A, Castellani G, Cavallini G, Scuro LA, et al (1991) Variations in time of serum pancreatic enzyme levels in chronic pancreatitis and clinical course of the disease. Int J Pancreatol 8: 279–287
3. Dominguez-Muñoz JE, Pieramico O, Büchler M, Malfertheiner P (1993) Ratios of different serum pancreatic enzymes in the diagnosis and staging of chronic pancreatitis. Digestion 54: 231–236
4. Fabris C, Del Favero G, Panucci A, Plebani M, Di Mario F, Piccoli A, Basso D, Burlina A, Naccarato R (1986) Serum elastase 1 and immunoreactive trypsin in chronic pancreatic disease: is there any relationship with trypsin inhibitors? Enzyme 35: 82–86
5. Funakoshi A, Yamada Y, Migita Y, Wakasugi H (1993) Simultaneous determinations of pancreatic phospholipase A2 and prophospholipase A2 in various pancreatic diseases. Dig Dis Sci 38: 502–506

6. Funakoshi A, Yamada Y, Ito T, Ishikawa H, Yokota M, Shinozaki H, Wakasugi H, Misaki A, Kono M (1991) Clinical usefulness of serum phospholipase A2 determination in patients with pancreatic diseases. Pancreas 6: 588-594
7. Kemmer TP, Malfertheiner P, Büchler M, Kemmer ML, Ditschuneit H (1991) Serum ribonuclease activity in the diagnosis of pancreatic disease. Int J Pancreatol 8: 23-33
8. Kitagawa M, Hayakawa T, Kondo T, Shibata T, Sakai Y, Sobajima H, Ishiguro H, Nakae Y (1991) The diagnostic value of serum pancreatic phospholipase A2 (PLA2) in pancreatic diseases. Gastroenterol Jpn 26: 62-68
9. Lankisch PG, Koop H, Otto J (1986) Estimation of serum pancreatic isoamylase: its role in the diagnosis of exocrine pancreatic insufficiency. Am J Gastroenterol 81: 365-368
10. LeMoine O, Devaster JM, Deviere J, Thiry P, Cremer M, Ooms HA (1994) Trypsin activity. A new marker of acute alcoholic pancreatitis. Dig Dis Sci 39: 2634-2638
11. Malfertheiner P, Bieger W, Trischler G, Ditschuneit H (1982) Diagnostische Bedeutung des pankreatischen Serumenzymmusters nach Stimulation mit Sekretin bei chronischer Pankreatitis. Dtsch Med Wochenschr 107: 849-853
12. Steinberg WM, Anderson KK (1984) Serum trypsinogen in diagnosis of chronic pancreatitis. Dis Dig Sci 29: 988-993
13. Ventrucci M, Pezzilli R, Gullo L, Plate L, Sprovieri G, Barbara L (1989) Role of serum pancreatic enzyme assays in diagnosis of pancreatic disease. Dig Dis Sci 34: 39-45
14. Ventrucci M, Pezzilli R, Montone L, Plate L, Buonamici L, Bergami R, Conci T (1992) Serum pancreatic enzyme assays in acute abdomen: a comparative prospective study. Ital J Gastroenterol 24: 115-118
15. Vezzadini P, Gullo L, Sternini C, Bonora G, Priori P, Labo G (1984) Serum immunoreactive trypsin response to secretin injection in patients with chronic pancreatitis. Am J Gastroenterol 79: 213-216

Table 1. Exocrine pancreatic function tests

	Validation	Clinical significance	Practicability
Direct tests			
Secretin-pancreozymin test	+++	++/--	--
Secretolin-cerulein test	+++	++/--	--
Lundh test	+++	+/--	--
Indirect tests			
NBT-PABA test	--	---	+++
Pancreolauryl test	++	+++	++
Enzyme estimation in serum			
Isoamylase	--	---	+++
IR-trypsin	--	---	+++
Fecal tests			
Fat and nitrogen determination	+	+++	+
Chymotrypsin	+	+++	+
Elastase-1	++	+++	++
Breath tests			
^{13}C-starch	---	---	+
^{13}C-hiolein	++	+/-	+
^{13}C-cholesteryl-octanoae	---	---	+
Plasma amino acid consumption test	+/-	+	-

Water content can be determined after freeze-drying or by the Karl Fisher method [12].

A method for routine analysis of fat, starch, and nitrogen using near-infrared reflectance analysis (NIRA) has recently been developed [13–17]. This technique, which is based on the measurement of radiation in the near infrared spectrum scattered by the surface of a spot sample, gives results in less than 1 min, without further processing of the feces and without use of any chemical reagents.

Principle

NIRA is based on the matrix- and substrate-specific relationship between reflectance intensity diffused by the fecal sample surface at a specific wavelength and the composition of the sample. Each component to be measured has typical functional groups (CH, NH, OH, etc.) possessing specific absorption bands in the near-infrared range (700–2500 nm). Therefore, the spectroscopic response (reflectance) of fecal samples is related to concentrations of the compounds (functional groups) as follows [18, 19].

$$X = Z - f_1 \log Rf_1 - f_2 \log Rf_2 - \ldots - f_n \log Rf_n$$

with X as the concentration of the analyte, Rf_n as the reflectance for the filter n, f_n as the scaling factor for each filter, and Z as a constant of bias correction. Wavelength and corresponding spectra structure for each filter are given in

Table 2. Spectra structure and results of calibration with selected filters

Filters	Corresponding wavelength (nm)	Specific corresponding structure	Scaling factors	t test
1	2336	—CH$_3$; >CH$_2$	−15.48	−5.69
5	2208	—CH—CH2 O	15.38	6.04
7	2100	>C=CH2	3.47	3.39
9	1940	—OH	21.34	8.29
10	1818	—CH	−19.48	−7.05
11	1680	>C=CH2; —CH	−5.19	−4.20

Table 2. Scaling factors corresponding to each selected filter were calculated by multilinear regression [20, 21] of results obtained from a training set consisting of samples analyzed by the routine chemical method covering the whole concentration range.

This method is based on the principle described by Peuchant et al. [20]. In summary: the sum of squares of the residual values (differences between referrence values and calculated values) must be as low as possible. The computer assessed every set of wavelength combinations from 1 to 12, via spectroscopic and statistical data based on a t test with t equal to the value of f/standard deviation (SD) value of F.

Each combination of wavelengths was characterized by the coefficient of multiple correlation (R) between the chemical and calculated values:

$$R = \sqrt{\frac{1 - \text{SEE}^2 (n - k - 1)}{\text{SD}^2 (n - 1)}}$$

where SEE is the standard error of estimate, n is the number of samples, and k is the number filters; and by the constant of Fisher (F ratio), which indicates the quality of regression:

$$\text{F ratio} = \frac{r^2 (n - k - 1)}{(1 - r^2) k}$$

As the number of wavelengths in the combination increased, the correlation coefficient approached 1 and the F ratio increased to values greater than 50.

Optical information is provided by a constantly rotating filter wheel fitted with 12 narrowband (10 nm) pass filters of fixed wavelength specification covering 1218–2345 nm (Table 2). The apparatus (Fig. 1) allowed measurement of reflectance (R_f) as the ratio of reflected energy from the sample and incident radiation. Since near-infrared reflectance measurements depend heavily upon the amount of scattering materials and pathlength, the 1940-nm water band was used to compensate effective path length difference [23]. The measurement of R_f was converted into log R_f, and the latter was measured at 1–12 wavelengths and entered into the computer.

Fig. 1. Principle compounds of near-infrared reflectance analysis (NIRA). *1*, Light source; *2*, lens; *3*, chopper; *4*, filter wheel with NIR filter; *5*, aperture; *6*, folding mirror; *7*, integrating sphere; *8*, detectors; *9*, diffuse reflectance; *10*, sample. (From [17])

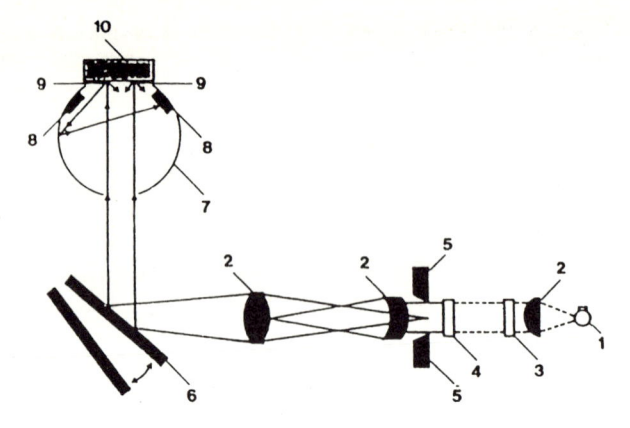

The manufacturer's software program was used to select the best combination of filters from a group of filters that were highly correlated spectroscopically by computer calculation [16]: wavelengths with clearly assignable spectral responses were included and those without were excluded. Wavelengths with low constants and poor correlations were excluded on statistical grounds by using student's test. The programm functioned with a combination of 1–12 wavelengths that provided for each combination the values of constants corresponding to each filter, the values of the correlation coefficient R, and the F ratio.

Clinical Validation

From January 1990 until December 1995, we studied 212 patients of all ages (3–71 years, mean 32 years) who were admitted to our hospital: (a) for the differential diagnosis of malabsorption syndromes (history of diarrhea, weight loss) or (b) with previously established causes of malabsorption or maldigestion (exocrine pancreatic insufficiency due to chronic pancreatitis or cystic fibrosis, inflammatory bowel disease, celiac sprue). A subgroup of extensively investigated patients with functional abdominal pain, but with entirely normal parameters of gastrointestinal function, who served as controls, was also admitted. In each case, final diagnoses were established after thorough investigation according to generally accepted criteria.

Fecal fat was measured by the titrimetric method of van de Kamer [9] which was preferred over the gravimetric method of Sobel and Bowers [24] for reasons of better reproducibility, and because we have more than 15 years of extensive practical experience with this technique. All measurements were performed in duplicate.

Fecal nitrogen was measured by the mineralometric method of Kjeldahl, which is based on strong acid digestion of total nitrogen [11, 12]. *Fecal water content* was analyzed by lyophilization: aliquots (2–3 g) of preweighed homogenized stools were freeze-dried over 72 h at $-24°$ and 10^{-2} mbar and reweighed. The difference in weight was taken as the fecal water content.

Fecal fat concentrations studied by NIRA in the 212 patients ranged from 0.32 to 13.4 g/100 g wet weight, *fecal nitrogen* values were within the range of 0.37–2.2 g/100 g wet weight, and *fecal water* content accounted for 55.2–100.0 g/100 g wet weight. For all three parameters, NIRA revealed linear regression when compared to conventional methods, with correlation coefficients of 0.934 for fecal fat (Fig. 2) 0.918 for nitrogen (Fig. 3) and 0.944 for water (Fig. 4). The respective standard errors of estimate (SEE) are 0.81, 0.175, and 3.075.

Table 3 shows the results of NIRA in stool from patients with diarrhea and/or steatorrhea of various etiologies in comparison to control subjects without diarrhea. Due to the different populations (age), this is not for statistical comparison, but for demonstration of clinical feasibility only. It is demonstrated that fecal water content is highly increased in patients with inflammatory bowel disease compared to controls (89.9 ± 5.2 % vs. 74.3 ± 4.3 %), although it may vary substantially in both groups.

Total nitrogen was significantly increased in patients with impaired pancreatic function, both in children with cystic fibrosis (1.26 % ± 0.13 %) and in adults with chronic pancreatitis (1.93 % ± 0.21 %) as compared to (adult) controls (0.93 % ± 0.17 %). Similarly, fecal fat concentration was elevated in adult patients with chronic pancreatitis (5.3 % ± 1.8 %) as well as in pediatric patients with cystic fibrosis (4.9 % ± 1.7 %; both with and without enzyme substitution) compared to controls (2.3 % ± 1.1 %).

Our data show near-infrared reflectance analysis to be a valuable practical alternative to conventional chemical methods for the measurement of fectal fat, nitrogen, and water. The absence of any potentially hazardous reagent (with the necessity of respective precautions), of homogenization, extraction; distillation, etc. allows this method to be applied in any hospital laboratory, not only in specialized centers. Moreover, the short analysis time of NIRA (less than 1 min) for all three parameters assessed makes the results rapidly available. Finally, comparison of NIRA in homogenized stools samples with traditional methods gives a precise correlation showing that NIRA is as accurate as conventional methods.

Fig. 2. Correlation between fecal fat concentration (g%) measured by near-infrared reflectance analysis (NIRA) and the method described by van de Kamer et al. in 212 stool samples ($y = 0.37 + 0.88\ x$, $r = 0.934$). (From [17])

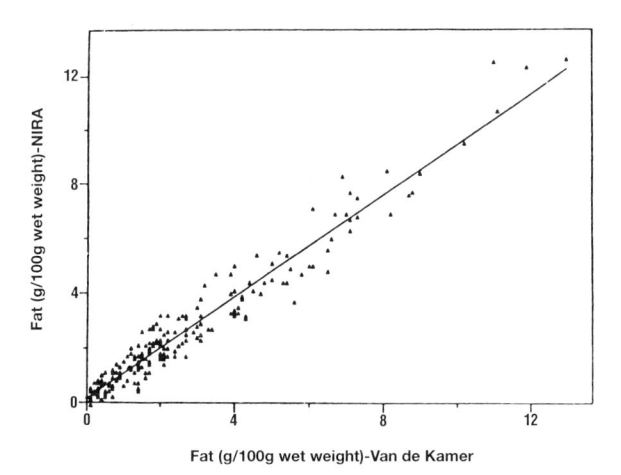

Fig. 3. Correlation between fecal nitrogen concentration (g%) measured by near-infrared reflectance analysis (NIRA) and the method described by Kjeldahl in 158 stool samples ($y = 0.15 + 0.88\,x$, $r = 0.918$) (From [17])

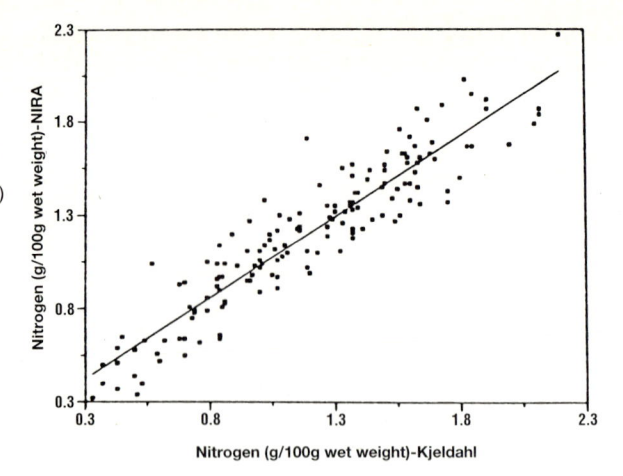

Repeated analysis of different portions of the same stool collection, performed in only a few minutes to avoid homogenization, is usually the most unpleasant part of classical methods. Five readings reduce the difference from the posthomogenized value for three parameters to less than 7%, but for clinical application three readings may fully suffice.

To avoid problems with NIRA, it should be emphasized that the assay is based on calibration with chemical methods, which is the first and indispensable step when starting measurements. This means that the reflectometric results depend on the availability and accuracy of reference methods in the respective laboratory as well as on the choice of biological matrix. Therefore, NIRA cannot be "more accurate" with respect to the true value than the reference methods. Benini et al. recently demonstrated that minimal changes of stool matrix (e.g., more liquid stools) may influence the results of nitrogen anal-

Fig. 4. Correlation between focal water content (g%) measured by near-infrared reflectance analysis (NIRA) and the lyophilization method in 154 stool samples ($y = 9.21 + 0.87\,x$, $r = 0.944$). (From [17])

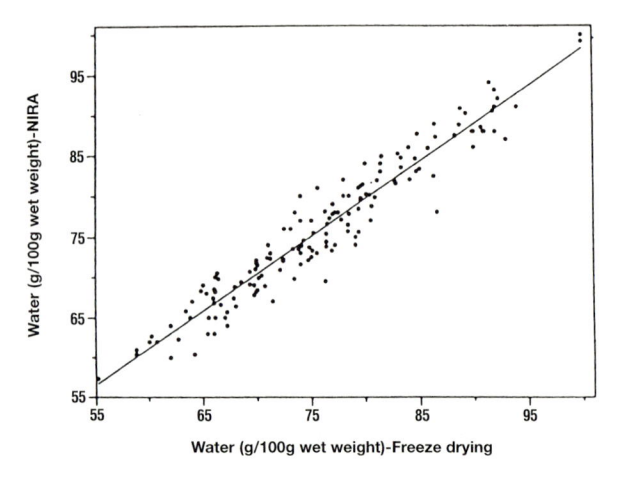

Table 3. Results of fectal fat, water, and nitrogen analysis by the near-infrared reflectance analysis (NIRA) method in patients with different gastrointestinal diseases (g/100 g wet weight)

	Total n	Total fat	Water
Controls (n = 64)			
Mean ± SD	0.93 ± 0.17	2.3 ± 1.1	74.3 ± 4.3
Range	0.54 – 1.65	0.3 – 3.8	66.8 – 82.7
Patients with CED (n = 12)			
Mean ± SD	0.93 ± 0.17	3.7 ± 0.08	89.9 ± 5.2
Range	0.61 – 1.54	0.41 – 3.60	79.4 – 94.6
Patients with impaired pancreatic function due to chronic pancreatitis (n = 22)			
Mean ± SD	1.93 ± 0.21	5.3 ± .8	72.3 ± 4.3
Range	1.23 – 2.23	2.1 – 7.6	60.1 –77.9
Patients with impaired pancreatic function due to cystic fibrosis (n = 47)			
Mean ± SD	1.26 ± 0.13	4.9 ± 1.7	77.3 ± 4.3
Range	0.76 – 1.86	2.3 – 7.8	63.7 – 81.9

ysis [25]. In such cases it would be necessary to adapt calibration by using an adapted stool matrix or to change the reference method. In this study we did not focus on this possibility, but throughout two years of investigation, there was no indication from our unselected patient groups, that this might be of clinical relevance for routine purposes. It should also be stated that, as Benini and colleagues found [25], NIRA can underestimate fat and nitrogen. This is of little consequence for a clinical screening method, but applying the NIRA method to balance studies would lead to systemic errors. The difference between reflectrometric and chemical values could also partly be explained by the imprecision of the methods. Thus, Grimble and colleagues [26] found that the Kjedahl method underestimated fecal nitrogen caused by acid-digestion-refractive nitrogen. Similary, the van de Kamer method may fail in detecting hydroxylated fatty acids if the appropriate extraction solvent is not used. Thus, by using different reference methods, improved correspondence of NIRA and chemical values could be expected.

Thus, for routine purposes in a clinical setting, we regard NIRA as an applicable and precise alternative to the van de Kamer method, to nitrogen determination according to the Kjedahl method, and to measurement of stool water content by lyophilization or heat-drying. Moreover, only one qualified person is required for running the apparatus. It is concluded that NIRA represents a useful replacement of the conventional laboratoy methods in the investigation of malabsorption.

Immunoreactive Elastase as a New Fecal Pancreatic Function Test

Since invasive diagnostic approaches of impaired pancreatic function, such as the secretin-pancreozymin test (SPT) with its several modifications or the Lundh test are time-consuming, invasive, unpopular with patients, and expen-

Fig. 5. Fecal immunoreactive elastase concentration in controls ranging from 136 to 4440 μg/g. Ninty-five percent of all values (2.5th–97.5th percentile) were within 175–2500 μg/g, with a mean value of 1083 ± 193 μg/g. (From [39])

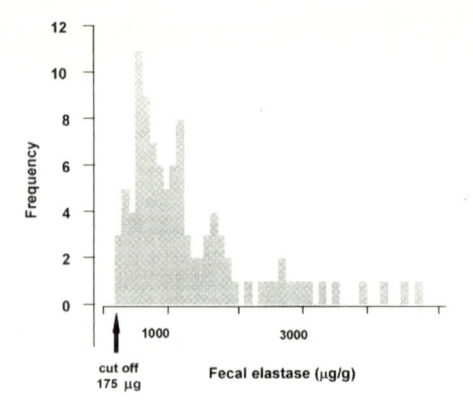

sive, numerous indirect or tubeless pancreatic function tests (fecal chymotrypsin, BT-PABA, pancreolauryl test) have been introduced as alternatives [27]. Among the tubeless pancreatic function tests, determination of fecal chymotrypsin has been accepted as an indirect test for pancreatic function for many years. As mentioned above, its sensitivity has been reported to range from 72% to 90%. The specificity reported in the literature ranges from 49% to 90% and appears to depend on the selection of control subjects studied [28–35].

Recently, Sziegoleit et al. detected human pancreatic elastase-1 [36], a member of the acidic elastase family, as a new endoprotease and sterol binding protein both in human pancreatic secretions and feces. Quantitative studies by rocket immunoelectrophoresis indicated that this enzyme was unaffected during intestinal passage. Concentrations in feces were five to six times higher than those determined in pancreatic juice [37, 38]. Therefore, we propose that concentrations of this enzyme in feces reflect pancreatic function. The aim of this prospective study was to evaluate the specificity and sensitivity of fecal immunoreactive elastase as an accurate test of exocrine pancreatic function by comparing the results with direct measurement of pancreatic enzyme secretion.

Fig. 6. Fecal excretion of chymotrypsin, fat, and immunoreactive elastase during a 24-h collection period in 12 patients with cystic fibrosis (CF) and steatorrhea with and without enzyme replacement therapy (mean values and SD). (From [39])

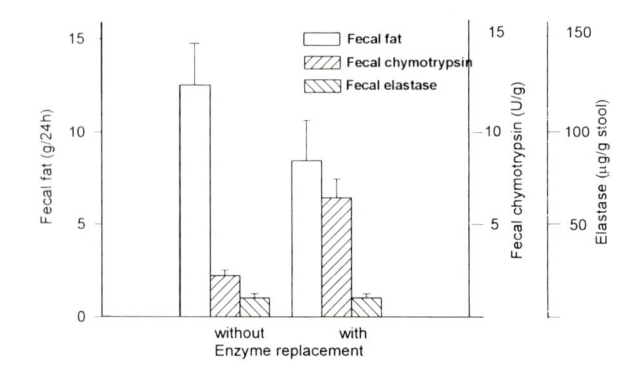

New Fecal Tests in the Diagnosis of Exocrine Pancreatic Insufficiency 285

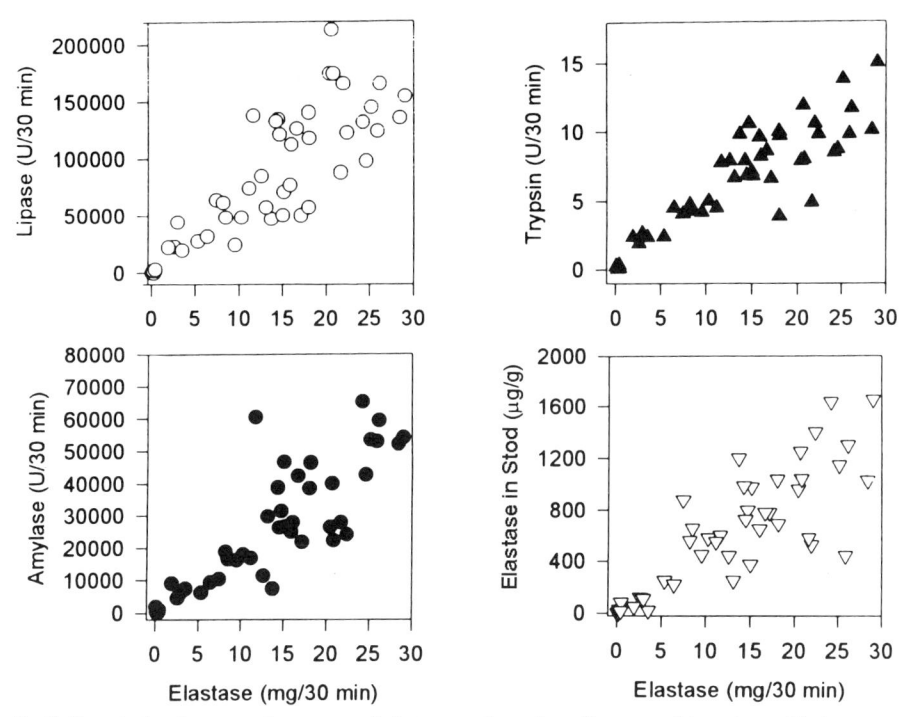

Fig. 7. Correlation between the output of elastase and amylase, lipase, and trypsin and between elastase in stool and elastase in pancreatic juice after stimulation in controls and in patients with pancreatic insufficiency. (From [39])

From August 1992 until December 1993, fecal elastase was measured in stool samples from 164 consecutive patients (84 males, 80 females) of 5–85 years of age (mean, 41 years) who were admitted to the hospital: (a) for the differential diagnosis of malabsorption syndromes (history of diarrhea, weight loss) or (b) with previously established causes of malabsorption or maldigestion (exocrine pancreatic insufficiency due to chronic pancreatitis or cystic fibrosis, inflammatory bowel disease, celiac sprue). A subgroup of extensively investigated patients with functional abdominal pain, but with entirely normal parameters of gastrointestinal functions, who served as controls, was also admitted. In each case, final diagnoses were established after thorough investigation according to generally accepted criteria.

Elastase was determined immunologically, using a new enzyme immunoassay following the sandwich technique. *Chymotrypsin, amylase, lipase*, and *trypsin activity* have been measured by the use of commercial test kits [39]. The *secretin-pancreozymin test (SPT)* was performed in the morning after overnight fasting according to Creutzfeldt and Lankisch [40, 41]. For evaluation of exocrine function, volume and concentration of bicarbonate were measured after stimulation with secretin. Amylase, lipase, and trypsin output were measured after cholecytokinin-pancreozymin (CCK-PZ).

Table 4. Fecal elastase 1 compared to secretin-pancreozymin test (SPT), fecal chymotrypsin, and fecal fat in pancreatic insufficiency with and without steatorrhea

SPT	Fecal elastase (n)	Abnormal (n)	(%)	Fecal chymotrypsin (n)	Abnormal (n)	(%)
Bicarbonate concentration, enzyme output abnormal, fecal fat normal	7	6	88	7	4	56
Bicarbonate concentration, enzyme output, fecal fat abnormal	22	21	96	22	20	91

Maximal concentration of bicarbonate: >70 mval/l (normal).
Amylase, trypsin, and lipase output 30 min after stimulation: amylase >12 000 units/30 min; trypsin >3 units/30 min; lipase >65 000 units/30 min (normal).
Normal stool fat <7 g/day.

Fecal immunoreactive elastase activity in controls ranged from 136 to 4440 µg/g. Ninety-five percent of all values (2.5th–97.5th percentile) were within 175–2500 µg/g with a mean value of 1083 ± 193 µg/g (Fig. 5).

Substitution replacement therapy in 12 patients with exocrine pancreatic insufficiency due to cystic fibrosis resulted in a significantly increased output of chymotrypsin activity and a significantly reduced fecal fat content, whereas fecal immunoreactive elastase was not affected by substitution therapy (Fig. 6).

There was a good correlation (Fig. 7) between the output of elastase compared to amylase, lipase, and trypsin with correlation coefficients of 0.83, 0.82, and 0.84, respectively, in normal subjects ($n = 25$), and 0.86, 0.91, and 0.91, respectively, in impaired pancreatic function ($n = 22$). Furthermore, there was a good correlation between the output of elastase in duodenal aspirate and elastase in feces ($r = 0.87, p < 0.01$). Calculating sensitivity and specificity at several cutoff values using a receiver-operating characteristic, the fecal elastase assay achieved optimal discrimination (defined as maximal likelihood ratio, i.e., true-positive rate divided by false-positive rate) when a cutoff value of 175 µg/g wet weight was used (specificity, 94%; sensitivity, 93%). When patients with pathological SPT were divided into groups with and without steatorrhea, correctly abnormal fecal elastase increased to 96% in severe exocrine pancreatic insufficiency. In less severely impaired patients without steatorrhea, diagnostic sensitivity decreased to 88%. It should be noted that diagnostic sensitivity for chymotrypsin in the same groups of patients with chronic pancreatitis was 91%, whereas diagnostic specificity was only 91% (with steatorrhea) and 56% (without steatorrhea), respectively (Table 4).

Immunoreactive elastase values in different diseases are shown in Fig. 8. Mean fecal values were significantly lower ($p < 0.001$) in patients with pancreatic insufficiency due to chronic pancreatitis (CP) and cystic fibrosis (CF) compared with healthy controls, celiac disease (with and without steatorrhea), inflammatory bowel disease, and patients with functional diarrhea.

Determination of fecal chymotrypsin has been accepted as an indirect test for pancreatic function. Measurement of fecal chymotrypsin can also be used to

Fig. 8. Values of fecal elastase in healthy controls (*N*), patients with chronic pancreatitis (*CP*), cystic fibrosis (*CF*), and with diseases of no pancreatic origin (*NPO*). (From [39])

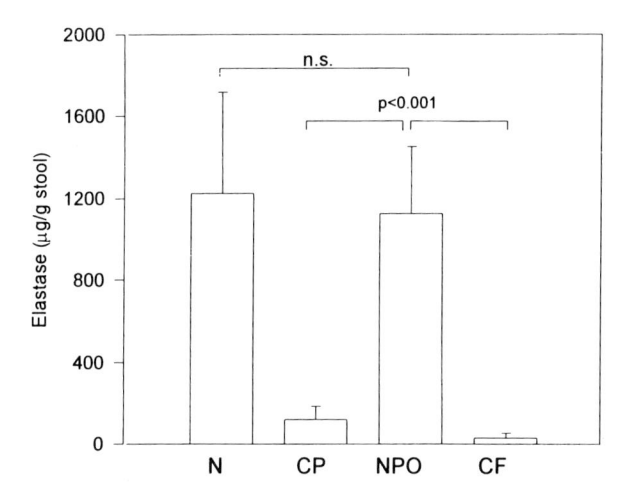

detect pancreatic insufficiency in children with cystic fibrosis. The test has some advantages over other tubeless tests. It is simple to perform when automatic titration is available. Stool samples from outpatients can be mailed to diagnostic centers that perform the assay because chymotrypsin activity is very stable over a number of days at room temperature. However, sensitivity of fecal chymotrypsin determination as a test for CP has been reported to range from 45% to 100%, with most studies reporting values of 72%–90% [30–34]. False-positive results have been reported in a variety of nonpancreatic diseases: liver cirrhosis, Billroth II gastrectomy, celiac spure, Crohn's disease, and other gastrointestinal diseases associated with diarrhea and malabsorption [42–45]. Studies comparing results of fecal chymotrypsin determination with those of the secretin-pancreozymin test (or analogous tests such as the secretin-cerulein test) showed that fecal chymotrypsin detects 85% of patients with advanced CP, but only 49% of those with mild or early manifestation of the disease [33–35].

Recently, Münch et al. [45] used fecal immunoreactive lipase (IRL) assay as a new tubeless test in the diagnosis of pancreatic exocrine insufficiency by means of a new enzyme-linked immunoabsorbant assay technique. In contrast to fecal chymotrypsin, the test results were unaffected by pancreatic enzyme replacement therapy. In spite of the excellent diagnostic specificity of 98%, the assay had the disadvantage of a very low sensitivity of 34%.

In contrast, measurement of fecal immunoreactive elastase has both high diagnostic sensitivity and specificity. All subjects with nonpancreatic diarrhea and celiac disease, except two patients with prior gastric resection (Billroth II) and two with severe secretoric diarrhea due to enzyme dilution (water content 98%), had immunoreactive elastase values within normal limits.

Overall sensitivity of immunoreactive elastase was also satisfactory, especially in patients with moderately or severely impaired pancreatic function. In patients with severe pancreatic insufficiency (steatorrhea) or cystic fibrosis, none had a falsely normal test result. Thus, compared with fecal chymotrypsin or fecal lipase, the fecal elastase test shows higher diagnostic sensitivity and specificity, which has also been confirmed by the recently published work of Dominguez et al. [46] and Löser et al. [47].

References

1. Lagerlöf HO (1942) Pancreatic function and pancreatic disease: studied means of secretin. Acta Med Scand Suppl 128: 1-289
2. Niederau C, Grendell JH (1985) Diagnosis of chronic pancreatitis. Gastroenterology 88: 1973-1995
3. Lankisch PG (1982) Exocrine pancreatic function tests. Gut 23: 777-798
4. DiMagno EP, Go VLW, Summerskill HJ (1973) Relations between pancreatic enzyme outputs and malabsorption in severe pancreatic insufficiency. New Engl J Med 288: 813-815
5. Bo-Linn G, Fordtran JS (1984) Fecal fat concentration in patients with steatorrhea. Gastroenterology 87: 319-322
6. Lembcke B, Grimm K, Lankisch PG (1987) Raised fecal fat concentration is not a valid indicator of pancreatic steatorrhea. Am J Gastroenterology 82: 526-531
7. Kjeldahl J (1883) Neue Methode zur Bestimmung des Stickstoffs in organischen Körpern. Anal Chem 22: 366-368
8. Archibald R, (1958) Nitrogen by the Kjeldahl method. Stand Methods. Clin Chem 2: 91-99
9. Van de Kamer JH, Huinik HB, Weyers HA. Rapid method for the determination of fat in feces.
10. Tomaszewski L (1975) Rapid and accurate method for determination of total lipids in feces. Clin Chem Acta 61: 113-120
11. Fales FW (1971) Evaluation of a spectrophotometric method for determination of total fecal lipid. Clin Chem 17: 1103-1108
12. Jensen R, Buffangeix D, Covi G (1976) Measuring water content of feces by the Karl Fisher method. Clin Chem 22: 1351-1346
13. Peuchant E, Salles C, Jensen R (1988) Value of a spectroscopic "fecalogram" in determining the etiology of steatorrhea. Clin Chem 34: 5-8
14. Benini L, Caliari S, Guidi GC, Brentegani MT, Castellani G, Sembenini C, Bardelli E, Vantini I (1989) Near infrared spectroscopy for fecal fat measurement: comparison with conventional gravimetric and titrimetric methods. Gut 30: 1165A-1167A
15. Stein J, Purschian B, Caspary WF, Lembcke B (1992) Validation of near-infrared reflectance analysis (NIRA) for assessment of fecal fat, nitrogen and water. A new approach to malabsorption syndromes [Abstract]. Gastroenterology 102: 243
16. Stein J, Purschian B, Bieniek U, Caspary WF, Lembcke B (1994) Near-infrared reflectance analysis (NIRA): a new dimension in the investigation of malabsorption syndromes. Eur J Gastroenterol Hepatol 6: 889-894
17. Stein J, Purschian B, Zeuzem S, Lembcke B, Caspary WF (1996) Quantification of fecal carbohydrates by near-infrared reflectance. Clin Chem 42: 309-312
18. Wetzel D (1983) Near-infrared reflectance analysis. Sleeper among spectroscopic techniques. Anal Chem 55: 1165A-1171A
19. Nyquist RA, Leugers MA, McKelvy ML, Papenfuss RR, Putzig CL, Yurga L (1990) Infrared spectroscopy. Anal Chem 62: 223-255R
20. Draper NM, Smith H (1981) Applied regression analysis, 2nd ed. New York: Wiley
21. Mark H, Workmann J (1986) Effect of repack on calibrations produced for near-infrared reflectance analysis. Anal Chem 58: 1454-1459
22. Peuchant E, Salles C, Jensen R (1987) Determination of serum cholesterol by near-infrared reflectance spectroscopy. Anal Chem 59: 1816-1819
23. Geladi P, MacDougall D, Martens H (1985) Linearization and scatter-correction for near-infrared reflectance spectra of meat. Appl Spectrosc 39: 491-500
24. Sobel W, Bowers A. (1964) In: Henry RJ, ed. Clinical chemistry: principles and techniques. New York: Harper and Row. 881-889
25. Benini L, Caliari S, Bonfate F, Guidi GC, Brentegani MT, Castellani G, Sembenini C, Bardelli E, Vantin I (1992) Near infrared reflectance measurement of nitrogen faecal losses. Gut 33: 749-752
26. Grimble GK, West MF, Acuti AB, Rees RG, Hunian MK, Webster JD, Frost PG, Silk DB (1988) Assessment of an automated chemiluminescence nitrogen analyzer for routine use in clinical nutrition. J Parent Ent Nutr 12: 100-106

27. DiMagno EP, Go VLW, Summerskill HJ (1973) Relations between pancreatic enzyme outputs and malabsorption in severe pancreatic insufficiency. New Engl J Med 288: 813–815
28. Ammann RW, Akovbiantz A, Haecki W, Largiader F, Schmid M (1981) Diagnostic value of the fecal chymotrypsin test in pancreatic insufficiency, particularly chronic pancreatitis: correlation with the pancreozymin-secretion test, fecal fat excretion and final clinical diagnosis. Digestion 21: 281–289
29. Adler G, Weidenbach F (1986) Fecal chymotrypsin in chronic pancreatitis disease. In: Malfertheiner P, Ditschuneit H, eds. Diagnostic procedures in pancreatic diseases. Berlin: Springer-Verlag, 231–241
30. Dyck WP (1967) Titrimetric measurements of fecal trypsin and chymotrypsin in cystic fibrosis. Am J Dig Dis 12: 310–317
31. Lami F, Callegari C, Miglioli M, Barbara L (1984) A single-specimen fecal chymotrypsin test in the diagnosis of pancreatic insufficiency: correlation with the secretion-cholecystokinin and NBT-PABA test. Am J Gastroenterol 79: 697–700
32. Duerr HK, Otte M, Forell MM, Bode JC (1978) Fecal chymotrypsin: a study on its diagnostic value by comparison with the secretin-cholecystokinin-test. Digestion 17: 404–409
33. Sale JK, Goldberg DM, Thjodleifson B, Wormsley KG (1974) Trypsin and chymotrypsin in duodenal aspirate and feces in response to secretin and cholecystokinin-pancreozymin. Gut 15: 132–138
34. Dyck W, Ammann RW (1965) Quantitative determination of fecal chymotrypsin as a screening test for pancreatic exocrine insufficiency. Am J Dig 10: 530–545
35. Müller L, Wisniewski ZS, Hansky J (1970) The measurement of fecal chymotrypsin: a screening test for pancreatic exocrine insufficiency. Aust Ann Med 19: 47–49
36. Sziegoleit A (1984) A novel proteinase from human pancreas. Biochemical J 219: 735–742
37. Sziegoleit A, Krause E, Klör HU, Kanacher L, Linder D (1989) Elastase and chymotrypsin B in pancreatic juice and feces. Clin Biochem 22: 85–89
38. Sziegoleit A, Linder D (1991) Studies on the sterol-binding capacity of human pancreatic elastase. Gastroenterology 100: 768–774
39. Stein J, Jung M, Sziegoleit A, Zeuzem S, Caspary WF, Lembcke B (1996) Fecal immunoreactive elastase-1: Clinical evaluation of a new tubeless pancreatic function test. Clin Chem 42: 222–226
40. Creutzfeldt W (1964) Funktionsdiagnostik bei Erkrankungen des exokrinen Pankreas. Verh Dtsch Ges Inn Med 70: 781–801
41. Lankisch PG, Schreiber A, Otto J (1983) Pancreolauryl-test. Evaluation of a tubeless pancreatic test in comparison with other indirect and direct tests for exocrine pancreatic function. Dig Dis Sci 28: 490–493
42. Dyck W, Ammann RW (1965) Quantitative determination of fecal chymotrypsin as screening test for pancreatic exocrine insufficiency. Am J Dig 10: 530–545
43. Ammann RW, Tagwercher E, Dashiwagi H, Roasenmund H (1968) Diagnostic value of fecal chymotrypsin and trypsin assessment for detection of pancreatic disease. Am J Dig Dis 13: 123–146
44. Ammann RW, Akovbiantz A, Haecki W, Lrgiader F, Schmid M (1981) Diagnostic value of fecal the fecal chymotrypsin test in pancreatic insufficiency, particularly chronic pancreatitis: correlation with the pancreozymin-test, fecal fat excretion and final diagnosis. Digestion 21: 261–269
45. Muench R, Ammann RW (1992) Fecal immunoreactive lipase: a new tubeless pancreatic function test. Scand J Gastroenterol 27: 289–294
46. Dominguez-Muñoz JE, Hieronymus C, Sauerbruch T, Malfertheiner P (1995) Fecal elastase test: Evaluation of a new noninvasive pancreatic function test. Am J Gastroenterol 90: 1834–1837
47. Löser C, Moligeard A, Fölsch U (1996) Fecal elastase 1-A novel, highly sensitive and specific tubeless pancreatic function test for easy routine application. Gastroenterology 110: A 31

Extracellular Matrix in Pancreatic Diseases

F. Müller-Pillasch · T. Gress · G. Adler

Pancreatic Cancer

It has been suggested that extracellular matrix (ECM) components play an important role in the strong desmoplastic reaction observed in pancreatic cancer, which is characterised by remarkable proliferation of interstitial connective tissue [1]. Quantitative analysis of collagen subtypes I, III and V in human pancreatic cancer, tumour-associated chronic pancreatitis (TACP) and alcoholic chronic pancreatitis (AICP) showed that mean collagen content was elevated in both pancreatic cancer and TACP tissue and to a lesser extent in AICP. The compositional proportions of type I, III and V appear to be similar in all tissues examined compared to normal pancreatic tissues [2]. In grade I and II tumours of the pancreas, collagen type I and fibronectin form small septa between tumorous structures whereas in grade III tumours, fibronectin and collagen type I were present as unoriented thick fibrous bundles. In large areas of the tumour, connective tissue was the main constituent of the ECM [3]. Laminin, a major component of basement membranes, was found only in well-differentiated pancreatic tumour tissue whereas, with progressive dedifferentiation, basal laminin was absent or discontinuously expressed [3, 4]. Similar expression patterns of basal laminar components were observed in colorectal carcinoma [5] and breast carcinoma [6]. In vitro cultivation of pancreatic carcinoma cell lines on laminin substrates resulted in an arrest of proliferation, while normal proliferation was found on collagen type I and fibronectin substrates [3]. Tumour progression starts with focal proliferation of cancer cells, often followed by invasion into the surrounding connective tissue supported by degradation of the extracellular matrix. In recent years, the role of extracellular matrix degrading proteases in tumour diseases has been the subject of intense studies. In this context, matrix metalloproteinases (MMPs) and their specific inhibitors (tissue inhibitors of metalloproteinases, TIMPs) were shown to be of major significance. Matrix metalloproteinases (MMPs) are enzymes which degrade the collagenous and non-collagenous components of extracellular matrix [7]. Their activity results in extensive tissue damage, and they have been associated with a variety of disease processes, including tumour cell invasion and inflammatory diseases. MMP-1, MMP-2, MMP-3 and MMP-9 are the most important matrix metalloproteinases with different substrate specificities. MMP-1 (interstitial collagenase) degrades type I, II and III collagens. MMP-3 (stromelysin) is responsible for the degradation of proteoglycans, laminin, fibronectin, gelatins and collagen type III, IV and V. MMP-2 (72-kDa collagenase type IV) and MMP-9 (92-kDa collagenase type IV) degrade collagens IV and V and, to a lesser extent, laminin and fibronectin [8]. MMPs are secreted as latent proenzymes in zymogen form and require removal of N-terminal peptides for activation [9, 10]. The activity of MMPs is regulated by endogenous proteins known as tissue inhibitors of metalloproteinases (TIMPs) [8]. Activated MMP-1 and MMP-3 and latent forms of MMP-2 and MMP-9 bind to and are inhibited by TIMP-1 and TIMP-2. However, TIMP-1 shows preferential binding to MMP-9 and TIMP-2 to MMP-2 [11, 12]. Alterations of the balance of expression between MMPs and TIMPs in inflammatory diseases has been shown, e.g. in active rheumatoid arthritis [13], Hashimoto's thyreoditis [14] and in chronic pancreatitis [15]. In most cases, expression of MMPs and TIMPs was shown to correlate with an increased metastatic and invasive potential of tumour cells [16-18].

Recently, Gress and coworkers presented a report describing the balance of expression between extracellular matrix genes and genes encoding ECM-degrading proteases and their specific inhibitors in human pancreatic cancer [19]. Elevated steady-state levels of mRNA of extracellular matrix components, including collagen types I, III and IV, fibronectin and laminin, were observed in all pancreatic cancer tissue samples examined. Expression of MMP-1 (interstitial collagenase) and MMP-3 (stromelysin) was too low in controls (healthy pancreas) and in pancreatic cancer tissue to allow detection by standard Northern blot analysis and in situ hybridisation. Increased mRNA levels of MMP-2 (72-kDa collagenase type IV), MMP-9 (92-kDa collagenase type IV), TIMP-1 and TIMP-2 were observed in all pancreatic cancer tissues (Fig. 1). Expression levels of MMPs, TIMPs and of genes coding for extracellular matrix proteins could not be correlated to tumour stage and differentiation, whereas there seemed to be a close correlation between these MMPs and TIMPs and the steady state levels of transcripts coding for extracellular matrix proteins, the amount of collagen protein and the extent of the desmoplastic reaction.

In-situ hybridisation was performed to clarify which cell type in pancreatic carcinoma tissue is responsible for elevated tanscripts of collagen I and III pro-

Fig. 1. Northern blots with total RNA from pancreatic cancer and control tissues (four lanes of each tissue; cancer, CA, and control, CO) hybridised with ^{32}P-labelled probes for: matrix metalloproteinases MMP-1 (interstitial collagenase), MMP-2 (72-kDa type IV collagenase), MMP-3 (stromelysin-1), MMP-9 (92-kDa type IV collagenase), tissue inhibitor of metalloproteinase TIMP-1, TIMP-2, COLI (collagen α_1 type I), COLIV (collagen type IV), LAM (Laminin), FIBRO (fibronectin), 18S (18S rNA)

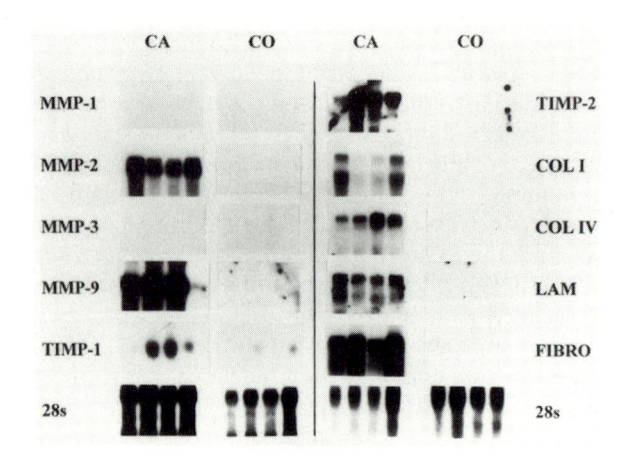

Fig. 2 a, b. Collagen histochemistry and in situ hybridisation. **a** Paraffin-embedded tissue from human pancreatic cancer tissue was stained with sirus red which binds selectively to collagenous protein. Note the *wide dark bands* of collagen fibres separating islands of acinar tissue. **b** Paraffin-embedded tissue was hybridised with an antisense probe for collagen type III mRNA. Silver grain label is predominantly located over connective tissue fibroblasts in the vicinity of tumour cells

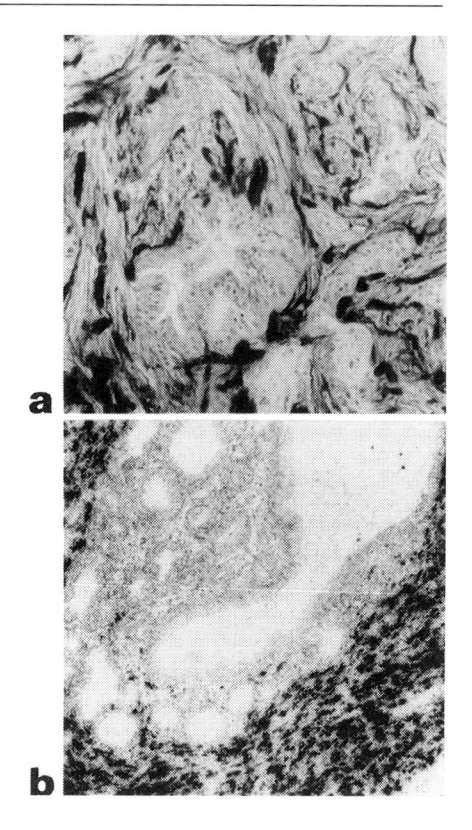

tein. As shown in Fig. 2, collagen transcription and protein synthesis are localised to spindle-shaped cells in the tumour stroma, due to the results of previous studies, which demonstrated an increased level of interstitial connective tissue components by immunohistochemical analysis [3]. Connective tissue cells in the neighbourhood of tumour cells appear to contain larger amounts of silver grains than stromal cells distant from the tumour. This phenomenon could be due to growth factors synthesised by pancreatic cancer cells, e.g. transforming growth factor TGF-β [20], which is known to stimulate the synthesis of extracellular matrix components [21, 22]. Gress and coworkers found collagen transcript and protein in acinar cells, duct cells, islet cells or inflammatory cells [19]. However, Löhr and coworkers [23] demonstrated by the use of expression studies in human ductal adenocarcinoma cell lines that human pancreatic cancer cells are capable of synthesising a variety of extracellular matrix proteins in vitro. However, based on the in vivo data reported above, stromal cells appear to be the main site of ECM-production in pancreatic cancer tissues.

It has been shown in vitro that tumour cell lines express MMPs and TIMPs at the transcript and protein levels [24, 25]. Using in situ hybridisation studies, we were able to demonstrate elevated transcript levels of MMP-2, MMP-9, TIMP-1 and TIMP-2 in both stromal and tumour cells in human pancreatic cancer tissues. MMP-2 transcripts appeared to be more abundant in stromal cells and MMP-9 transcripts were found predominantly in tumour cells. TIMP-1 and TIMP-2 transcripts were evenly distributed among stromal and tumour cells. Although the differences in MMP-2 and MMP-9 observed among stromal and tumour cells were consistent, they were too discrete to allow any valid conclusion concerning the biological significance of this observation. Therefore, we have to assume that in pancreatic cancer tissue both stromal and tumour cells are the source of the designated MMPs and TIMPs. The fact that MMP-2, MMP-9, TIMP-1 and TIMP-2 are overexpressed in pancreatic cancer tissues indicates that these proteins may be major players in processes leading to the strong desmoplastic reaction observed in these tumours.

Chronic Pancreatitis

It has been suggested that extracellular matrix components play an important role not only in the strong desmoplastic reaction in pancreatic carcinoma, but also in fibrosis of chronic pancreatitis. Chronic inflammatory diseases of the pancreas are characterised by destruction of acinar tissue and replacement by connective tissue. An increase and disorganisation of extracellular matrix (ECM) components including laminin, collagen IV and fibronectin in the basal lamina and collagens I, III and IV, procollagen III and fibronectin in the interstitial tissue was visualised by immunohistochemistry in chronic pancreatitis tissue samples [26, 27]. As in pancreatic cancer, we performed expression studies for genes encoding extracellular matrix components and for genes encoding extracellular matrix degrading proteases (MMPs) and their specific inhibitors (TIMPs) in tissues from patients with chronic pancreatitis [15]. Transcripts for interstitial collagenase (MMP-1) and stromelysin (MMP-3) were not detectable in all examined tissues from chronic pancreatitis and healthy pancreatic tissues by standard Northern blot hybridisation. Steady state levels of transcripts encoding extracellular matrix components, MMP-2 (72-kDa collagenase IV), TIMP-1 and TIMP-2 were elevated in seven out of eight chronic pancreatic tissue samples and showed a large degree of variation among the different chronic pancreatitis tissue samples (Fig. 3).

The magnitude of MMP/TIMP transcript levels could not be correlated to the degree of fibrosis and inflammation detectable by histological analysis or to the total amount of deposited collagen protein, which was high in all chronic pancreatitis tissue samples examined. With in situ hybridisation, the connective tissue cells could be identified as the main site of collagen I and III transcription in chronic pancreatitis. Deposition of collagen protein into the extracellular matrix may reflect fibrosis as a result of chronic and repeated acute inflammation, whereas collagen transcripts localised in fibroblasts of the ECM may be an indicator for the ongoing activity of processes leading to pancreatic fibrosis. Whereas in the case of interstitial extracellular matrix components, such as collagens type I and III and fibronectin, increased expression appears to be the major alteration in chronic pancreatitis, the main alterations observed for basal lamina components (collagen type IV and laminin) were changes of distribu-

Fig. 3 A–H. Northern blots with total RNA from chronic pancreatitis (*P*) and control tissues (*C*) hybridised with ^{32}P-labelled probes for **A** collagen type I, **B** collagen type III, **C** collagen type IV, **D** laminin, **E** fibronectin, **F** matrix metalloproteinase (MMP)-2, **G** tissue inhibitor of metalloproteinase (TIMP)-2, **H** 18S rRNA

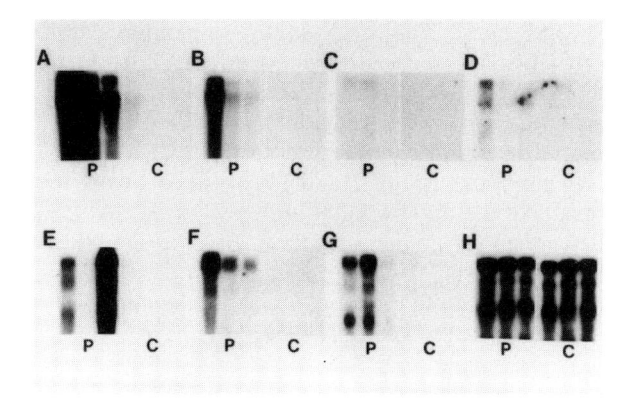

tion pattern within the tissue (extension from basal lamina into the adjacent interstitial matrix or absence from the basal lamina of ducts containing precipitates) [4, 27]. As shown in Fig. 3, it appears that transcripts of genes encoding extracellular matrix-degrading proteases with a substrate specificity for interstitial extracellular matrix components (MMP-1 and MMP-3) were not elevated in chronic pancreatitis despite the enormous increase in interstitial extracellular matrix components [15]. Possibly, the lack of MMP-1 and MMP-2 expression contributes to the deposition of ECM components in the interstitial space. In contrast, the 72-kDa collagenase type IV (MMP-2) with a substrate specificity for collagens type IV and V, gelatin and fibronectin showed increased transcript levels in chronic pancreatitis. In addition, we were able to demonstrate that MMP-2 overexpression in chronic pancreatitis was accompanied by a parallel rise of TIMP-2 transcript levels. TIMP-2 has been described to bind preferentially to MMP-2 in a 1:1 molar ratio [11, 12]. This parallel increase of a protease and its specific inhibitor in chronic pancreatitis may be part of an autoregulatory mechanism of extracellular matrix degradation and remodelling.

Serum Levels of Extracellular Matrix Components in Acute and Chronic Pancreatitis

Useful tools for the diagnosis of chronic pancreatitis are the conventional imaging methods such as ultrasonography, computed tomography and endoscopic retrograde pancreatography. Morphological and biochemical processes leading to pancreatic fibrosis are still poorly understood. The detection of markers that reflect pancreatic fibrogenetic activity in chronic pancreatitis could be useful in the follow-up of patients with chronic pancreatitis, as parameters for the prediction of disease progression.

Monitoring of the serum levels of connective tissue components was suggested as a useful approach to follow the involvement of extracellular matrix components in repair processes in response to inflammatory events in liver, lung, skin and other organs [28]. The aminoterminal procollagen type III peptide (PIIINP) is released from procollagen III during the extracellular synthesis of collagen and thereafter circulates in the plasma [29]. Circulating PIIINP is elevated in many fibrosing diseases, including liver [30] and rheumatic [31] diseases. In addition, increased serum PIIINP levels have been correlated with inflammation, necrosis and fibrogenesis in the liver [32]. Figure 4 shows the results of a study by Adler and coworkers [33] designed to examine the time-dependent serum concentrations of extracellular matrix proteins (PIIINP, laminin, hyaluronic acid) in patients with severe and moderate acute pancreatitis and in those with an acute attack of chronic pancreatitis. Only in severe acute pancreatitis all three parameters increased. In patients who died as a conse-

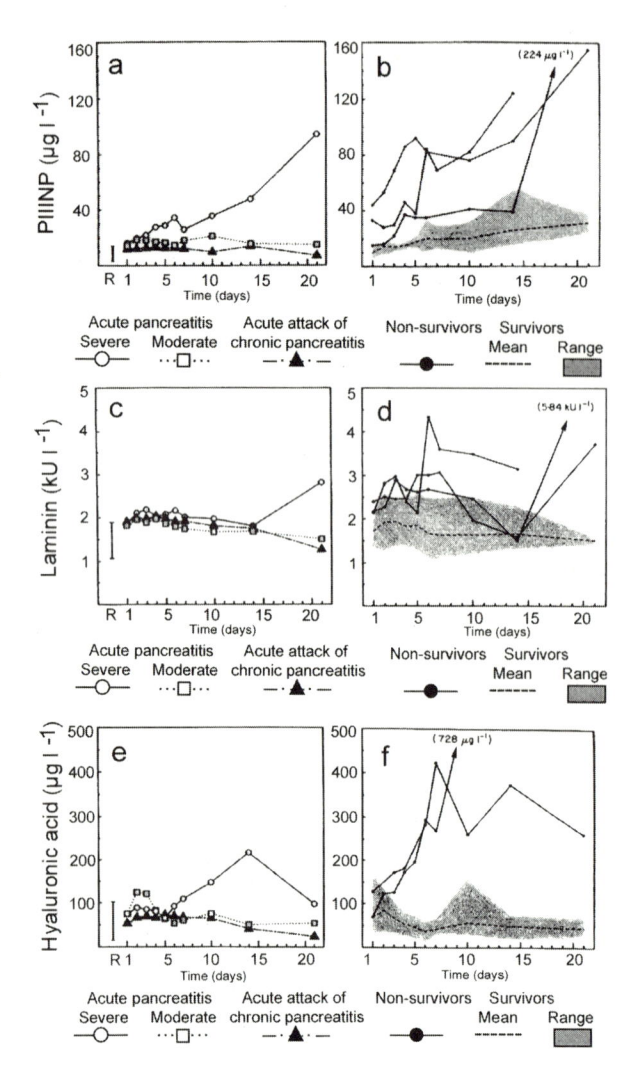

Fig. 4 a–f. Mean serum concentrations of **a, b** procollagen type III peptide (PIIINP), **c, d** laminin and **e, f** hyaluronic acid within different disease groups in relation to the time after onset of acute pancreatitis. **a, c, e** Total population of the study. Mean values are given for each patient group. **b, d, f** Differentiation between survivors and non-survivors within the severe acute pancreatitis group. Individual values are shown for non-survivors and compared with the concentration range (*shaded area*) found for survivors

quence of sepsis and multi-organ failure, the increase in PIIINP, laminin and hyaluronic acid was more pronounced. There seems to be a relationship between the severity of acute pancreatitis and the increase in serum concentrations of PIIINP.

Others authors have described elevated levels of PIIINP in patients with chronic pancreatitis, although PIIINP did not correlate with the duration and morphological and functional stage of the disease [34]. Navarro and coworkers also investigated the serum PIIINP level in patients with chronic pancreatitis and evaluated the relationship between the PIIINP level and pancreatectomy, pancreatic fibrogenesis and exocrine pancreatic function [35]. In this study, serum PIIINP values were significantly higher in patients with chronic pancreatitis without liver disease than in the control group. Moreover, they found a correlation between the PIIINP serum level and the severity of pancreatic fibrogenetic activity, but no relationship between pancreatic exocrine function and duration of disease and PIIINP. Thus, it has been suggested that PIIINP could be a useful marker for chronic pancreatitis without liver disease.

However, metabolic clearance rates of extracellular matrix components may be influenced by the severity of the common complications in acute pancreatitis, such as multi-organ failure in acute pancreatitis. In addition, the reported data on serum levels of ECM components in chronic pancreatitis is slightly variable. Further studies including a larger number of patients are required to confirm the prognostic value of serum levels of matrix components in inflammatory pancreatic diseases.

Caerulein-Induced Acute Pancreatitis in Rats

Data on the dynamic processes of biosynthesis, deposition and breakdown of extracellular matrix proteins during pancreatitis is available only from animal studies. In rat, acute pancreatitis induced by intraductal injection of trypsin was combined with increased deposition of extracellular matrix proteins and a rise in hydroxyproline concentration [36]. A similar time course of deposition and regression of collagen was observed during regeneration of caerulein-induced pancreatitis in the rat. Pancreatic regeneration from caerulein-induced pancreatitis is characterised by proliferation of acinar and centroacinar cells, an increase in mitotic activity of fibroblasts and stimulation of synthesis and deposition of collagen [37, 38]. Approximately 2 weeks after induction of pancreatitis, histology, organ weight and collagen content of the pancreas returned to normal control values, indicating complete regeneration [38]. One day after induction of caerulein-pancreatitis in rats, fibroblast proliferation was increased 30-fold [37]. Twenty-four hours later, collagen protein synthesis was stimulated 15-fold [38] and was accompanied by a significant, but transient, deposition of interstitial collagen. A similar time course could be observed for collagen I and III transcript levels, indicating the involvement of transcriptional mechanisms either by increased transcription rates or by inhibition of collagen mRNA degradation [39]. The rapid changes in fibroblast function observed during regeneration result from the complex regulation of this cell type by a broad spectrum of mediators [40, 41], TGF-β being one of the most potent and best defined. TGF-β was found to be present in cells of nearly every origin, with a prevalence of mesenchymal-derived cells, and to be highly pleiotropic by modulating a variety of different biological processes [42]. It stimulates proliferation of connective tissue cells, while it is a potent inhibitor of cell proliferation in others, such as lymphocytes and most epithelial cells [40, 42]. TGF-β has been shown to be an important modulator of the extracellular matrix (ECM) by interfering with a number of essential processes such as synthesis of ECM components [21, 22]. Excessive production of TGF-β or abnormal sensitivity of target cells to its actions has been suggested to contribute to the pathogenesis of a number of diseases characterised by aberrant inflammation, hyperproliferation and fibrosis [43, 44].

We determined the expression pattern of TGF-β1, as the most potent regulator of the extracellular matrix, during regneration from caerulein-induced pancreatitis in the rat, in particular in comparison with the well-studied alterations of the pancreatic extracellular matrix. Active TGF-β protein content in total pancreas reached peak values after one day, with protein levels remaining high throughout the second day and returning to normal on the seventh day of regeneration. In situ hybridisation revealed only low levels of TGF-β1 mRNA in acinar cells, islets cells and duct cells of control animals. Two days after the end of maximal caerulein infusion, the amount of TGF-β1 mRNA was approximately three times higher than in controls (Fig. 5), with exocrine acinar cells and stromal cells containing the largest amount of TGF-β1 transcripts. Seven days after the end of caerulein infusion, TGF-β1 protein levels dropped to control values, whereas TGF-β1 mRNA remained slightly elevated. The time course

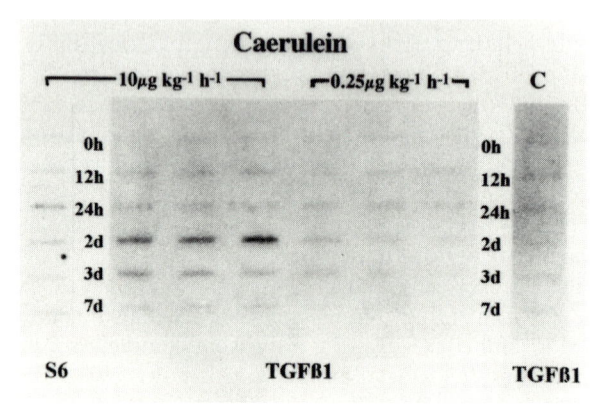

Fig. 5. Slot-blot hybridisations for transforming growth factor *TGF-β1* illustrating representative results observed at different time points after induction of pancreatitis (10 μg kg^{-1} h^{-1}; 0 h to 7 days) and after submaximal stimulation (0.25 μg kg^{-1} h^{-1}; 0 h to 7 days). *S6*, hybridisation with a cDNA probe for the S6 gene onto slot-blots from caerulein-treated animals at different time points to normalise eventual unequal loading of RNA. The single lane on the *right side* shows the transcript level of TGF-β1 in pancreata of control animals (*C*) infused with saline. Each slot contains 15 μg total RNA from rat pancreata. Exposure was 7 days at −70 C°C for TGF-β1, and 5 h at −70 °C for S6 hybridisations

of TGF-β1 transcript levels was similar to the time course observed for collagen α_1 (I) and α_1 (III) transcripts.

The early maximal increase in TGF-β1 protein content 24 h after induction of pancreatitis could not be correlated with an equivalent rise of specific mRNA, reaching peak values at earliest 24 h later. TGF-β1 released from α-granules of platelets found as aggregates in pancreatic blood vessels may be the source of this early rise of protein. Alternatively, inflammatory cells such as macrophages and leukocytes could be responsible for the early increase in TGF-β1 protein content as shown, for example for the model of bleomycin-induced lung fibrosis [45]. As TGF-β1 is known to induce its own synthesis in an autoregulatory way, it is possible that TGF-β1 protein initially released from platelets or inflammatory cells during regeneration of pancreatitis may induce its own de novo synthesis in the rat pancreas. In summary, expression of TGF-β1 in acinar and stromal cells of the rat pancreas is enhanced during regeneration from caerulein-induced pancreatitis, which may indicate an involvement of TGF-β1 in the regulation of extracellular matrix regeneration in the rat pancreas after caerulein-induced pancreatitis. In addition, it has been shown that TGF-β1 transcript levels are elevated in patients with chronic pancreatitis. These studies demonstrated that TGF-β1 is mainly located in mononuclear cells in fibrotic areas and ductal epithelium [46, 47]. Finally, pancreatic tissue of transgenic mice expressing TGF-β1 in pancreatic β-islet cells under the control of the human insulin promoter was characterised by fibrosis, infiltration of monocytes and neutrophils, developmental dysregulation and induction of ECM protein synthesis [48]. Thus TGF-β1 has been suggested to be involved in the development of fibrosis in chronic pancreatitis.

The Influence of TGF-α Expression on the Extracellular Matrix

As another member of the superfamily of transforming growth factors, TGF-α has been suggested to be involved not only in carcinogenesis in the pancreas but in fibrosis of chronic pancreatitis as well. Transgenic mice that overexpress TGF-α exhibit an increase in size of the pancreas which has been suggested to be the result of extensive ECM production. Except for the absence of inflammatory cells, morphology of the pancreas of transgenic mice is similar to that found in patients with chronic pancreatitis [49]. It is not known yet whether TFG-α overexpression is responsible for the histological changes observed in the pancreas of transgenic mice. Binding of TGF-α to its cellular receptor EGFR (epidermal growth factor receptor) may result in the activation of subsequent signal transduction pathways which in turn may alter cellular function to induce the histopathological changes in the pancreas of mice overexpressing TGF-α. To study the influence of TGF-α on the expression of genes encoding extracellular matrix components and genes encoding extracellular matrix degrading proteases and their specific inhibitors, we used transgenic mice overexpressing TGF-α under the control of the mouse elastase promoter. We were able to show that in the pancreas of these transgenic mice the mRNA level of collagen types III and IV, laminin B_1 and B_2 and fibronection were approximately 1.5 to two times higher than those in the pancreas from control mice. A similar increase of transcript levels was observed for the tissue inhibitor of metalloproteinases TIMP-1 and TIMP-2. It appears that TGF-α has no or only little influence on the transcription of genes encoding ECM-degrading proteases (unpublished data). These alterations of gene expression may be a primary direct or secondary effect of TGF-α overexpression, indicating that this growth factor may be involved in processes leading to fibrosis of the pancreas. Interestingly, mRNA concentrations of EGFR and TGF-α were increased in the pancreas of patients with chronic pancreatitis. EGFR as well as TGF-α appear to be expressed at high concentrations in pancreatic ducts and acinar cells in chronic pancreatitis tissues [50]. It has been suggested that TGF-α overexpression in these cells leads to duct cell proliferation, modulation of acinar cell function and enhancement of collagen production. These processes may participate in the development of fibrosis in chronic pancreatitis. This hypothesis is supported by the observation that transcript levels of TGF-α and EGFR are elevated in pancreatic cancer tissue and may thus be partly responsible for formation of the strong desmoplastic reaction found in these cancer tissues [51].

References

1. Klöppel G (1993) Pathology of nonendocrine pancreatic tumors. In: Go VLW, DiMagno EP, Gardner JD, Lebenthal E, Reber HA, Scheele GA (eds). The Pancreas: biology, pathobiology and disease. Raven, New York; 2nd ed: 871–897
2. Imamura T, Iguchi H, Manabe T, Ohshio G, Yoshimura T, Wang Z, Suwa H, Ishigami S, Imamura M (1995) Quantitative analysis of collagen and collagen subtypes I, III, and V in human pancreatic cancer, tumor-associated chronic pancreatitis and alcoholic chronic pancreatitis. Pancreas 11: 357–364
3. Mollenhauer J, Roether I, Kern H (1987) Distribution of extracellular matrix proteins in pancreatic ductal adenocarcinoma and its influence on tumor cell proliferation in vitro. Pancreas 2: 14–24
4. Shimoyama S, Gansauge F, Gansauge S, Takeshi O, Beger HG (1995) Altered expression of extracellular matrix molecules and their receptors in chronic pancreatitis and pancreatic adenocarcinoma in comparison with normal pancreas. Int J Pancreatol 18: 227–234
5. Havenith MG, Arends JW, Simon R, Volovics A, Wiggers T, Bosman FT (1988) Type IV collagen immunoreactivity in colorectal cancer. Cancer 62: 2207–2211
6. D'Ardenne AJ, Richman PI, Horton MA, Mcaulay AE, Jordan S (1991) Coordinate expression of alpha-6 integrin laminin receptor subunit and laminin in breast cancer. J Pathol 165: 213–220
7. Matrisian LM (1990) Metalloproteinases and their inhibitors in matrix remodeling. TIG 6: 121
8. Chen WT (1992) Membrane proteases: roles in tissue remodeling and tumour invasion. Curr Opinon Cell Biol 4: 802–809
9. Stetler-Stevenson W, Krutzsch HC, Wacher MP, Margulies IMK, Liotta LA (1989) The activation of human type IV collagenase proenzyme. J Biol Chem 264: 1353–1356
10. Howard EW, Bullen EC, Banda MJ (1991) Regulation of the autoactivation of human 72 kDa progelatinase by tissue inhibitor of metalloproteinase-2. J Biol Chem 266: 13064–13069
11. De Clerck YA, Yean TD, Lu HS, Ting J, Langley KE (1991) Inhibition of autoproteolytic activation of interstitial procollagenase by recombinant metalloproteinase inhibitor MI/TIMP-2. J Biol Chem 266: 3893–3899
12. Goldberg GI, Marmer BL, Grant GA, Eisen AZ, Wilhelm S, He C (1989) Human 72 kDa type IV collagenase forms a complex with a tissue inhibitor of metalloproteinases designated TIMP-2. Proc Natl Acad Sci USA 86: 8207–8211

13. Unemori EN, Hibbs MS, Amento EP (1991) Constitutive expression of 92 kd gelatinase (type V collagenase) by rheumatoid synovial fibroblasts and its induction in normal human fibroblasts by inflammatory cytokines. J Clin Invest 88: 1656–1662
14. Campo E, Merino MJ, Liotta L, Neumann R, Stetler-Stevenson W (1992) Distribution of the 72kd type IV collagenase in nonneoplastic thyroid tissue. Hum Pathol 23: 1395–1401
15. Gress TM, Müller-Pillasch F, Lerch MM, Friess H, Büchler M, Beger HG, Adler G (1994) Balance of expression of genes coding for extracellular matrix proteins and extracellular matrix degrading proteases in chronic pancreatitis. Z Gastroenterol 32: 211–225
16. Levy AT, Cioce V, Sobel ME, Spiridone G, Grigoioni WF, Liotta A (1991) Increased expression of the Mr 72,000 type-IV collagenase in human colonic adenocarcinoma. Cancer Res 51: 439–444
17. Muller D, Wolf C, Abecassis J, Millon J, Engelmann A, Bonner G, Rouyer N, Rio MC, Eber M, Methlin G, Chambon P, Basset P (1993) Increased stromelysin 3 gene expression is associated with increased local invasiveness in head and nack squamous cell carcinomas. Cancer Res 53: 165–169
18. Stearns ME, Wang M (1993) Type IV collagenase (Mr72000) expression in human prostate: benign and malignant tissue. Cancer Res 53: 878–883
19. Gress TM, Müller-Pillasch F, Lerch MM, Friess H, Büchler M, Adler G (1995) Expression and in-situ localization of genes coding for extracellular matrix proteins and extracellular matrix degrading proteases in pancreatic cancer. Int J Cancer 62: 407–413
20. Friess H, Yamanaka Y, Büchler M, Ebert M, Beger HG, Gold LI, Korc M (1993) Enhanced expression of transforming growth factor β isoforms in pancreatic cancer correlates with decreased survival. Gastroenterology 105: 1846–1856
21. Roberts AB, Sporn MB, Assoian RK, Smith JM, Roche NS, Wakefield LM, Heine UI, Liotta LA, Falanga V, Kerhl JH, Fauci AS (1986) Transforming growth factor type-beta: Rabit induction of fibrosis and angiogenesis in vivo and stimulation of collagen formation in vitro. Proc Natl Acad Sci 83: 4167–4171
22. Ishikawa O, Yamakage A, LeRoy EC, Trojanowska M (1990) Persistent effect of TGFβ1 on extracellular matrix gene expression in human dermal fibroblasts. Biochem Biophys Res Commun 169: 232–238
23. Löhr M, Trautmann B, Göttler M, Peters S, Zauner I, Maillet B, Klöppel G (1994) Human ductal adenocarcinomas of the pancreas express extracellular matrix proteins. Br J Cancer 69: 144–151
24. Stetler-Stevenson WG, Krutzsch HC, Liotta LA. Tissue inhibitor of metalloproteinase (TIMP-2) (1989) A new member of the metalloproteinase inhibitor family. J Biol Chem 264: 17374–17378
25. Sato H, Takino T, Okada Y, Cao J, Shinagawa A, Yamamoto E, Seiki M (1994) A matrix-metalloproteinase expressed on the surface of invasive tumor cells. Nature 370: 61–65
26. Bedossa P, Lemaigre G, Bacci J, Martin E (1989) Quantitative estimation of the collagen content in normal and pathological pancreatic tissue. Digestion 44: 7–13
27. Kennedy RH, Bockmann DE, Usganga L, Choux R, Grimaud JA, Sarles H (1987) Pancreatic extracellular matrix alterations in chronic pancreatitis. Pancreas 2: 61–72
28. Risteli L, Risteli J (1986) Radioimmunoassays for monitoring connective tissue metabolism. Rheumatology 10: 216–245
29. Smedsröd B (1988) Aminoterminal propeptide of type III procollagen is cleared from the circulation by receptor-mediated endocytosis in liver endothelial cells. Collagen Rel Res 8: 375–388
30. Torres-Salinas M, Parés A, Caballería J, Jiménez W, Heredia J, Bruguera M, Rodés J (1986) Serum procollagen type III peptide as a marker of hepatic fibrogenesis in alcoholic hepatitis. Gastroenterology 90: 1241–1246
31. Horsley-Petersen K (1990) Circulating extracellular matrix components as markers for connective tissue response to inflammation. A clinical and experimental study with special emphasis on serum aminoterminal type III procollagen peptide in rheumatic disease. Dan Med Bull 37: 308–329
32. Plebani M, Burlina A (1991) Biochemical markers fibrosis. Clin Biochem 24: 219–239
33. Adler G, Kropf J, Grobe E, Gressner AM (1990) Follow-up the serum level of extracellular matrix components in acute and chronic pancreatitis. Eur. J Clin Invest 20: 494–501
34. Domínguez-Muñoz JE, Manes G, Büchler M, Malfertheiner P (1993) Assessment of the fibrogenetic activity in chronic pancreatitis. Int J Pancreatol 14: 253–259
35. Navarro S, Valderrama R, Lopez J, Giménez A, Caballería J, Parés A, Fernandez-Cruz L (1996) Serum amino-terminal propeptide of type III procollagen levels in chronic pancreatitis. Pancreas 12: 153–158

36. Uscanga L, Kennedy RH, Choux R, Druguet M, Grimaud JA, Sarles H (1987) Sequential connective matrix changes in experimental acute pancreatitis. An immunohistochemical and biochemical assessment in the rat. Int J Pancreatol 2: 33-45
37. Elsässer HP, Adler G, Kern HF (1986) Time course and cellular source of pancreatic regeneration following acute pancreatitis in the rat. Pancreas 1: 421-429
38. Elsässer HP, Adler G, Kern HF (1989) Fibroblast structure and function during regeneration from hormone-induced acute pancreatitis in the rat. Pancreas 4: 169-178
39. Gress TM, Müller-Pillasch F, Elsässer HP, Bachem M, Ferrara C, Weidenbach H, Lerch M, Adler G (1994) Enhancement of transforming growth factor β1 expression in the rat pancreas during regneration from caerulein-induced pancreatitis. Eur J Clin Invest 24: 679-685
40. Sporn MB, Roberts AB (1988) Peptide growth factors are multifunctional. Nature 332: 212-219
41. Roberts AB, Heine UI, Flanders KC, Sporn MB (1990) Transforming growth factor-β. Major role in regulation of extracellular matrix. Ann NY Acad Sci 593: 226-232
42. Sporn MB, Roberts AB, Wakefield LM, de Crombrugghe B (1987) Some recent advances in the chemistry and biology of transforming growth factor-β. J Cell Biol 105: 1039-1045
43. Broekelmann TJ, Limper AH, Colby TV, Mc Donald JA (1991) Transforming growth factor β1 is present at sites of extracellular matrix gene expression in human pulmonary fibrosis. Proc Natl Acad Sci USA 88: 6642-6646
44. Castilla A, Prieto J, Fausto N (1991) Transforming growth factor β1 and α in chronic liver disease. New Engl J Med 324: 933-940
45. Khalil N, Greenberg AH (1991) The role of TGF-β in pulmonary fibrosis. Ciba Foundation Symposium 157: 194-211
46. van Laethem J-L, Deviere J, Resibois A, Rickaert F, Vertongen P, Ohtani H, Cremer M, Miyazono K (1995) Localization of transforming growth factor β1 and its latent binding protein in human chronic pancreatitis. Gastroenterology 108: 1873-1881
47. Slater SD, Williamson RCN, Foster CS (1995) Expression of transforming growth factor-β1 in chronic pancreatitis. Digestion 56: 237-241
48. Lee M-S, Gu D, Feng L, Curriden S, Arnush M, Krahl T, Gurushanthaiah D, Wilson C, Loskutoff DL, Fox H, Sarvetnick N (1995) Accumulation of extracellular matrix and developmental dysregulation in the pancreas by transgenic production of transforming growth factor-β1. Am J Pathol 147: 42-52
49. Bockman DE, Merlino G (1992) Cytological changes in the pancreas of transgenic mice overexpressing transforming growth factor α. Gastroenterology 103: 1883-1892
50. Korc M, Friess H, Yamanaka Y, Kobrin MS, Buechler M, Beger HG (1994) Chronic pancreatitis is associated with increased concentrations of epidermal growth factor receptor, transforming growth factor α, and phospholipase Cγ. Gut 35: 1468-1473
51. Korc M, Chandrasekar B, Yamanaka Y, Friess H, Buechler M, Beger HG (1992) Overexpression of the epidermal growth factor receptor in human pancreatic cancer is associated with concomitant increases in the levels of epidermal growth factor and transforming growth factor alpha. J Clin Invest 90: 1352-1360

Endocrine Pancreatic Function in the Diagnosis and Staging of Chronic Pancreatitis

B. Glasbrenner · C. v. Tirpitz · P. Malfertheiner · G. Adler

Introduction

Diabetes mellitus is a frequent complication in chronic pancreatitis (CP) that occurs with progressive atrophy of the gland. Ammann and coworkers have shown in their large population of patients with chronic-calcifying pancreatitis that the incidence of diabetes mellitus goes in parallel with exocrine insufficiency and pancreatic calcifications. In patients with noncalcifying chronic pancreatitis, the incidence of impaired glucose tolerance and of overt diabetes is lower. In the majority of patients, the time between diagnosis of chronic pancreatitis and onset of pancreatic diabetes ranges from 7 to 15 years [1–3].

Morphology of the Endocrine Pancreatic Compartment in Chronic Pancreatitis

The qualitative morphological changes of the endocrine pancreas in chronic pancreatitis are characterized by focal accumulation of islets in sclerotic tissue, occasional neoformation of islets through ductuloinsular proliferation (nesidioblastosis), and perisinusoidal fibrosis of the sclerotic islets. Perisinusoidal fibers often split the islets into separate lobules [4].

In an immunocytochemical and ultrastructural study in 12 diabetic and nondiabetic patients with chronic pancreatitis, Klöppel and coworkers have found that the proportion of B cells was reduced to about 60% of control values. A cells appeared to be more resistant to pancreatic sclerosis than B cells, resulting in a shift in the A/B ratio from 1:3 to 1:3.5 in controls to 1:0.4 to 1:1.7 in patients with chronic pancreatitis. The relative number of PP cells was increased in this study, whereas the number of D cells was found to be normal [4]. Table 1 summarizes the quantitative changes of islet cells in CP patients according to [4]. The morphological changes contrast with the functional studies presented in this paper, and this might be due to further factors such as local circulation or due to the heterogeneity of the populations studied.

Table 1. Quantitative changes of islet cells in chronic pancreatitis (see [4])

Cell type	Hormone	Relative number
B	Insulin	Decreased
A	Glucagon	Increased
PP	PP	Increased
D	Somatostatin	Normal

Studies on Insulin and C Peptide in Chronic Pancreatitis

Various studies have investigated B cell function by different types of stimulation and have compared patients with chronic pancreatitis to healthy controls and to other types of diabetes. The most relevant findings can be summarized as follows:

1. C peptide plasma concentrations are superior to insulin in reflecting B cell function in chronic pancreatitis. The major reason seems to be that insulin metabolism in the liver is reduced in chronic alcoholics [5].
2. B cell function in patients with chronic pancreatitis is correlated to exocrine pancreatic function in most studies. This was found for the C peptide response to various types of stimulation and for direct and indirect exocrine pancreatic function tests [6-11].
3. No consistent abnormality of B cell function has been found in patients with early chronic pancreatitis, e.g., endoscopic retrograde cholangiopancreatography (ERCP) stage I patients [12]. The incidence of abnormal B cell responses following stimulation is significant only in patients with ERCP stage II or III (unpublished data, see below) or with at least moderate exocrine insufficiency when staged according to the secretin-ceruletide test [7].
4. B cell function tests cannot reliably distinguish diabetes secondary to chronic pancreatitis from other types of diabetes [6, 13].
5. The "incretin effect" is preserved in patients with chronic pancreatitis and impaired glucose tolerance [14].

We compared the sensitivity of different endocrine stimulation tests in the diagnosis and staging of chronic pancreatitis. Eighteen patients with different ERCP stages of chronic pancreatitis (Table 2) and fasting normoglycemia (blood glucose < 120 mg/dl) and ten healthy control subjects underwent three standardized endocrine stimulation tests: (1) an oral glucose load (75 g); (2) an intravenous glucose load (0.5 g/kg bw); and (3) an intravenous arginine infusion test (0.5 g/kg bw).

Blood glucose concentrations and insulin, C peptide, and glucagon plasma levels were measured before and in standardized time intervals after stimulation. Exocrine pancreatic function was assessed by the pancreolauryl serum test [15].

We found that the C peptide response to arginine infusion was the only B cell function test that was already significantly impaired in ERCP stage II (Fig. 1). However, none of these function test is helpful in the early diagnosis of chronic

Table 2. Clinical data from patients with chronic pancreatitis (see Figs. 1–3)

Patient no.	Age (years)	Sex	ERCP stage	Etiology	Duration of chronic pancreatitis (years/months)	Calcifications
1	35	M	I	Idiopathic	0/5	Neg
2	38	M	I	Alcohol	2/5	Neg
3	54	M	I	Alcohol	9/0	Neg
4	56	F	I	Obstruction	3/0	Neg
5	41	M	I	Alcohol	1/5	Neg
6	54	M	I	Alcohol	14/0	Neg
7	42	M	II	Alcohol	14/0	Pos
8	34	M	II	Alcohol	0/7	Neg
9	42	M	II	Alcohol	5/0	Pos
10	33	M	II	Alcohol	9/0	Pos
11	46	M	II	Alcohol	3/5	Pos
12	40	M	III	Alcohol	1/5	Neg
13	43	M	III	Alcohol	0/7	Pos
14	35	M	III	Alcohol	3/0	Pos
15	15	W	III	Idiopathic	2/0	Pos
16	66	M	III	Alcohol	13/0	Pos
17	27	M	III	Obstruction	5/0	Pos
18	30	M	III	Obstruction	11/0	Pos

ERCP, endoscopic retrograde cholangiopancreatography; Neg, negative; Pos, positive.

pancreatitis (ERCP stage I). Furthermore, C peptide response to arginine does not distinguish diabetes secondary to chronic pancreatitis from other types of diabetes [6].

We also found that there is a relationship between exocrine pancreatic function (as assessed by the pancreolauryl serum test) and endocrine function in chronic pancreatitis without overt diabetes. The strongest correlation was calculated for the C peptide response following arginine infusion (Fig. 2).

Fig. 1. C peptide response (*AUC,* area under curve) following arginine infusion in healthy controls and patients with different, endoscopic retrograde cholangiopancreatography (*ERCP*) stages of chronic pancreatitis. **$p < 0.01$ versus healthy controls. For further details, see text and Table 2

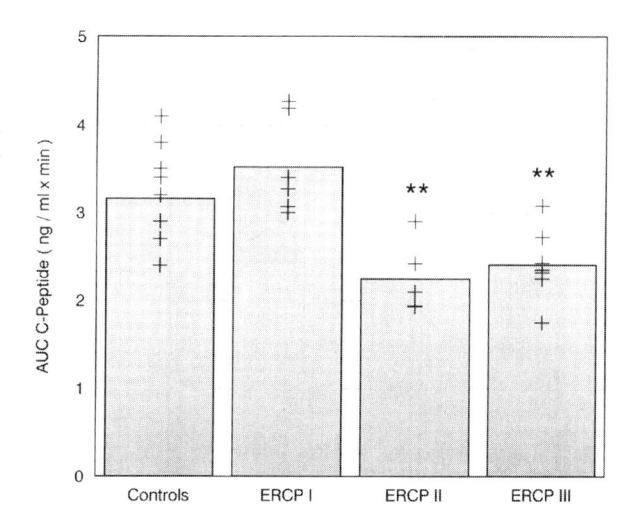

Fig. 2. Correlation between C peptide response (*AUC*, area under curve) following arginine infusion and peak fluorescein serum concentration in the pancreolauryl serum test (*PLT*) in patients with chronic pancreatitis. $r = 0.845$; $p < 0.001$. For further details, see text and Table 2

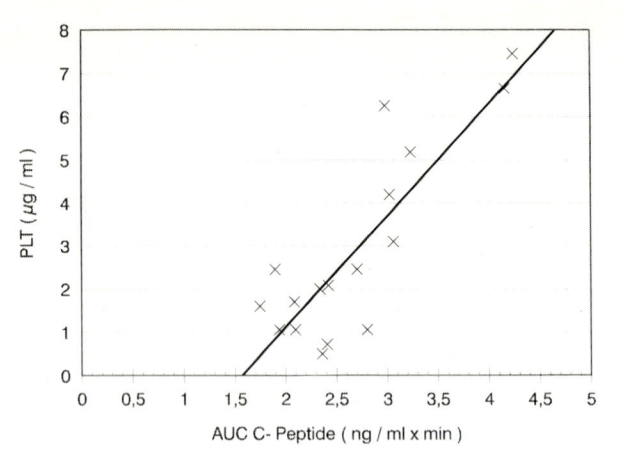

Studies on Glucagon in Chronic Pancreatitis

In insulin-dependent diabetes mellitus (IDDM), glucagon response to a protein meal or following arginine infusion is primarily increased [16, 17]. Glucagon release in chronic pancretitis has been investigated by Keller and coworkers [13]. They have shown that glucagon release following arginine infusion is impaired in diabetic CP patients but also in CP patients without overt diabetes. In contrast, glucagon release in idiopathic diabetics was normal, and the major conclusion of this paper was that glucagon release following arginine infusion could distinguish the two types of diabetes.

In our own study in 18 CP patients and ten healthy control subjects (Table 2), we also measured glucagon, and we found that the glucagon response to arginine tends to decrease earlier than C peptide (Fig. 3). However, the difference between ERCP stage I patients and healthy control subjects was not significant, leading to the conclusion that neither C peptide nor glucagon response following arginine infusion are helpful in the early diagnosis of chronic pancreatitis.

Studies on Pancreatic Polypeptide in Chronic Pancreatitis

Pancreatic polypeptide in chronic pancreatitis was investigated in various studies with various types of stimulation. There is agreement that the PP response to hormonal or test-meal stimulation is impaired in CP patients with severe exocrine insufficiency [18-20]. In contrast, data on the correlation between PP release and the degree of exocrine pancreatic insufficiency are controversial [21].

In our patients with mild to moderate CP (i.e., ERCP stage I and II or patients without steatorrhea), the PP response following stimulation is normal [20, 22]. Therefore, we focused on interdigestive PP release, and Fig. 4 shows the mean PP plasma concentrations during different phases of interdigestive gastroduo-

Fig. 3. Glucagon response (*AUC*, area under curve) following arginine infusion in healthy controls and patients with different, endoscopic retrograde cholangiopancreatography (*ERCP*) stages of chronic pancreatitis. ***$p < 0.001$ versus healthy controls. For further details, see text and Table 2

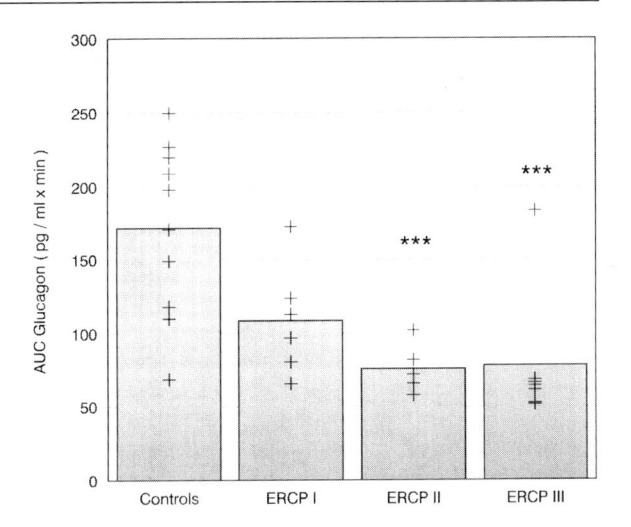

denal motility (phase I, II, III) in healthy controls and patients with different stages of chronic pancreatitis [22]. We found a progressive decrease in interdigestive PP release with increasing severity of disease, and the decrease in PP plasma concentrations in patients with mild to moderate CP was significant during phase III but not already during phase I and II. We conclude that there is a disorder of interdigestive PP release in early stages of CP, but it is inconvenient to investigate and not practicable in clinical routine.

Studies on Somatostatin in Chronic Pancreatitis

The number of D cells in chronic pancreatitis is normal [4], and only few functional data are available. One study has reported on elevated somatostatin plasma concentrations in patients with chronic pancreatitis without residual B

Fig. 4. PP plasma concentrations (mean ± SEM) during different phases of interdigestive gastroduodenal motility (I, II, III) in 17 healthy controls, nine patients with mild to moderate chronic pancreatitis (*MCP*), endoscopic retrograde cholangiopancreatography (*ERCP*) stage 1–2 and eight patients with severe chronic pancreatitis (*SCP*), ERCP stage 3. *$p < 0.05$, ***$p < 0.001$ versus healthy controls. (From [21])

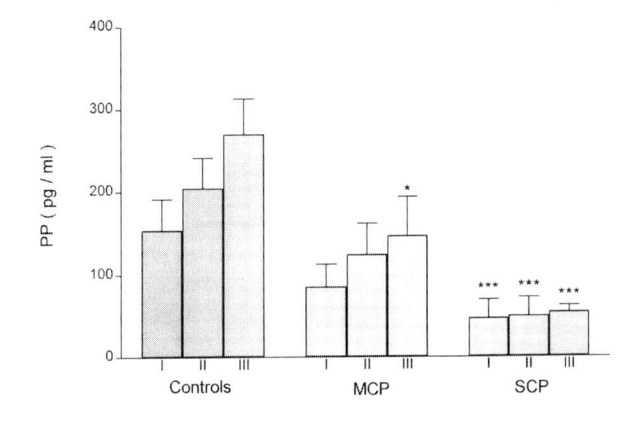

cell function [23]. However, it is unclear whether this is somatostatin of pancreatic or extrapancreatic origin. It is also a methodological problem that determination of somatostatin plasma concentration is not a useful diagnostic tool in chronic pancreatitis.

Conclusions

In our opinion, the following conclusions must be drawn at the present state of knowledge:

- In the *diagnosis* of chronic pancreatitis, B cell function tests are not helpful (poor sensitivity and poor specificity). Glucagon release following arginine infusion may help to distinguish different types of diabetes if necessary. Investigation of interdigestive PP release is not practicable in clinical routine, whereas stimulated PP release is not helpful.
- With regard to the *staging* of chronic pancreatitis, it seems appropriate to distinguish between normal and abnormal glucose tolerance and overt diabetes. Although it might be possible to stage chronic pancreatitis according to glucagon or PP release, the question arises: Why should we? It is not helpful in the clinical management of these patients.

References

1. Ammann R, Akovbiantz A, Largiader F, Schueler G (1984) Course and outcome of chronic pancreatitis. Gastroenterology 86: 820–828
2. Bank S, Marks IN, Vinik AI (1975) Clinical and hormonal aspects of pancreatic diabetes. Am J Gastroenterol 64: 13–22
3. Bank S (1986) Chronic pancreatitis: clinical features and medical management. Am J Gastroenterol 81: 153–166
4. Klöppel G, Bommer G, Commandeur G, Heitz PU (1978) The endocrine pancreas in chronic pancreatitis: immunocytochemical and ultrastructural studies. Virchows Arch [A] 377: 157–174
5. Bonora E, Rizzi C, Lesi C, Berra P, Coscelli C, Butturuni U (1988) Insulin and C-peptide plasma levels in patients with severe chronic pancreatitis and fasting normoglycemia. Dig Dis Sci 33: 732–736
6. Andersen BN, Krarup T, Pedersen NT, Faber OK, Hagen C, Worning H (1982) B-cell function in patients with chronic pancreatitis and its relation to exocrine pancreatic function. Diabetologia 23: 86–89
7. Cavallini G, Bovo P, Zamboni M, Bosello O, Filippini M, Riela A, Brocco G, Rossi L, Pelle C, Chiavenato A, Scuro LA (1992) Exocrine and endocrine functional reserve in the course of chronic pancreatitis as studied by maximal stimulation tests. Dig Dis Sci 37: 93–96
8. Domschke S, Stock KP, Pichl J, Schneider MU, Domschke W (1985) Beta-cell reserve capacity in chronic pancreatitis. Hepatogastroenterol 32: 27–30
9. Kalk WJ, Vinik AI, Jackson PU, Bank S (1979) Insulin secretion and pancreatic exocrine function in patients with chronic pancreatitis. Diabetologia 16: 355–358
10. Larsen S, Hilsted J, Tronier B, Worning H (1987) Metablic control and B cell function in patients with insulin-dependent diabetes mellitus secondary to chronic pancreatitis. Metabolism 36: 964–967
11. Stock KP, Domschke S, Pichl J, Schneider MU, Domschke W (1985) Einschränkung von Insulinreserven und exokriner Pankreassekretion bei chronischer Pankreatitis. Dtsch med Wschr 110: 134–136
12. Axon ATR, Classen M, Cotton PB, Cremer M, Freeny PC, Lees WR (1984) Pancreatography in chronic pancreatitis: international definitions. Gut 25: 1107–1112

13. Keller U, Szöllösy E, Varga L, Gyr K (1984) Pancreatic glucagon secretion and exocrine function (BT-PABA test) in chronic pancreatitis. Dig Dis Sci 29: 853–857
14. Fölsch UR, Stöckmann F, Nauck M, Creutzfeldt W (1990) Endocrine pancreatic function during atrophy of the exocrine gland in rats and patients with chronic pancreatitis. In: Beger HG, Büchler M, Ditschuneit H, Malfertheiner P (eds) Chronic pancreatitis. Springer, Berlin Heidelberg New York, pp 235–244
15. Malfertheiner P, Büchler M, Müller A, Ditschuneit H (1987) Fluorescein dilaurate (FDL) serum test – a rapid tubeless pancreatic function test. Pancreas 2: 53–60
16. Raskin P, Aydin I, Yamamoto T, Unger RH (1978) Abnormal alpha cell function in human diabetes. The response to oral protein. Am J Med 64: 988–997
17. Unger RH, Aguilar-Parade E, Müller WA (1970) Studies of pancreatic alpha cell function in normal and diabetic subjects. J Clin Invest 49: 837–848
18. Sive A, Vinik AI, Tonder SV, Lund A (1978) Impaired pancreatic polypeptide secretion in chronic pancreatitis. J Clin Endocrinol Metab 47: 556–559
19. Adrian TE, Besterman HS, Mallinson CN, Garalotis C, Bloom SR (1979) Impaired pancreatic polypeptide release in chronic pancreatitis with steatorrhea. Gut 20: 98–101
20. Glasbrenner B, Dominguez-Muñoz JE, Nelson DK, Riepl RL, Büchler M, Malfertheiner P (1994) Relationship between postprandial release of CCK and PP in health and in chronic pancreatitis. Regul Pept 50: 45–52
21. Owyang C, Scarpello JH, Vinik AI (1982) Correlation between pancreatic enzyme secretion and plasma concentration of human pancreatic polypeptide in health and in chronic pancreatitis. Gastroenterology 83: 55–62
22. Pieramico O, Nelson DK, Glasbrenner B, Malfertheiner P (1994) Impaired interdigestive pancreatic polypeptide release: early hormonal disorder in chronic pancreatitis? Dig Dis Sci 39: 69–74
23. Larsen S, Hilsted J, Tronier B, Worning H (1988) Pancreatic hormone secretion in chronic pancreatitis without residual beta-cell function. Acta Endocrinol (Copenh) 118: 357–364

IV
Chronic Pancreatitis: Guidelines

Diagnostic Standards for Chronic Pancreatitis

P. DiMagno

Introduction

Diagnosis of chronic pancreatitis begins by suspecting the presence of the disease based on the clinical presentation of the patient and substantiated by laboratory testing (which may include function tests), and imaging of the pancreas. There are many definitions of chronic pancreatitis. One of the more commonly accepted definitions is that of Sarner [1]: "Chronic pancreatitis is a continuing inflammatory disease of the pancreas characterized by irreversible morphological change and typically causing pain and/or causing permanent impairment of function." This definition covers the pathological, clinical, and functional changes characteristic of the disease. Further, Sarner elaborated upon this definition by stating that the standard for exocrine insufficiency should be permanent impairment of exocrine function two standard deviations below the normal for the test and that the morphologic change must be permanent.

I will discuss the standards to establish the diagnosis of chronic pancreatitis that we have used in our studies and briefly review of the natural history of the various forms of chronic pancreatitis we have established based on the these standards and the criteria that should be required to establish new tests to diagnose chronic pancreatitis; further, I will review the results of function and imaging tests in the diagnosis of chronic pancreatitis and arrive at an algorithm to establish which tests should be used by different practitioners to establish the diagnosis of this disease.

Criteria for Diagnosis

In our clinical and epidemiologic studies [2–4], we have used a scoring system based on clinical, morphologic, and functional characteristics of chronic pancreatitis (Table 1). The scoring system has been validated. In a large epidemiologic study, the mean scores of patients with early-onset or late-onset chronic pancreatitis and alcoholic chronic pancreatitis were 8.4, 7.5, and 9.1, respectively [3] (a score of 4 or more indicates presence of chronic pancreatitis). The weakest combination of items of the scoring system is the combination of pain and abnormal exocrine function, which would occur in patients who have other gastrointestinal diseases, such as nontropical sprue [5], or other pancreatic disease, such as pancreatic cancer. Differentiation between chronic pancreatitis

Table 1. Criteria for diagnosis of chronic pancreatitis

Criterion	Score
Pain, weight loss	2
Calcification	4
Histology	4
Major duct abnormalities (operation, ERCP, US, CT, or EUS)	3
Abnormal exocrine function	2
Abnormal endocrine function	1

A score of 4 or more indicates a diagnosis of chronic pancreatitis.
ERCP, endoscopic retrograde cholangiopancreatography; US, ultrasound; CT, computed tomography; EUS, endoscopic ultrasonography.

and pancreatic cancer is particularly problematic. All clinical features of chronic pancreatitis may be present in both diseases. Even the tissue diagnosis of chronic pancreatitis may be made in patients with pancreatic cancer, because small tumors obstructing the pancreatic duct may not be detected and the biopsy is taken from an area of chronic pancreatitis cause by the obstructing tumor. In addition, intraductal papillary mucinous tumor (IPMT), an increasingly recognized lesion [6], has abnormalities of the ducts and a clinical history that may mimic chronic pancreatitis.

Nevertheless, this scoring system, if used after exclusion of other gastrointestinal disease, is very accurate to establish the diagnosis of chronic pancreatitis for clinical studies [2-6].

It is also important to recognize that the accuracy of any test to diagnose chronic pancreatitis, and thus the accuracy of any scoring system or set of standards, is affected by the natural history of the different forms of chronic pancreatitis. The rates for developing morphologic and functional abnormalities among the forms of chronic pancreatitis vary, but usually take years. This characteristic of chronic pancreatitis is not so important in epidemiologic or other clinical studies when patients are either followed over many years or only patients with definite chronic pancreatitis are selected for the studies. However, this characteristic of chronic pancreatitis is the major reason why it is difficult to make the diagnosis of chronic pancreatitis early in the course of the disease.

Natural History

We [3] and others [7] have identified several forms of chronic pancreatitis. In a large epidemiologic study, we found that, besides alcoholic chronic pancreatitis, there were two forms of idiopathic chronic pancreatitis. The idiopathic forms occurred in patients aged 35 years or younger (early onset) or in patients older than 35 years (late onset). The early-onset form is characterized by a long, painful course and late occurrence of morphologic (calcification) and functional (exocrine and endocrine function) changes (Fig. 1-3). Late-onset chronic pancreatitis, however, often is painless, but patients may have exocrine insuffi-

Diagnostic Standards for Chronic Pancreatitis

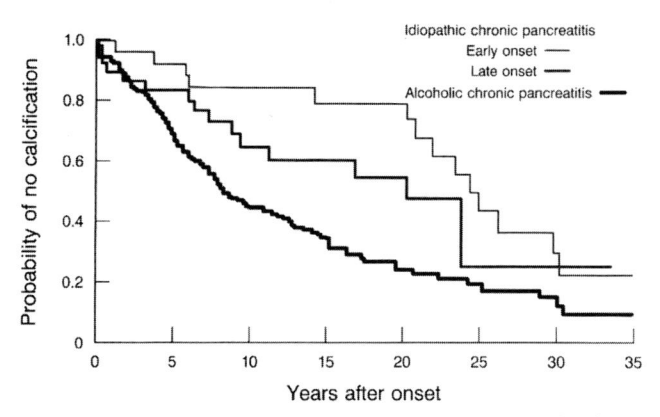

Fig. 1. Probability of remaining free of calcification for patients with early-onset (*thin line*) or late-onset (*medium line*) idiopathic chronic pancreatitis or alcoholic pancreatitis (*thick line*). Differences were significant between early-onset idiopathic chronic pancreatitis and alcoholic chronic pancreatitis ($p = 0.0001$) and between late-onset idiopathic chronic pancreatitis and alcoholic chronic pancreatitis ($p = 0.01$). (Reprinted with permission from [3])

ciency at onset and have more rapid development of morphologic and functional abnormalities of chronic pancreatitis. Patients with alcoholic chronic pancreatitis (≥ 50 g alcohol/day), the most common form (55% of patients), develop calcification (Fig. 1) much faster than patients with other forms of chronic pancreatitis and develop functional abnormalities (Fig. 2, 3) as fast as patients with late-onset idiopathic chronic pancreatitis. In this study, we did not include patients with a daily alcohol intake of less than 50 g or an unknown daily alcohol intake – about 25% of our patients – with chronic pancreatitis. Currently, we are analyzing these patients, and it appears that their natural his-

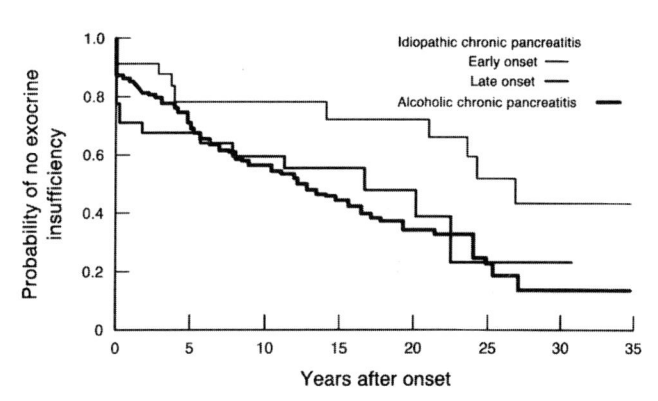

Fig. 2. Probability of remaining free of exocrine insufficiency for patients with early-onset (*thin line*) or late-onset (*medium line*) idiopathic chronic pancreatitis and alcoholic pancreatitis (*thick line*). Differences were significant between early-onset idiopathic chronic pancreatitis and late-onset idiopathic chronic pancreatitis ($p = 0.024$) and between early-onset idiopathic chronic pancreatitis and alcoholic chronic pancreatitis ($p = 0.0008$). (Reprinted with permission from [3])

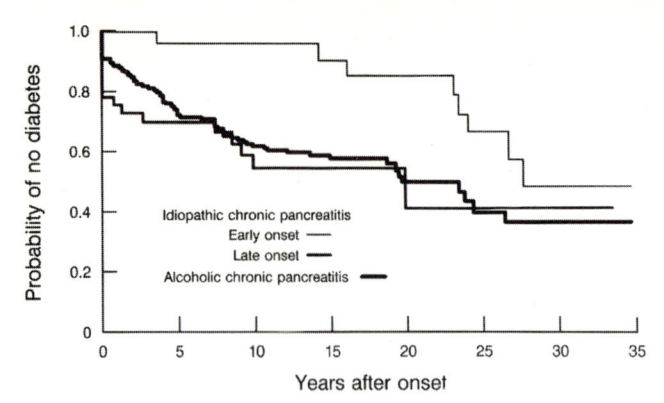

Fig. 3. Probability of remaining free of diabetes mellitus for patients with early-onset (*thin line*) or late-onset (*medium line*) idiopathic chronic pancreatitis and alcoholic chronic pancreatitis (*thick line*). Differences were significant between early-onset idiopathic chronic pancreatitis and late-onset idiopathic chronic pancreatitis ($p = 0.01$) and between early-onset idiopathic chronic pancreatitis and alcoholic chronic pancreatitis ($p = 0.0025$). (Reprinted with permission from [3])

tory most resembles that of late-onset and alcoholic chronic pancreatitis patients.

Because the rates for developing morphologic and functional abnormalities are more rapid in the late-onset idiopathic chronic pancreatitis and alcoholic pancreatitis groups than in the early-onset idiopathic group (and these abnormalities are sometimes present at the onset of disease), the diagnosis is much easier. Patients with early-onset idiopathic pancreatitis may take 25–30 years to develop morphologic and functional abnormalities, and thus diagnosis may be delayed. However, it is important to test for functional abnormalities in these patients if morphologic abnormalities (imaging tests) are normal, because there may not be congruence between the development of morphologic and functional abnormalities within a patient.

Criteria To Establish New Diagnostic Tests

From the foregoing discussion, it is apparent that there is a wide range of forms of chronic pancreatitis that will be in various stages at the time of presentation. For this reason, new tests must detect the entire spectrum of chronic pancreatitis, from early to late disease and the different forms. Inclusion of this wide spectrum of disease will also ensure a realistic measure of sensitivity; a high sensitivity for a test is often claimed for chronic pancreatitis after the test has been evaluated in a group of patients with end-stage disease, a population in which the diagnosis is obvious and in which special tests are not required to make the diagnosis. In addition, to validate the specificity of new tests, they should be assessed in control groups suspected of having the disease, but which turn out in prospective studies to have other conditions. Lastly, new tests must be compared to existing standard tests (gold standard test), if possible. For example, if tests of pancreatic function are being evaluated, they must be compared to invasive tests of pancreatic function.

Evaluation of Tests of Pancreatic Function

Tests of exocrine pancreatic function may be used to answer three clinical questions:

1. Is malabsorption present?
2. Is malabsorption due to exocrine insufficiency?
3. Is there chronic pancreatitis?

The gold standard test to determine whether malabsorption is present is the quantitative fecal fat test. However, the quantitative fecal fat test is time consuming; it requires a 48- to 72-h collection and a minimum of 24 h to carry out the laboratory measurement. Unfortunately, other tests such as the serum carotene test are relatively insensitive [8]; the qualitative stool fat test and triolein breath test are surprisingly sensitive and specific (Table 2), but are not frequently used because the test depends on the experience of the operator, requires the use of radiolabeled materials, and may give false-positive results in patients with diabetes mellitus and liver disease and/or pulmonary disease, respectively. However, recent advances such as NMR near-infrared reflective analysis (NIRA) [9–11] may be sensitive and only require the collection and analysis of a single small stool specimen.

The gold standard test to answer the question of whether malabsorption is caused by pancreatic insufficiency is an invasive test of pancreatic function that involves duodenal intubation and quantification of pancreatic exocrine secretion during stimulation with a secretagogue such as cholecystokinin octapeptide (CCK-OP) or secretin or a test meal. For these different stimulants, pancreatic enzymes are usually measured with CCK-OP stimulation, bicarbonate with secretin stimulation, and enzymes, bile acids, and duodenal pH when a test meal is the stimulus. These tests measure the entire range of pancreatic secretion and can detect mild to severe exocrine pancreatic insufficiency. However, to answer this question, noninvasive tests of pancreatic secretion are satisfactory, since they have a sensitivity of 80%–90% when malabsorption is present.

These tests include the following:

- Nitroblue tetrazolium *p*-aminobenzoic acid (NBT-PABA) test
- Pancreolauryl test

Table 2. Summary of tests of malabsorption (from [8])

Test	Sensitivity (%)	Specificity (%)
Carotine	60	96
Quantitative stool fat	92	96
Triolein breath test	100	96

Table 3. Sensitivity and specificity of pancreatic function tests

Tubeless tests	Sensitivity (%)	Specificity (%)
Bentiromide test	85	90
Pancreolauryl test	90	82
Trypsin RIA	33–65	?
Serum PP	48–76	86–93
Fecal chymotrypsin	78	94
Fecal elastase	?	?
Quantitative stool fat	30	?

Higher values are generally obtained in studies with end-stage chronic pancreatitis patients. Values are much less with "early" chronic pancreatitis.
RIA, radioimmunoassay.

- Dual-labeled Schilling test
- Fecal analyses (chymotrypsin, elastase)
- Cholesteryl octanoate breath test
- Plasma amino acid consumption (AACT)

However, the AACT test lacks accuracy for the detection of exocrine pancreatic insufficiency or the diagnosis of chronic pancreatitis [12].

To answer the question of whether there is chronic pancreatic disease, exocrine pancreatic function tests are usually used if imaging tests are negative. Necessarily, therefore, the criterion for these tests in this clinical setting is that they must have a high sensitivity and specificity and measure the entire range of function. Only invasive pancreatic tests meet this criterion; they are 90% sensitive and specific [13, 14]. False-negative results occur rarely in diseases such as calcific pancreatitis [13], nontropical spure [5], and gastrointestinal malignancies [14]. Noninvasive tests are too insensitive to determine whether there exocrine pancreatic disease is present if there is no exocrine insufficiency (Table 3).

Evaluation of Imaging Tests

Multiple studies have been peformed to evaluate this sensitivity and specificity of imaging tests. The sensitivities of the various imaging tests vary from 60% to 100% (Table 4). The current sensitivity and specificity for endoscopic ultrasonography (EUS) is under evaluation, but in our experience there is difficulty in differentiating pancreatic cancer from chronic pancreatitis in the presence of a mass complicating chronic pancreatitis. However, our current strategy for imaging tests in chronic pancreatitis is to perform the computed tomography (CT) examination and, if this is negative, to proceed with either endoscopic retrograde pancreatography and or EUS. Specifically we perform EUS if we suspect there is a pancreatic cancer. If these tests are negative, then a pancreatic function test is performed.

Diagnostic Standards for Chronic Pancreatitis

Table 4. Sensitivity and specificity of imaging tests in chronic pancreatitis

Test	Sensitivity (%)	Specificity (%)
Ultrasound[a]	60–70	80–90
CT	74–90	85–90
ERP	67–93	89–100
EUS	?	?
MRI	?	?
PET	?	?

CT, computed tomography; ERP, endoscopic retrograde pancreatography; EUS, endoscopic ultrasound; MRI, magnetic resonance imaging; PET, positron emission tomography.
[a] Ultrasound + transcutaneous ultrasound.

Table 5. Order of tests, site of testing, and costs of tests for diagnosis of chronic pancreatitis

Test	Site	Cost[a]
Serum enzymes	CH	55
Indirect test of pancreatic function	CH	22
US	CH	201
CT	CH/TC	720
EUS	TC	1000
ERCP	TC	1288
Direct test of pancreatic function (CCK stimulation)	TC	610
Follow-up evaluations	CH/TC	

Cost for serum enzyme is for serum amylase, for indirect test for fecal chymotrypsin.
US, ultrasound + transcutaneous ultrasound; CT, computed tomography; ERP, endoscopic retrograde pancreatography; EUS, endoscopic ultrasound; CH, community hospital (family practitioner); TC, tertiary center (gastroenterologist).
[a] Costs are estimates in US $ (1995).

Conclusion: Algorithm and Costs of Diagnostic Tests

Based on these data, the first test (Table 5) in patients suspected of having chronic pancreatitis should be serum pancreatic enzymes, plain abdominal roentgenogram, an indirect pancreatic function test, and an abdominal ultrasound. These tests can be performed at the direction of a family practitioner and at a community hospital. If the diagnosis is still in doubt, CT is the next test. Although CT can be performed and may be available at a community hospital, subtle changes of chronic pancreatitis may be missed unless the CT is interpreted by an expert pancreatic radiologist. Therefore, at this point in the workup, it is probably better for the patient to be evaluated at a tertiary center that has expert pancreatologists. Certainly, if the diagnosis of chronic pancreatitis is not made with CT and is still suspected, EUS and endoscopic retrograde cholangiopancreatography (ERCP) should be performed by a gastroenterologist. Finally, an invasive test of exocrine pancreatic function should be done if the diagnosis is still suspected and no imaging tests are diagnostic of chronic pancreatitis.

The costs of tests needed to diagnose chronic pancreatitis can be minimal if the diagnosis is relatively easy and requires tests that are relatively easily performed and inexpensive (Table 5). However, the costs can rapidly mount if the diagnosis requires expensive imaging and function tests and special consultations. Based on 1995 estimates, the costs of tests (in US dollars) to make the diagnosis of chronic pancreatitis could range from $278 (for serum amylase, fecal chymotrypsin, and abdominal ultrasound) to more than $4000 of diagnosis depends upon tests such as CT, EUS, ERCP, and a direct test of exocrine function.

References

1. Sarner M (1993) Pancreatitis definitions and classification. In: Go VLW, DiMagno EP, Gardner JD, Lebenthal E, Reber HA, Scheele GA (eds) The pancreas. New York, Raven Press, pp 575–580
2. Riela A, Zinsmeister AR, Melton LJ, Weiland LH, DiMagno EP (1992) Increasing pancreatic cancer incidence in women over five decades in Olmsted County, Minnesota. Mayo Clin Proc 67: 839–845
3. Layer P, Yamamoto H, Kalthoff L, Clain JE, Bakken LJ, DiMagno EP (1994) The different courses of early and late onset idiopathic and alcoholic chronic pancreatitis. Gastroenterology 107: 1481–1487
4. Maringhini A, Nelson DK, Jones JD, DiMagno EP (1994) Is the plasma amino acid consumption test an accurate test of exocrine pancreatic insufficiency? Gastroenterology 106: 488–493
5. Regan PT, DiMagno EP (1980) Exocrine pancreatic insufuciency in celiac spure: a cause of treatment failure. Gastroenterology 78: 484–487
6. Loftus EV Jr, Olivares-Pakzad BA, Batts KP, Adkins MC, Stephens DH, DiMagno EP, Members of the Pancreas Clinic, and Pancreatic Surgeons of Mayo Clinic (1996): Intraductal papillary-mucinous tumors of the pancreas – clinicopathologic features, outcome, and nomenclature. Gastroenterology 110: 1909–1918
7. Amman RW, Akobiantz A, Largiader F, Schueler G (1984) Course and outcome of chronic pancreatitis. Longitudinal study of a mix medical-surgical series of 245 patients. Gastroenterology 86: 820–828
8. Newcomer AD, Hofmann AF, DiMagno EP, Thomas PJ, Carlson GL (1979) Triolein breath test: a sensitive and specific test for fat malabsorption. Gastroenterology 76: 6–13
9. Benini L, Caliari S, Bonfante F, Guidi GC, Brentegani MT, Castellani G, Sembenini C, Bardelli E, Vantini I (1992) Near infrared reflectance measurement of nitrogen faecal losses. Gut 33: 749–752
10. Picarelli A, Greco M, Di Giovambattista F, Ramazzotti A, Cedrone C, Corazziari E, Torsoli A (1995) Quantitative determination of faecal fat, nitrogen and water by means of a spectrophotometric technique: near infrared reflectance analysis (NIRA). Assessment of its accuracy and reproducibility compared with chemical methods. Clin Chim Acta 234: 147–156
11. Stein J, Purschian B, Zeuzem S, Lembcke B, Caspary WF (1996) Quantification of fecal carbohydrates by near-infrared reflectance analysis. Clin Chem 42: 309–312
12. Maringhini A, Nelson DK, Jones JD, DiMagno EP, Is the plasma amino acid consumption test an accurate test of exocrine pancreatic insufficiency? GASTROENTEROLOGY 1994; 106: 488–493.
13. DiMagno EP, Go VLW, Summerskill WHJ (1973) Relations between pancreatic enzyme outputs and malabsorption in severe pancreatic insufficiency. N Engl J Med 288: 813–815
14. DiMagno EP, Malagelada J-R, Moertel CG, Go VLW (1977) Prospective evaluation of the pancreatic secretion of immunoreactive carcinoembryonic antigen, enzyme, and bicarbonate in patients suspected of having pancreatic cancer. Gastroenterology 73: 457–461

Standards in Surgical Treatment of Chronic Pancreatitis

M. Siech · H. G. Beger

Introduction

Treatment of chronic pancreatitis has improved over the past decades, with the result that 50% of patients with chronic inflammation of the pancreas live for more than 20 years (Ammann 1984). The natural course leads to autodestruction of the gland and frequently to spontaneous relief of pain (Ammann 1984). The prognosis of chronic pancreatitis is listed in Table 1. Pedersen et al. (1982) showed that patients with chronic pancreatitis have a 5-year survival of 65%, a 10-year survival of 43%, and a 20-year survival of 50%. In 19%, the mortality related to the patients disease; however, in the other 81%, the causes of death are related to factors other than chronic pancreatitis, such as malignancies, alcohol hepathopathy, and severe infections (Table 1). About 58%–67% of these patients need surgery during the course of pancreatitis (Levy 1989). The most frequent indications for surgery are listed in Table 2. As shown in Table 2, 97% of patients suffer from severe intractable pain. Bockman et al. (1988) demonstrated that patients with inflammatory mass of the head of the pancreas had increased diameter of nerves in this area. Additionally, the perineural sheet was damaged by inflammatory cells. The diameter of the nerves was increased and the mean area which is served per nerve was diminished. These mechanisms might be responsible for the severe pain attacks in patients with inflammatory mass of the head of the pancreas due to chronic pancreatitis. In 79% of patients, the inflammatory mass within the head of the pancreas was larger than 4 cm (Beger 1990). Büchler et al. (1992) demonstrated within the head of the pancreas increased neuropeptide Y, substance P, and calcitonin gene-related peptide by immunostaining of neuropeptides in patients with chronic pancreatitis when compared to organ donors. Both investigations argue for the responsibility of the inflammatory mass of the head of the pancreas for severe pain attacks. Forty-nine percent of patients with chronic pancreatitis additionally had common bile duct stenosis within the lower third of common bile duct and 6% of those patients had severe duodenal stenosis (Table 2). Both mechanical problems are also caused by enlargement of the head of the pancreas. Seventeen percent of these patients had vascular obstruction, which was mainly caused by infiltration of the superior mesenteric vein and portal vein (Table 2). This latter complication is also due to enlargement and inflammatory mass of the head of the pancreas. Therefore, inflammatory enlargement of the head of the pancreas is the major problem in chronic pancreatitis, and the surgical procedure should

Table 1. Prognosis in chronic pancreatitis (CP)

Factor		Reference
Survival after onset of CP (cumulative survival)		
5-year	65 %	(Pedersen 1982)
10-year	43 %	(Pedersen 1982)
20-year	50 %	(Ammann 1984)
	50 %	(Levy 1989)
Mortality related to CP	13 %	(Lankisch 1996)
	19.3 %	(Levy 1989)
	19.0 %	(Ammann 1984)
Causes of death not related to CP	Malignancies	
	Cardiovascular disease Alcohol hepatopathy Severe infections	(Levy 1989)
Surgical treatment	66.7 %	(Bernardes 1983)
	58.0 %	(Levy 1989)

focus on this problem. As shown by Nealon et al. (1988), Beger et al. (1989), and Bittner et al. (1992), surgical treatment of chronic pancreatitis improves or delays impairment of endocrine and exocrine function.

At the present time the following procedures for chronic pancreatitis are most frequently employed in different hospitals: partial duodenopancreatectomy (Whipple procedure), pylorus-preserving partial duodenopancreatectomy, left resection or combined with drainage (Puestov type), duodenum-preserving pancreatic head resection (Beger et al. 1980), and drainage operations of Partington-Rochelle modification. In the following, we try to discuss the advantages and drawbacks of the different operations.

Resectional Procedures

Pylorus-Preserving Partial Duodenopancreatectomy

The technique of preserving the pylorus in resections of the head of the pancreas including the duodenum was developed by Watson in 1944 and introduced into the clinical routine by Traverso et al. (1978). This technique was described for small periampullary carcinomas and allows a sufficient distance to be left between the tumour and the pylorus of the stomach. This operation avoids the typical problems of gastric dumping. Later, surgeons tried to use this technique for patients with chronic pancreatitis. It was shown that the mortality (1.7 %) is lower than in patients undergoing a classic Whipple operation. In addition, the pain relief in those patients is better than in patients undergoing the classic Whipple operation (74 % vs. 64 %), the rate of surgical diabetes is 15.6 %, also lower than in patients undergoing a classic Whipple operation (24.5%). The typical postoperative complications after a pylorus-presserving

Table 2. Indications for surgical treatment in 141 patients with inflammatory mass of the head of the pancreas in chronic pancreatitis

	n	(%)
Pain		
Daily severe	94	67
Frequently severe	42	30
Common bile duct stenosis	84	59.6
Cholestasis ($n = 37$)		
Jaundice ($n = 47$)		
Stenosis of the duodenum	48[a]	36.4
Slight/moderate ($n = 33$)		
Severe ($n = 15$)		
Portal hypertension	25	17.7
Portal vein compression ($n = 16$)		
Portal vein thrombosis ($n = 2$)		
Liver cirrhosis ($n = 7$)		
Stenosis of the main pancreatic duct	141	100
Single head ($n = 53$)		
Multiple ($n = 88$)		

From Beger et al. 1990
[a] Out of 132 patients.

Whipple operation are delayed gastric emptying the first 4 weeks after operation in 12%–32% and anastomotic ulcerations in 2%–11% of patients (Traverso 1993; Warshaw 1985; Pellegrini 1989). In summary, the pylorus-preserving Whipple procedure has advantages compared to the classic Whipple procedure. However, the early and late postoperative results are not as good as in duodenum-preserving pancreatic head resection (see below). Therefore, we believe this technique is indicated in patients with chronic pancreatitis in whom malignancy is additionally suspected.

Duodenum-Preserving Pancreatic Head Resection

The duodenum-preserving resection of the head of the pancreas is a surgical procedure which was specially developed for chronic pancreatitis with inflammatory mass of the head of the pancreas by Beger et al. (1980). The first reference appeared in *Der Chirurg* 1980. In our institution, more than 400 patients have been operated upon so far, and this procedure is now a standard procedure worldwide. In our experience, this method is best to treat almost all patients with mechanical problems of chronic pancreatitis for the following reasons. Duodenum-preserving resection of the head of the pancreas allows a local resection of the inflammatory mass of the head of the pancreas with preservation of all other surrounding organs (especially duodenal passage). It decompresses the common bile duct and preserves the integrity of the common bile duct at the same time. It leads to a decompression of the main pancreatic duct and to restoration of the normal secretion flow into the upper jejunum. It decompresses the duodenum and the major vessels (e.g., portal vein). Table 3

Table 3. Early and late results after different types of operations for chronic pancreatitis (CP)

	Whipple[a] (%)	PP Whipple[b] (%)	DPHR[c] (%)
Mortality (30 days)	3.2	1.2	0.6
Late mortality	20.7	n.d.	5
Pain relief	64	74	76
Professional rehabilitation	n.d.	67	80
New diabetes, late	24.5	15.6	3.7

PP, pylorus-preserving; DPHR, duodenum-preserving pancreatic head resection; n.d., not determined.
[a] Howard 1990, Frick 1987, Gall 1990, Stone 1988, Morel 1990.
[b] Traverso 1993, Braasch 1990, Büchler 1995, Morel 1990.
[c] Beger 1990, Büchler 1995.

Table 4. Results after duodenum-preserving head resection of the pancreas in 141 patients with severe chronic pancreatitis

Hospitalisation (postoperative)	15.5 days (range, 7–52)
Relaparotomy	9/41 patients (6.4%)
Hospital mortaliy	1/141 patients (0.6%)
Late mortality	7/140 patients (5%)

From Beger et al. 1990.

shows that the duodenum-preserving pancreatic head resection has the lowest mortality rate of all resectional procedures. Pain relief was best after this procedure, when compared to the conventional Whipple or pylorus-preserving Whipple procedure (Table 3). The early and late postoperative results are shown in Tables 4 and 5. To evaluate advantages of duodenum-preserving pancreatic head resection for pylorus-preserving Whipple procedure, a controlled randomized trial has been performed which was published by Büchler and Beger in 1995. This study demonstrated that patients after duodenum-preserving pancreatic head resection had less pain, a greater weight gain, better glucose tolerance, and a higher insulin secretion capacity. These results are widely confirmed by other groups (Klempa et al. 1995).

Table 5. Late results after duodenum-preserving head presection of the pancreas in 109 patients with severe chronic pancreatitis

	Patients (n)	(%)
Abdominal pain[a]		
No	84	77
Seldom	13	12
Frequent	12	11
Professional rehabilitation[b]		
Complete	68	67
Unemployed	13	13
Retired	20	20

From Beger et al. 1990.
[a] Assessed in 109 patients.
[b] Assessed in 101 patients.

Table 6. Pain relief in 205 patients after pancreaticojejunostomy (5-year follow-up)

Complete pain relief (%)	Paint, but improved (%)	Failure
44	31	25

From White 1979, Prinz 1981, Morrow 1984, Bradley 1987.

Drainage Procedures

Drainage operations are performed as lateral side-to-side pancreaticojejunostomy (Partington and Rochelle 1960) or in combination with pancreatic tail resection (Puestow-type drainage operation; Puestow and Gillesby 1958). The disadvantage of this procedure is that inflammatory mass of the head of the pancreas is not treated. Because 79% of all patients suffer from mechanical problems due to inflammatory mass of the head of the pancreas, the use of a drainage operation alone is limited to a few cases. Single drainage operations are of value in patients without inflammatory mass of the head of the pancreas, but with dilatation of the main pancreatic duct of at least 6–8 mm. However, single drainage procedures fail to decompress the pancreatic duct branches and the tissue and cannot sufficiently drain the pancreatic duct within the head (Table 6). Additionally, restoration of normal bile flow or vascular problems cannot be resolved by a drainage operation. Patients with drainage operations and inflammatory mass of the head of the pancreas cannot be expected to become pain-free (Table 6). However, drainage operations sometimes may be helpful additionally as a combined procedure with duodenum-preserving pancreatic head resection. Drainage of the main pancreatic duct by lateral pancreaticojejunostomy in combination with limited resection of inflamed tissue of the head of the pancreas has been described by Frey et al. (1987). This procedure is a modification of the Partington-Rochelle drainage of the pancreatic main duct. The late outcome of the Frey procedure needs to be evaluated.

Procedures of Limited Indication

Kausch-Whipple Procedure

The Kausch-Whipple procedure was first described by Kausch in 1912 and then by Whipple in 1935 and was introduced for treatment of periampullary carcinomas. Because of the wide safety margin, the lower part of the common bile duct and part of the stomach is also removed in this procedure. Chronic pancreatitis, however, is a benign disease, and radical resection is not necessary. Therefore, different authors studied the perioperative mortality and morbidity of Whipple procedure in chronic pancreatitis patients (Howard and Zhang 1990; Frick et al. 1987; Stone et al. 1988; Morel et al. 1990). In these studies, the overall mortality was 3.2%, which was much higher than in other surgical procedures for chronic pancreatitis. Additionally, the postoperative so-called surgical diabetes was much higher than in other techniques (24.5%). Another problem of the Whipple operation is the dumping syndrome, which is caused by partial resection of the stomach. In summary, the classic Whipple operation constitutes overtreatment in patients with chronic pancreatitis, with unnecessary increased mortality and morbidity (Table 3).

Pancreatic Left Resection

Because left resection of the pancreas is much easier to perform than all other resections of the right pancreas, the postoperative morbidity and mortality is much lower. Therefore, many authors have performed pancreatic left resections in patients with chronic pancreatitis. The postoperative results, however, are rather discouraging. In diffuse pancreatitis, pancreatic left resection failed to improve pan in 48%-66%. Even patients with segmental left chronic pancreatitis had a failure of improvement or recurrence in 8%-33% (Table 7). Because of the poor results of pancreatic left resection, we see an indication for this procedure only in segmental pancreatitis in the left pancreas with otherwise normal parenchyma. This is a very rare constellation, usually only occurring after pancreatic trauma. For these patients, the spleen-preserving left resection should be the procedure of choice.

Drainage of Pancreatic Pseudocysts in Chronic Pancreatitis

The first option in the treatment of pancreatic pseudocysts due to chronic pancreatitis is ultrasound (US)- or computed tomography (CT)-guided drainage. In the case of small pseudocysts of 4–6 cm, spontaneous disappearance may occur. Larger pseudocysts should, if possible, be punctured quantitatively by US-guided fine-needle aspiration. The possibiliy of cystic tumor must always be excluded by additional diagnostic procedures. Our own experience with pancreatic pseudocysts and their symptoms and locations is that most of the pseudocysts larger than 4–6 cm cause severe pain. Other symptoms are weight loss, compresssion of duodenum, common bile duct, and obstruction of the superior mesenteric vein or portal vein. As shown by Washaw and Torchiana (1985), the rate of spontaneous resolution of pseudocysts larger than 4–6 cm in only 7%. Even under conservative management of chronic pancreatic pseudocysts, complications have to be taken into account in upt to 41% (Bradley et al. 1979; O'Malley et al. 1985). The mortality rate in pancreatic pseudocyst patients with nonsurgical management is 12%–14% (Wade 1985; Bradley et al. 1979). Therefore, we think that pseudocysts larger than 4–6 cm should be drained surgically. This is usually performed by cystojejunostomy with a blinded loop and Roux-Y reconstruction. In 1991, all pseudocyst treatments in the literature (1142 patients) were summarized and it was demonstrated that the mortality rate after surgical treatment was as high as 9%. The incidence was 9%, and the complication rate 35%. Many of those patients with pseudocyst and chronic pancreatitis

Table 7. Late results after left resection in chronic pancreatitis (CP) patients

	Patients (n)	Failure of improvement or recurrence (%)
Segmental left CP (n = 54)		
Partial	24	33.3
Subtotal	34	8
Diffuse CP (n = 67)		
Partial	24	66.7
Subtotal	43	48.8

From Gebhardt et al. (1981)

need additional resection of the head of the pancreas later on. In smaller cysts, duodenum-preserving pancreatic head resection can be performed simultaneously. Pseudocysts larger than 4 cm should first be drained surgically, and resection of the head of the pancreas might be performed as a second procedure after an interval of 6–12 months.

References

Amann RW, Akovbiantz A, Largiader F, Schueler G (1984) Course and outcome of chronic pancreatitis. Longitudinal study of a mixed medical-surgical series of 245 patients. Gastroenterology 86: 820–828

Beger HG, Witte C, Kraas R, Bittner R (1980) Erfahrung mit einer das Duodenum erhaltenden Pankreaskopfresektion bei chronischer Pankreatitis. Chirurg 51: 303–307

Beger HG, Krautzberger W, Bittner R, Büchler M, Limmer J (1985) Duodenum preserving resection of the head of the pancreas in patients with severe pancreatitis. Surgery 97: 467–473

Beger HG, Büchler M, Oettinger W, Roscher R (1989) Duodenum-preserving resection of the head of the pancreas in severe chronic pancreatitis. Ann Surg 209: 273–278

Beger HG, Büchler M (1990) Duodenum-preserving resection of the head of the pancreas in chronic pancreatitis with inflammatory mass in the head. World J Surg 14: 83–87

Bittner R, Büchler M, Butters M, Leibl B, Nägele S, Roscher R, Beger HG (1992) The effect of duodenum preserving pancreatic head resection on the endocrine pancreatic function in patients with chronic head pancreatitis. Z Gastroenterol 30: 12–16

Bockmann DE, Büchler M, Malfertheiner P, Beger HG (1988) Analysis of nerves in chronic pancreatitis. Gastroenterology 94: 1459–1469

Braasch JW, Vito L, Nugent FW (1978) Total pancreatectomy for end-stage chronic pancreatitis. Ann Surg 188: 317–322

Bradley EL (1987) Long-term results of pancreatojejunostomy in patients with chronic pancreatitis. Am J Surg 153: 207–213

Bradley EL, Clements JL, Gonzalez AC (1979) The natural history of pancreatic pseudocysts: an unfied concept of management. Am J Surg 137: 135–141

Büchler M, Weihe E, Friess H, Malfertheiner P, Bockmann D, Müller S, Nohr D, Beger HG (1992) Changes in peptidergic innervation in chronic pancreatitis. Pancreas 7: 183–192

Büchler MW, Friess H, Müller MW, Wheatley AM, Beger HG (1995) Randomized trial of duodenum-preserving pancreatic head resection versus pylorus-preserving Whipple in chronic pancreatitis. Am J Surg 169: 65–69

Cattell RB (1947) Anastomosis of the duct of Wirsung; its use in palliative operations for cancer in the head of the pancreas. Surg Clin North Am 27: 636–642

Frey CF, Child CG, Frey W (1976) Pancreatectomy for chronic pancreatitis. Ann Surg 184: 403–414

Frey CF, Smith G (1987) Description an rationale of a new operation for chronic pancreatitis. Pancreas 2: 701–712

Frick S, Jung K, Rückert K (1987) Chirurgie der chronischen Pankreatitis. Dtsch med Wochschr 112: 629-635

Gall FP, Mühe E, Gebhardt Ch (1981) Results of partial and total pancreaticoduodenectomy in 117 patients with chronic pancreatitis. World J Surg 5: 269-275

Gebhardt C, Zirngibl H, Gossler M (1981) Pankreaslinksresektion zur Behandlung der chronischen Pankreatitis. Langenbecks Arch Chir 354: 209-220

Howard J, Zhang Z (1990) Pancreaticoduodenectomy (Whipple resection) in the treatment of chronic pancreatitis. World J Surg 14: 77-82

Izbicki JR, Bloechle C, Knoefel WT, Wilker DK, Dornschneider G, Seifert H, Passlick B, Roiers X, Busch, C, Broelsch CE (1994) Complications of adjacent organs in chronic pancreatitis managed by duodenum-preserving resection of the head of the pancreas. Brit J Surg 81: 1351-1355

Kausch W (1912) Das Carcinom der Papilla duodeni und seine radikale Entfernung. Beitr Klin Chir 78: 439-486

Klempa I, Spatny M, Menzel J, Baca I, Nustede R, Stockmann F, Arnold W (1995) Pankreasfunktion und Lebensqualität nach Pankreaskopfresektion bei der chronischen Pankreatitis. Eine prospektive, randomisierte Vergleichsstudie nach duodenumerhaltender Pankreaskopfresektion versus Whipple'scher Operation

Lankisch PG, Lohr-Happe A, Otto J, Creutzfeldt W (1995) Natürlicher Verlauf der chronischen Pankreatitis – Schmerz, exokrine und endokrine Pankreasinsuffizienz und Prognose der Erkrankung. Zentralbl Chir 120: 278-286

Leger L, Lenriot JP, Lemaigre G (1974) Five to twenty year follow-up after surgery for chronic pancreatitis in 148 patients. Ann Surg 180: 185-191

Levy P, Milan C, Pognon JP, Baetz A, Bernardes P (1989) Mortality factors associated with chronic pancreatitis. Unidimensional and multidimensional analysis of a medical-surgical series of 240 patients. Gastroenterology 96: 1165-1172

Morel P, Mathey P, Corboud H, Huber O, Egeli RA (1990) Pylorus-preserving duodenopancreatectomy: long-term complications and comparison with the Whipple procedure. World J Surg 14: 642-647

Morrow CE, Cohen JI, Sutherland DER, Najarian JS (1984) Chronic pancreatitis: Longterm surgical results of pancreatic duct drainage, pancreatic resection, and near-total pancreatectomy and islet autotransplantation. Surgery 96: 608-615

Nealon WH, Townsend CJ, Thompson JC (1988) Operative drainage of the pancreatic duct delays functional impairment in patients with chronic pancreatitis. Am Surg 208: 321-329

Nealon WH, Thompson JC (1993) Progressive loss of pancreatic function in chronic pancreatitis is delayed by main pancreatic duct decompression. A longitudinal prospective analysis of the modified Puestow procedure. Ann Surg 217: 458-468

O'Malley V, Cannon JP, Postier RG (1985) Pancreatic pseudocysts: cause, therapy, and results. Am J Surg 150: 680-682

Partington PF, Rochelle REL (1960) Modified Puestov procedure for retrograde drainage of the pancreatic duct. Ann Surg 152: 1037-1043

Pellegrini CA, Heck CF, Raper S, Way LW (1989) An analysis of the reduce morbidity and mortality rates after pancreaticoduodenectomy. Arch Surg 124: 778-781

Prinz RA, Greenlee HB (1981) Pancreatic surgical drainage of pancreas for chronic relapsing pancreatitis. Arch Surg 76: 194: 313-320

Pueston CB, Gillerby WJ (1958) Retrograde surgical drainage of pancreas for chronic relapsing pancreatitis. Arch Surg 76: 898-906

Stone WM, Sarr MG, Nagorney DM, McIlrath DC (1988) Chronic pancreatitis. Results of Whipple's resection and total pancreatectomy. Arch Surg 123: 815-819

Thorsgaard-Pedersen N, Nyboe-Andersen B, Pedersen Worning H (1982) Chronic pancreatitis in Copenhagen. A retrospective study of 64 consecutive patients. Scand J Gastroenterol 17: 925-931

Traverso LW, Longmire WP (1978) Preservation of the pylorus during pancreaticoduodenectomy. Surg Gynecol Obstet 146: 959-962

Traverso LW, Abou Zam-Zam AM, Longmire WP (1981) Human pancreatic cell autotransplantation following total pancreatectomy. Ann Surg 193: 191-195

Traverso WL, Kozarek RA (1993) The Whipple procedure for severe complications of chronic pancreatitis. Arch Surg 128: 1047-1053

Wade JW (1985) Twenty-five year experience with pancreatic pseudocysts. Are we making progress? Am J Surg 149: 705-708

Warshaw AL, Torchiana DL (1985) Delayed gastric emptying after pylorus-preserving pancreaticoduodenectomy. Surg Gynecol Obstet 160: 1-4

Watson K (1944) Carcinoma of ampulla of Vater: Successful radical resection. Br J Surg 31: 368–373
Whipple AO, Pearson WB, Mullins CR (1935) Treatment of carcinoma of the ampulla of Vater. Ann Surg 102: 763–769
Whipple AO (1946) Radical surgery for certain cases of pancreatic fibrosis associated with calcareous deposits. Ann Surg 124: 991–1006
White TT, Hart MJ (1979) Pancreaticojejunostomy versus resection in the treatment of chronic pancreatitis. Am J Surg 138: 129–135

Pancreatic Cancer

Langerhans Islets Are the Origin of Ductal-Type Adenocarcinoma

P. M. Pour · L. Weide · G. Liu · K. Kazakoff · M. Scheetz
I. Toshkov · W. Sanger

Pancreatic exocrine adenocarcinoma has remained a mysterious disease. The short survival, late clinical manifestation, lack of early symptoms, a high recurrence rate after surgery, and its resistance to conventional therapy have contributed to its high mortality. Reasons for these characteristics can be attributed, in part, to its unknown etiology and histogenesis. Recent studies have shown hormonal abnormalities (altered glucose tolerance, diabetes, serological changes in pancreatic hormones) in pancreatic cancer patients, and these alterations precede the clinical symptoms [1]. We have observed proliferation of endocrine cells in many human pancreatic cancers and alterations in hormonal content of islet cells in pancreatic islets around pancreatic cancer [2, 3]. More recently, elevation of islet amyloid polypeptide has been found in patients with pancreatic cancer but not with other gastrointestinal cancers [1]. Morphological evidence for participation of pancreatic islets and endocrine abnormalities in pancreatic cancer in humans and experimentally induced pancreatic ductal adenocarcinomas was brought about by the proliferation of malignant cells within the islets near or remote from the primary pancreatic tumors [2-4]. In the hamster pancreatic cancer model, which mimics the human disease morphologically, biologically, and clinically [4-7], the first morphological change during carcinogenesis is the appearance of intrainsular ductular structures which either progress to form patterns resembling human pancreatic microcystic adenomas or become increasingly hyperplastic and culminate in the formation of malignant glands that gradually destroy the islets and invade the surrounding tissues [8]. Characteristically, and analogous to our findings in human tissues, almost all induced pancreatic cancers contain foci of islets or retain the ability to produce islet hormones even in their metastatic sites [9]. These observations indicate that, in addition to pancreatic ducts, some components of islets (most probably the stem cells) are the origin of pancreatic ductal-type adenocarcinoma. Support for this hypothesis comes from the observation that destruction of β-cells by the diabetogenic compounds alloxan and streptozotocin (STZ), prior to carcinogen treatment, inhibits or prevents pancreatic cancer induction, but not when the STZ-treated hamsters receive nicotinamide, which prevents islet cell destruction by STZ [10, 11]. Moreover, genetically diabetic hamsters with atrophic islets are resistant to the pancreatic carcinogenic effect of N-nitrosobis(2-oxopropyl)amine (BOP), whereas the pancreas of nondiabetic strains with intact islets are susceptible to this effect [12]. However, convincing proof for the role of islets in pancreatic exocrine cancer induction has been hampered by the complex structure of the pancreas with its interacting endocrine and exocrine components.

Given that islets are important for pancreatic cancer induction, tumors should be inducible in any nontarget tissue of BOP, where homologous islets could be transplanted. Because the submandibular glands (SMG) of hamsters were found to be a suitable site for islet transplantation [13], in our recent study, when freshly isolated pancreatic islets were transplanted into the SMG of recipient hamsters which were subsequently treated with BOP, ductal/ductular lesions developed within the SMG [14]. However, no frank carcinoma was seen, and the origin of the lesions from either the SMG or islets could not be determined. Therefore, in the present study we examined the effect of BOP in female hamsters after transplantation of islets from male hamsters (Eppley colony) into their SMG. By transplanting male hamster islets into the SMGs of females, we could identify the tissue of tumor origin as either male (islets) or female (SMG) by examining the marker for Y chromosome in the induced lesions.

Islets were isolated by a modified procedure of Lacy and Kostianovsky [15] and were hand-picked under a dissecting microscope fitted with a green light filter according to the method of Finke and colleagues [16] to ensure a pure population of islets. The purity was substantiated by histological and electron microscopy examination of samples from each batch. Under pentobarbital anesthesia (50 mg/kg bw), 750 purified islets were injected into the right SMG of female hamsters in the direction of the lower median to upper lateral poles of the gland. Two million immortal pancreatic ductal cells, which were established from pancreatic ductal cells of a male hamster [17, 18], and cellulose powder were injected into their left SMG in the lower median to upper lateral direction, and digested thyroid gland tissue from three donor male hamsters was injected in the lower left to upper median poles of the SMG. One week later, when the growth of the transplants is usually well established [13], all hamsters were treated with BOP (40 mg/kgbw) weekly for 3 weeks.

Between 4 and 12 weeks after BOP treatment, 18 hamsters developed bulky, encapsulated nodular tumors ranging in size from 2 to 30 mm in diameter (13 ± 7 mm, Fig. 1). In ten out of 18 hamsters, tumors were in the right SMG, in

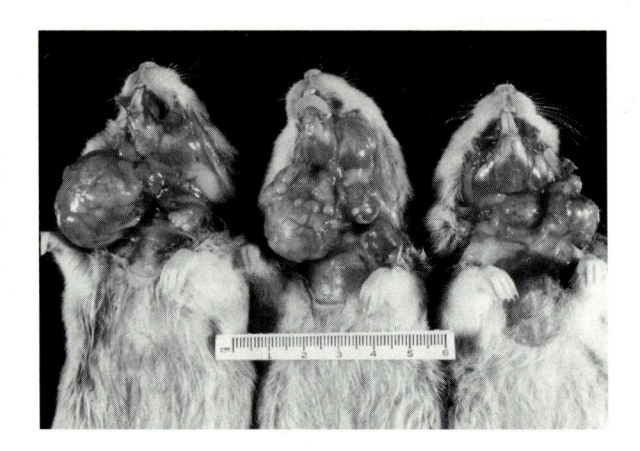

Fig. 1. Tumors in the submandibular glands (SMG) of three hamster, 6 weeks after the last *N*-nitrosobis(2-oxopropyl) amine (BOP) injection. The bulky neoplasms developed at the site of islet transplantation. Two had tumors in the right SMG and one in the left SMG where islets were injected

seven hamsters they were in the fatty tissue between the left and right SMG, and in one hamster the mass was in the left SMG region (Fig. 1). Histologically, all 18 tumors presented the same morphology of moderately to poorly differentiated adenocarcinoma (Fig. 2) that had invaded the surrounding SMG tissue, and 11 of them showed lymph node, lymphatic, and vascular invasion and lung metastases. Aggregation of islets was detectable in the vicinity of 14 tumors, including tumors that were located in the fatty tissue between the SMG (presumably as a result of leakage after transplantation) and the one in the left SMG, where islets were transplanted by error. Within some islet aggregates, single or multiple cysts, immunoreactive with antiblood group A antigen, were found (Fig. 3). On the border between tumor cells and islet aggregates, some cancer cells were immunoreactive with anti-insulin (Fig. 4). In other areas, normal-appearing or atypical ductular structures, where some cells showed a weak reactivity with anti-insulin (Fig. 5), were within these islets. All cancer cells were immunoreactive with anti-BGA antibody, which is a marker for pancreatic cancer [2, 4], while no immunoreactivity was seen in the surrounding SMG tissue.

In the left SMG of all hamsters, well-preserved thyroid tissue fragments and foreign body granulomas (in response to cellulose powder) were present. Remnants of injected immortal ductal cells could not be identified.

From one of the large tumors, a cell culture was prepared for cytogenetic analysis as reported [17, 18]. The tumor cells were hyperdiploid/pseudotetraploid with one to five extra copies of chromosomes numbers 1–17, and 19–21.

Fig. 2. Poorly differentiated adenocarcinoma in the submandibular gland (SMG) showing desmoplastic reaction

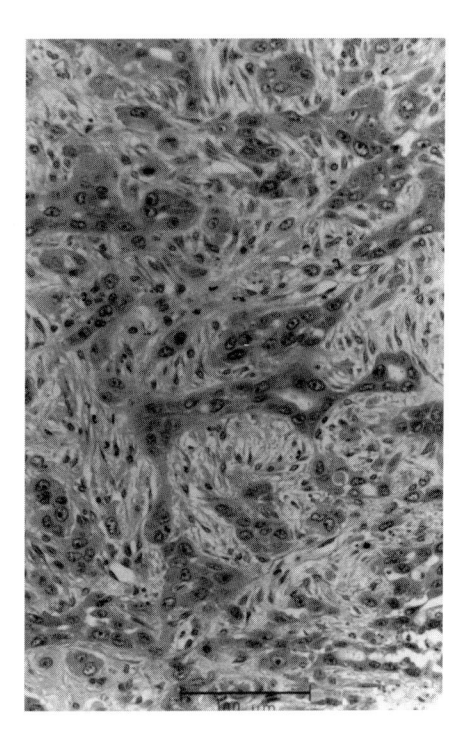

Fig. 3. Formation of cysts within an islet conglomerate (*dark area*) within the submandibular gland (SMG). The wall and the contents of the cysts were immunoreactive with antibody against blood group A. ABC, multilabeling technique, ×200.

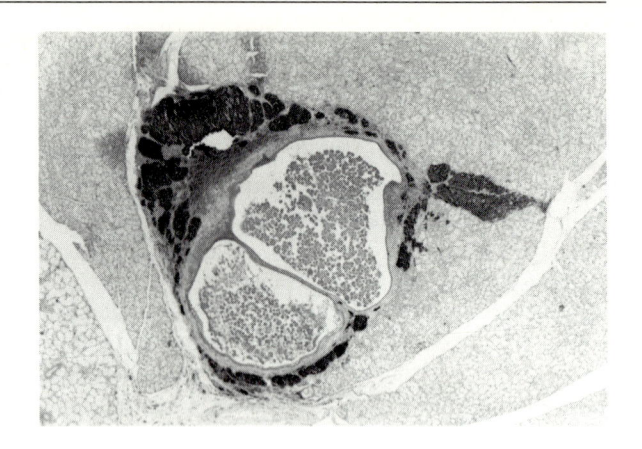

An X or Y chromosome was missing (Fig. 6). Amplification of the sex-determining region Y by PCR, however, yielded a positive result in one of the three tumors examined (data not shown). All three tumors that were examined by polymerase chain reaction (PCR) technique and DNA sequencing with a fluorescent detection method [17, 18] had a c-ki-ras mutation at codon 12.

The results of the present study validate the hypothesis that islets are the source of induced adenocarcinomas of ductal phenotype [19]. This conclusion is based on the following findings: the development of tumors only at the site of islet transplantation, the association of the transplanted islets with tumor cells, some of which were immunoreactive with anti-insulin, expression of blood group antigen, and the mutation of the c-Ki-*ras* oncogene, all of which are characteristic of induced pancreatic cancers [6, 7, 20, 21]. Our inability to detect the Y chromosome by cytogenetic analysis of one tumor cell line is not surprising because loss or gain of chromosomes frequently occurs in some aggressive and fast growing tumors. Specifically, a missing Y chromosome (-Y) has been

Fig. 4. An invasive cancer in the submandibular gland (SMG) in the immediate area of islet aggregate. Some of the pleomorphic cancer cells contain a few granules immunoreactive with anti-insulin. All tumor cells also expressed blood group A antigen (not shown). ABC method, ×400

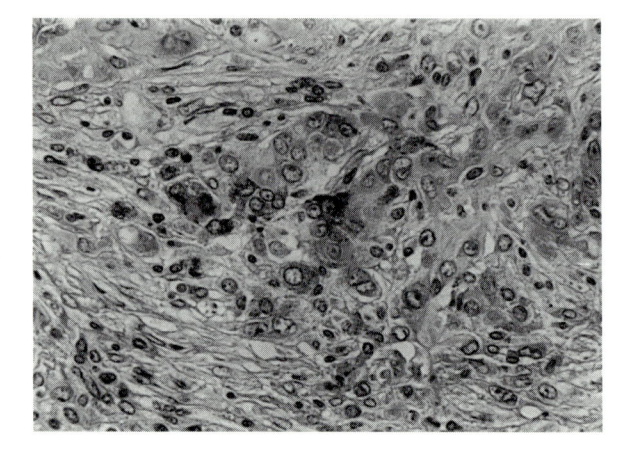

Fig. 5. A large islet conglomerate in the right submandibular gland (SMG) is composed primarily of β-cells (*dark areas*) and contains atypical ductular structures, where some cells show a weak immunoreactivity with anti-insulin. The lumen of the ductular structures expressed BGA antigen (*light area, center*). ABC method, ×400

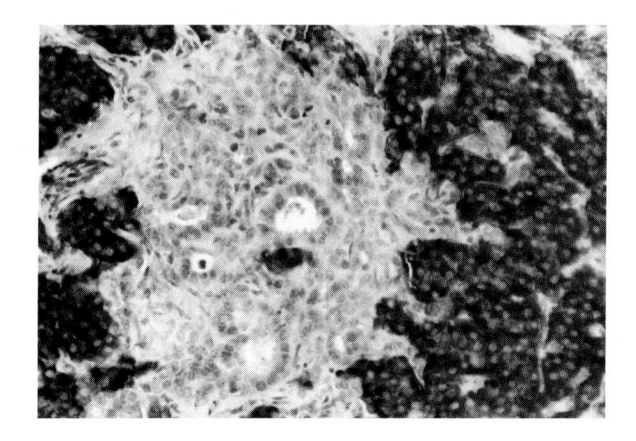

reported as one of the most common numerical abnormalities in human pancreatic adenocarcinoma [22, 23]. However, the Y chromosome message by PCR indicates that in some tumors Y chromosome DNA is maintained.

Evidence for the participation of islets in pancreatic ductal carcinogenesis opens a revised avenue for research into understanding this malignant disease. The expression of carbohydrate antigens in the islets [3] and the presence of malignant intrainsular ductal structures in the pancreas of pancreatic cancer patients [4] indicate that the above observation is not unique to the hamster. The assumption that most human pancreatic cancers derive from ductal epithelium is based only on anecdotal cases. It has been well established that both in humans and hamsters, tumors deriving from ductal epithelium are slow-growing lesions that remain within the ductal boundary for a considerable time [24], whereas the common pancreatic cancers are highly invasive even if they are small. We believe that pancreatic cancer in both humans and hamsters derives from stem cells that populate the ductal tree and islets. The greater susceptibility of intrainsular stem cells for malignancy and growth could be due to their local exposure to many growth factors, including insulin, insulin-like

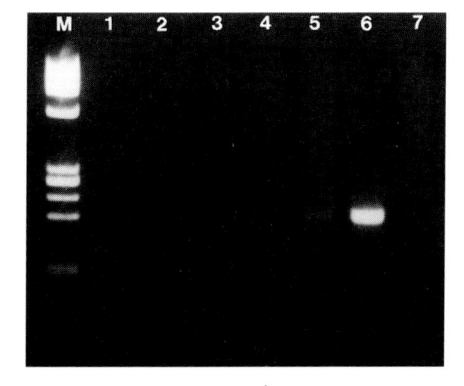

Fig. 6. Amplification of the sex-determining region Y by polymerase chain reaction (PCR). The primers used in PCR to amplify the Syrian hamster Y chromosome were designed according to the conserved region among humans, rabbits, and mice [27, 28]. Mixed bases were used in the region where the difference exists among the species. The sequences of the primers were as follows: upstream primer: 5' CAT GAA TGC TGC ATT TAT S(G and C)GT GTG GTC 3'; downstream primer: 5' TTT ATA GTT TGG GTA TTT CTC TY(C and T)T GT 3'. The lanes are: *M*, marker; *1*, negative control (H$_2$O); *2*, female liver; *3–5*, submandibular gland (SMG) tumors; *6*, male liver; *7*, female SMG

growth factor (IGF)-1, and transforming growth factor (TGF)-α [25]. Our concept is in line with the alteration of islet hormones in pancreatic cancer. The elevation of islet amyloid polypeptide in hamsters with pancreatic cancer [26] and particularly in pancreatic cancer patients, but not in patients with any other gastrointestinal cancers [1], may just be the beginning of the search for hormonal abnormalities associated with pancreatic cancer, data that can help early diagnosis and possibly prevention of this dismal disease.

Acknowledgment. This work was supported by the NIH/NCI 5R01 CA60479, by the NCI Laboratory Cancer Research Center support grant CA36727 and ACS Special Institutional Grant.

References

1. Permert J, Larsson J, Westermark GT, Herrington M, Christmanson L, Pour PM, Adrian TE (1994) Islet amyloid polypeptide in patients with pancreatic cancer and diabetes. New Engl J Med 330: 313-318
2. Pour PM, Permert J, Mogaki M, Fujii H, Kazakoff K (1993) Endocrine aspects of exocrine cancer of the pancreas. Their patterns and suggested biological significance. Am J Clon Pathol 100: 223-230
3. Pour PM, Morohoshi T (1994) Ductal adenocarcinoma. In: Atlas of Exocrine Pancreas. Morphology, Biology and Diagnosis with an International Guide for Tumor Classification. Pour PM, Konishi Y, Klöppel G, Lonnecker DS (eds), Springer Verlag, Toyko 1994, pp 117-154
4. Pour PM, Wilson R (1980) Experimental pancreas tumor. In: Cancer of the Pancreas (Moossa, AR ed). Williams and Wilkins, Baltimore, London, pp 37-158
5. Pour PM, Egami H, Takiyama Y (1991) Patterns of growth and metastases of induced pancreatic cancer in relation to the prognosis and its clinical implications. Gastroenterology 100: 1-7
6. Takiyama Y, Egami H, Pour PM (1990) Expression of human tumor-associated antigens in pancreatic cancer-induced in Syrian hamsters. Am J Pathol 136: 707-715
7. Fujii H, Egami H, Chaney W, Pour PM, Pelling J (1990) Pancreatic ductal adenocarcinomas induced in Syrian hamsters by N-nitrosobis(2-oxopropyl)amine contain a c-Ki-ras oncogene with a point-mutated codon 12. Molecular Carcinogenesis 3: 296-301
8. Pour PM (1989) Experimental pancreatic cancer. Am J Surg Pathol 13: 96-103
9. Pour PM, Bell RH (1989) Alteration of pancreatic endocrine cell patterns and their secretion during pancreatic carcinogenesis in the hamster model. Cancer Res 49: 6396-6400
10. Pour PM, Kazakoff K, Carlson K (1990) Inhibition of Streptozotocin-induced islet cell tumors and BOP-induced exogenous pancreatic tumors in Syrian hamsters. Cancer Res 50: 1634-1639
11. Bell RH, Sayers HJ, Pour PM, Ray MB, McCullough PJ (1989) Importance of diabetes in inhibition of pancreatic cancer by streptozotocin. J Surg Res 46: 515-519
12. Bell RH, Pour PM (1987) Induction of pancreatic tumors in genetically non-diabetic but not in diabetic Chinese hamster. Cancer Lett 34: 221-230
13. Pour PM, Weide LG, Ueno K, Corra S, Kazakoff K (1992) Submandibular gland as a site for islet transplantation. Int J Pancreatol 12: 187-191
14. Ishikawa O, Ohigashi H, Imaoka S, Nakai I, Mitsuo M, Weide L, Pour PM (1995) The role of pancreatic islets in experimental pancreatic carcinogenicity. Am J Pathol 147: 1456-1464
15. Lacy PE, Kostianovsky M (1967) Method for the isolation of intact islets of Langerhans from the rat pancreas. Diabetes 16(1): 35-39
16. Finke EH, Lacy PE, Ono J (1979) Use of reflected green light for specific identification of islets in vitro after collagenase isolation. Diabetes 28: 612-613
17. Takahashi T, Moyer MP, Cano M, Wang QJ, Mountjoy CP, Sanger W, Adrian TE, Sugiura H, Katoh H, Pour PM (1995) Differences in molecular biological, biological and growth characteristics between the immortal and malignant hamster pancreatic ductal cells. Carcinogenesis 16: 931-939

18. Takahashi T, Moyer MP, Cano M, Wang QJ, Adrian TE, Mountjoy CP, Sanger W, Sugiura H, Katoh H, Pour PM (1995) Establishment and characterization of a new, spontaneously immortalized, pancreatic ductal cell line from the Syrian golden hamster. Cell Tissue Res 282: 163–174
19. Pour PM (1978) Islet cells as component of pancreatic ductal neoplasm. I. Experimental study. Ductular cells, including islet cell precursors, and primary progenitor cells of tumors. Am J Pathol 90: 295–316
20. Egami H, Chaney WG, Takiyama Y, Pour PM (1991) Subcellular localization of blood group A substance produced by pancreatic adenocarcinoma induced in hamsters by N-nitrosobis(2-oxopropyl)amine (BOP) and by its cell line (PC-1). Carcinogenis 12: 509–514
21. Pour PM (1984) Histogenesis of exocrine pancreatic cancer in the hamster model. Envir Health Persp 56: 229–243
22. Bardi G, Johansson B, Pandis N, Mandahl N, Bak-Jensen E, Andrén-Sandberg Å, Mitelman F, Heim S (1993) Karyotypic abnormalities in tumors of the pancreas. Br J Cancer 67:1106–1112
23. Johansson B, Bardi G, Heim S, Mandahl N, Mertens F, Bak-jensen E, Andrén-Sandberg Å, Mitelman F (1992) Nonrandom chromosomal rearrangements in pancreatic carcinomas. Cancer 69: 1674–1681
24. Yamao K, Nakazawa S, Fujimoto M, Milchgrub S, Albores-Saavedra J (1994) Intraductal papillary mucinous tumors. Nob-invasive and invasive. In: Atlas of Exocrine Pancreas. Morphology, Biology and Diagnosis with an International Guide for Tumor Classification. Pour PM, Konishi Y, Klöppel G, Lonnecker DS (eds), Springer Verlag, Tokyo, pp 67–82
25. Tomioka T, Toshkov I, Kazakoff K, Andrén-Sandberg Å, Takahashi T, Büchler M, Friess H, Vaughn R, Pour PM (1995) Cellular and subcellular localization of transforming growth factor-α and epidermal growth factor receptor in normal and diseased human and hamster pancreas. Teratogenesis, Carcinogenesis, and Mutagenesis 15: 231–25
26. Adrian TE, Permert J, Westermark G (1994) Islet hormones in pancreatic cancer. The association between islet amyloid polypeptide level and diabetes. Int J Pancreatol 16: 274–277

I
Imaging Procedures

Ultrasound and Endoscopic Ultrasound in the Diagnosis of Pancreatic Tumors

H. Meier · H. Friebel

Introduction

Due to the increasing number of new imaging techniques and tumor markers, it is difficult to establish which method or combination of methods may provide the greatest amount of information for diagnosis of pancreatic carcinoma. The accuracy of different imaging methods in the detection of pancreatic tumors depends mainly on the size of the tumor and the involvement of the main pancreatic duct and common bile duct. Endoscopic retrograde cholangiopancreatography (ERCP) has a very high sensitivity in the diagnosis of tumors because of the frequent involvement of the main pancreatic duct; the specificity in cases of chronic pancreatitis is, however, limited. Small tumors of less than 2 cm in diameter are hardly demonstrated by ultrasound (US) or even computed tomography (CT); in these cases, the sensitivity of endoscopic ultrasound (EUS) is clearly superior (higher than 90%).

Most patients with pancreatic cancer are first identified on the basis of their symptoms. Pain, jaundice, or both are present in over 80% of patients at the time of diagnosis [1]. Weight loss is reported by almost 100% of subjects. Fatigue, nausea, palpable mass, hepatomegaly, and ascites are other relatively frequent associated symptoms and clinical signs. Carcinomas of the body and tail of the pancreas do not produce jaundice until they metastasize, and they may remain painless until advanced stages of the disease. In these cases, weight loss and fatigue are the symptoms which may lead to the diagnosis. Acute pancreatitis is occasionally the first manifestation of pancreatic cancer. The new onset of diabetes mellitus can also direct to pancreatic cancer. All these symptoms, however, are not specific either to cancer or to a particular type of cancer.

US and CT are the methods most frequently used to confirm a clinical suspicion of pancreatic cancer. Both can detect pancreatic masses as small as 2 cm, dilation of the pancreatic and bile ducts, hepatic metasases, and extrapancreatic spread of the tumor [2]. US is cheap, generally available, and accurate in distinguishing obstructive from nonobstructive jaundice, which is the presenting feature in 50% of patients [3]. CT provides better definition of the tumor and its surrounding structures than US and relies less on the experience of the observer and on the body habitus [4]. In advanced pancreatic cancer, CT provides all the information needed for a complete assessment, including staging if metastases are observed. US, apart from the absence of ionizing radiation, also has the advantage of being able to distinguish changes in echogenicity, which in some cases can make a small tumor apparent before it changes the contour of the gland, a condition required for detection by CT. Neither of these techniques is capable of differentiating pancreatic adenocarcinoma from other solid tumors of the pancreas.

Ultrasonographic Signs in Pancreatic Tumors

Tumefaction. The mass and the associated bulge in the contour result in a loss of the harmony of the outline of the pancreas. Localized swelling may be due to a tumor that is smaller than the apparent swelling. The maximum thickness of the normal gland is 30–35 mm. A pathological thickness, of 40 or 50 mm, for example, corresponds to the normal thickness of the gland with the addition of tumor tissue. The diameter of the tumor may thus be less than 2 cm. These small tumors are practically all located in the head of the pancreas and are discovered because of their close relationship to the common bile duct and the early appearance of jaundice. Small caudal tumors are rarely found.

Contours. Pancreatic contours are well demarcated. In large tumors, expansions of the gland are evident. Most small tumors have smooth borders.

Echotexture. Carcinomas are practically always hypoechoic and have a semisolid appearance with few echoes. A dilatation of the pancreatic duct behind the tumor is usually observed in cases in which the tumor obstructs the duct (Fig. 1). An associated dilatation of the common bile duct may also be present in cases of obstruction of the ampulla of Vater or tumoral infiltration of the bile duct.

Associated Signs and Spread. The vena cava may be compressed. The mesenteric vein is usually completely flattened, but the superior mesenteric artery and the celiac trunk escape usually compression until late in the disease. Involvement of the wall and invasion of the lumen indicate that the prognosis is poor and that

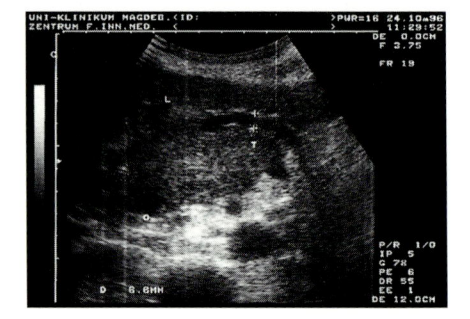

Fig. 1. Adenocarcinoma of the head of the pancreas with dilatation of the main pancreatic duct behind the tumor (6.6 mm). *L,* liver; *C* common bile duct; *T,* tumor

the chances of successful curative surgery are low. CT shows invasion of perivascular fat better than US. Intraoperative US shows better the boundaries of the tumor and its spread to the surrounding anatomic structures. A systematic search for hepatic metastasis and for signs of peritoneal carcinomatosis (ascites) should be carried out. Tumors of the uncinate process displace the normal pancreatic tissue forwards, along with the mesenteric vessels, in a fashion similar to retroperitoneal adenopathies.

Endocrine Tumors

Secreting endocrine tumors (insulinomas gastrinomas) give rise to onset of functional symptoms when their volume is still quite small. Davies (1993) reported a success rate of 33 % in the preoperative US diagnosis of tumors over 5 mm in diameter. A success rate of 50 % was achieved by Zeiger (1993). The pattern of small endocrine tumors is that of hypoechoic nodules with smooth borders (Fig. 2). Attention must be paid to gastrinomas, since 30 % are multiple, 30 % ectopic, and 60 % malignant. Most ectopic gastrinomas are located within the duodenal wall and are thus accessible to intraoperative US. Nonsecreting neuroendorcine tumors become clinically apparent much later as a result of mechanical compression due to their volume. Thus they are much more accessible to US.

Cystic Tumors

Cystic tumors can be different in appearance depending on the size of cystic formations. When the cysts are large, cystic tumors have the appearance of a liquid collection and can be confused with pseudocysts. The configuration of the tumors is quite different when the cysts are small. The multiple interface between the cyst walls in microcystic adenomas result in multiple hyperechoic foci that give the tumor a solid appearance. Morphological analysis associated with biopsy by guided puncture is required to differentiate between microcystic adenomas, mucinous cystoadenocarcinomas, and mucinous cystadenomas.

Fig. 2. Carcinoid of the body-tail of the pancreas (30.9 mm). *LL,* liver; *P,* pancreas; *MV,* splenic vein

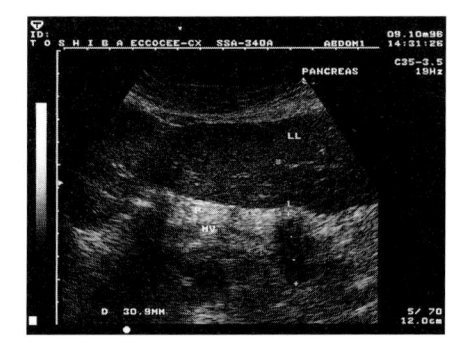

Ultrasound-Guided Fine-Needle Biopsy

Despite the progress and refinement of imaging modalities (ERCP, US, CT, EUS), the precise diagnosis of pancreatic masses continues to be a problem in many instances [5-8]. The best approach to surgical or nonsurgical treatment of pancreatic cancer can be only undertaken on the basis of a cytologically or cytohistologically confirmed diagnosis. Percutaneous fine-needle biopsy (FNB) guided by means of real-time US has become an increasingly important diagnostic tool for tumor diagnosis before therapeutic decisions. FNB can be performed with a high-resolution electronic linear tranducer with a central biopsy slit or with a lateral biopsy attachment, which allows a needle to be placed into the tumor target during real-time cross-sectional viewing of the area of interest, favoring the shortest distance to the target whenever possible. Biopsy is performed using commercially available spinal-type needles or cutting needles with an internal stylet and an outer diameter of 20-22 gauge. The procedure is performed during suspended respiration without local anesthesia [9-10].

The sensitivity of US-guided FNB of pancreatic cancer is as high as 86%-100% [11, 12]. Possible complications that may arise in connection with the transperitoneal biopsy include bleeding, peritonitis, septicemia, and general dissemination of tumor cells or malignant seeding along the puncture channel. However, in experienced hands this method is safe and of great value for cytohistological diagnosis of malignancy.

Endoscopic Ultrasonography

EUS provides direct ultrasonic imaging of pancreatic tumors and lymph nodes through the gastrointestinal lumen and has been reported to be accurate in the demonstration and differential diagnosis of pancreatic cancer [13], as well as being an additional method of staging [14, 15]. The goal of preoperative staging of pancreatic cancer should be to ascertain the optimal treatment for each patient. The aim is to determine which tumors are potentially resectable, which cannot be resected but are still localized, and which have metastasized to distant sites. The extent of preoperative staging depends on the treatment options available to the patient [16]. Mortality of less than 5% for pancreatoduodenectomy in specialized centers are being reported. On the other hand, patients with metastatic disease are probably best served if spared an operation.

EUS allows images of the pancreas and adjacent organs with a degree of resolution superior to other imaging modalities in current use [17]. Tumors are seen as hypoechoic nodules. Heterogeneous or infiltrative nodules may be more difficult to delineate. EUS readily shows the relationship of the mass to the pancreatic and bile ducts. In particular, it is possible to evaluate the local tumor extension. Resectability requires the absence of posterior venous invasion and of extension to the celiac region and mesenteric root. The search for adenopathies is another step in the evaluation of patients with pancreatic tumors. Criteria of malignancy for adenopathies are hypoechoic echotexture, rounded shape, and clear delineation. Invasion of the celiac and mesenteric regions is encountered in large infiltrative tumors, and EUS shows such infiltration as hypoechoic areas and streaks within the echogenic retroperitoneal fat. With regard to detection of pancreatic carcinomas, the sensitivity of EUS (95%), as reported in recent studies, is superior to that of conventional US (65%) or CT (70%) [18]. It is similar to that of ERCP, but EUS has the advantage of direct nodular display. EUS is particularly useful for the detection of tumors less than 2 cm in diameter.

Staging of pancreatic tumors based on EUS yields accurate results in 90% of patients regarding extention of the tumor, in 75% regarding adenopathies, and in 90% regarding venous invasion.

Endocrine Tumors

EUS shows endocrine tumors as well-delineated hypoechoic nodules and has a sensitivity of 82% and a specificity of 95%, which is superior to that of conventional procedures.

Ampullar Tumors

Most ampullar tumors are adenomas or adenocarcinomas. They induce a hypoechoic thickening of the duodenal wall over 5 mm. The dilated bile duct and pancreatic duct may be followed down to the lesion. EUS gives a correct evaluation of the local tumor extension in 70%-90% of patients. T1 tumors, limited to the ampulla, are differentiated from T2 tumors, which invade the duodenal wall down to the muscularis propria.

References

1. Classen M (1987) Erkrankungen des Pankreas. In: Siegenthaler W. Lehrbuch der inneren Medizin. Thieme Stuttgart, S 1061-1072
2. Hessel SJ (1982) A prospective evaluation of CT and US of the pancreas. Radiology 143: 129-133
3. Campbell JP (1988) Pancreatic neoplasm: how useful is evaluation with US? Radiology 167: 341-344
4. Smith KJ (1989) Is US equivalent to CT in the diagnosis of pancreatic cancer? Gastroenterology 96: A480
5. Tao (1990) The pancreas. In: Transabdominal fine-needle aspiration biopsy. Igaku-Shoin, New York, pp 133-178
6. Hal-Craggs (1986) FNAB: pancreatic and biliary tumors. AJR 1986: 399-403
7. Glenthoj (1990) Us guided histological and cytological fine needle biopsie of the pancreas. Gut 31: 930-933
8. Elvin (1990) Biopsy of the pancreas with a biopsy gun. Radiology 176: 677-679
9. Charboneau (1990) CT and US guided needle biopsy: current techniques and new innovations. AJR 154: 1-10
10. Schwerk (1986) US guided FNB in the diagnosis of pancreatic tumors. Diagnostic procedures in pancreatic disease. P. Malfertheiner (ed) Springer, Berlin
11. Fornari (1992) US guided FNAB of gastrointestinal organs. Dig Dis 10: 121-133
12. Parson (1989) How accurate is FNAB of the pancreas? Arch Surg 124: 681-686

13. Dancygier (1988) Pancreatic cancer. In: Kawai (ed) Endoscopic ultrasonography in Gastroenterology. Igaku-Shoin, Tokyo, pp 72-78
14. Roesch (1992) Staging of pancreatic and ampullary carcinoma by EUS. Gastroenterology 102: 188-199
15. Roesch (1990) Endosonographische Diagnostik bei Pankreastumoren. Dtsch med Wschr 115: 1339-1347
16. Tio (1986) Endoscopic ultrasonography in staging local resectability of pancreatic and periampullary malignancy. Scand J Gastroenterol 21, Suppl. 123: 135-142
17. Yasuda (1988) The diagnosis of pancreatic cancer by EUS. Gastrointest Endoscopy 34: 1-8
18. Kaufmann (1989) EUS in the differential diagnosis of pancreatic disease. Gastrointest. Endosc 35: 214-219

Computed Tomography and Magnetic Resonance Imaging in Pancreatic Cancer

J. M. Friedrich

Introduction

Modern imaging modalities in pancreatic cancer include computed tomography (CT) and magnetic resonance imaging (MRI). While CT is widely accepted as the gold standard in the screening and follow-up of pancreatic disease, MRI did not primarily appear to have a significant role in the evaluation of pancreatic disorders. Susceptibility to respiratory and bowel motion, confusion with surrounding bowels, and inferior spatial resolution seemed to limit the role of MRI vis-à-vis CT. In the last 2 years, both techniques have improved dramatically: CT with the introduction of high-speed spiral acquisition (Fig. 1a, b) and MRI with the introduction of the phased array technique and ultrafast sequences allowing imaging in breathhold modalities.

Both modalities can differentiate between the different histologic types in pancreatic cancer, provide helpful information about tumor staging, and help to optimize surgical treatment according to prognosis.

With an incidence of about 80%, the most commonly diagnosed pancreatic tumor is ductal adenocarcinoma, which is classically found in the head of the

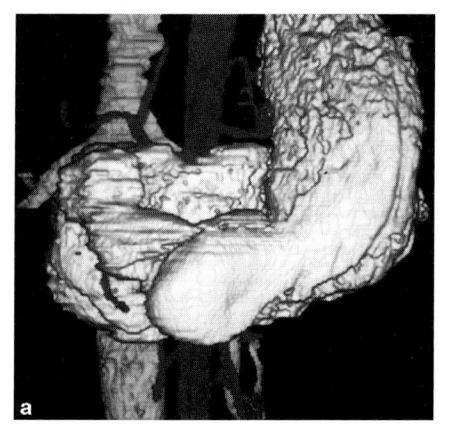

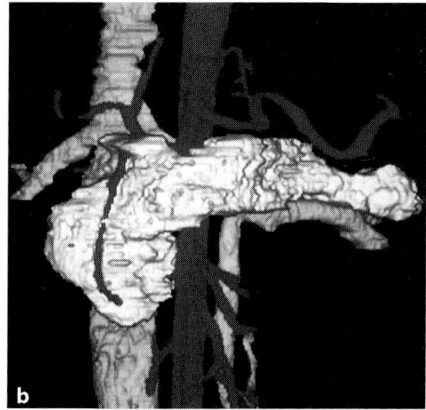

Fig. 1a, b. Reconstruction of the pancreas and the retroperitoneal vessels in high resolution spiral technique (Elscint twin) with and without the stomach. Excellent topographic resolution is achieved (Courtesy Dr. Sokiranski, Ulm)

pancreas. Mucinous cystadenocarcinomas are characterized by their partly cystic appearance. Islet cell tumors have the highest incidence of endocrine neoplasm; they usually measure less than 2 cm in diameter and may cause symptoms due to their hormonal activity. Ampullary carcinomas are usually diagnosed early because of occlusive jaundice. Metastases and lymphomas are rarely localized in the pancreas, and their features are generally nonspecific.

Early diagnosis of pancreatic cancer is rare despite recent advances in imaging; this is because clinical symptoms appear late after lymph nodes and liver metastases have occurred [1-5]. The diagnostic challenge in pancreatic tumor imaging is currently high.

Technique of Computed Tomography

The *conventional technique* has the following features:

- Clusters of two scans with an interscan delay of 3.5 s
- Slice thickness of 5 mm
- Total scan time of 200 s
- 120 ml nonionic contrast agent

Features of the *spiral technique* include the following:

- All slices acquired during one breathhold
- Slice thickness of 5 mm
- Total scan time of 15 s
- 80 ml non ionic contrast agent

With the spiral technique, it is possible to distinguish early arterial from late parenchymatous and venous phases; three-dimensional reformation of CT arteriography or CT venography is also possible.

Diagnostic Features

The main diagnostic feature of pancreatic cancer is evidence of a hypodense pancreatic mass in the contrast study (Fig. 2a, b). Local infiltration in the surrounding fatty tissues, retroperitoneal structures, and infiltration of the mesenterial or splenic vessels are important features. Vascular involvement of mesenterial and portal vein indicates nonresectability. Pancreatic dilatation is seen in 50%, and biliary duct dilatation in 40% of patients. Liver metastases are present in about 15%.

Lymph node metastases may be difficult to image in the periportal field, but can be imaged more easily in the retroperitonium. Ascites may indicate peritoneal extension.

The features of pancreatic cancer seen on CT are shown in Table 1 [15]
Endocrine tumors are frequently hypervascular [13]. Mucinous cystadenocarcinoma demonstrates low attenuation and septation. Typically less then six

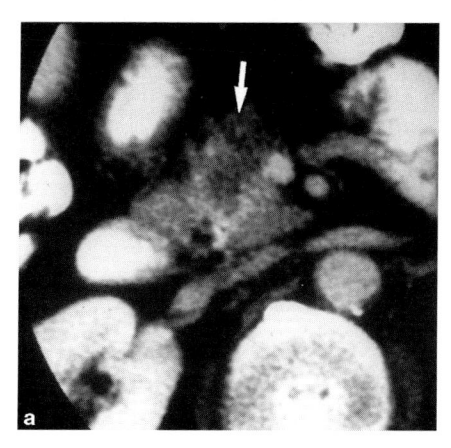

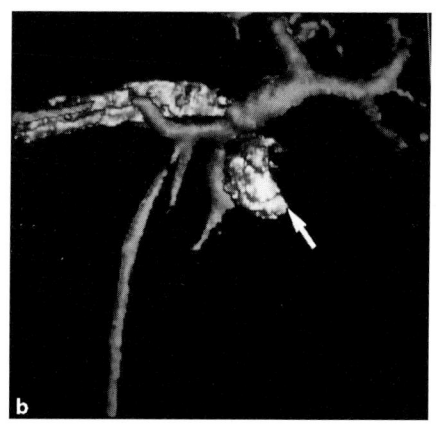

Fig. 2a, b. Small carcinoma of the head of the pancreas (*arrow*) with infiltration of mesenteric fatty tissue. Three-dimensional reconstruction (**b**) shows the displacement of the superior mesenteric vein by the tumor (*arrow*) (posterior view)

cysts with a diameter greater than 2 cm are found [6]. Sometimes tumor calcifications are demonstrated. Obstructive jaundice due to distal obstruction of the biliary duct may be an early sign of pancreatic cancer, while obstruction at the level of the liver hilus duct may be an early sign of pancreatic cancer, while obstruction at the level of the liver hilus provides evidence of extended disease. CT and CT angiography are very sensitive in the diagnosis of thrombotic lesions of the portal vein. Endoscopic retrograde cholangiography (ERC) or MR cholangiography may establish exactly the site of obstruction, while thin-sliced CT is helpful in differentiating a prepapillary encrusted gallstone from a prepapillary tumor. Dilatation of the pancreatic duct without any other signs of chronic pancreatitis strongly suggests pancreatic neoplasm.

Evidence of dilated pancreaticoduodenal veins is a very strong indication of vascular involvement by infiltrating tumor [8, 11]. CT demonstrates an increasing number of vessels in the peripheral part of the tumor caused by occlusion of central vessels.

Table 1. Features of pancreatic cancer seen on CT

Feature	Detected in Patients (%)
Pancreatic mass	95
Low attenuation	75
Vascular involvement	60
Pancreatic duct dilatation	50
Biliary duct dilatation	38
Liver metastases	30
Gland atrophy	20
Lymph node metastases	15
Ascites	10
Calcifications	20

In extended disease, severe compression of the inferior caval vein or renal vein may occur. Sensitivity of CT in detecting lymph node metastases in low (38%) [11]. In comparison to ultrasound, CT is clearly the modality with the optimal clinical impact in pancreatic cancer.

The spiral technique allows a significantly shorter acquisition time to be used and provides the possibility of higher resolution two- or three-dimensional reformation (Fig. 3a, b).

As a result of the most recent results using the best spiral technology available, a tremendous improvement in tumor depiction related to higher-contrast resolution may be expected.

Due to its volumetric nature, helically acquired image data can be reconstructed in smaller increments, thus improving the quality of two- or three-dimensional reconstruction. With the same slice thickness, a substantially larger volume of data may be acquired within one single breathhold, thus avoiding respiratory-related artifacts. Structures with different timing of peak contrast enhancement such as liver and pancreas may be imaged more appropriately during their optimal enhancement, e.g., 30 s for pancreas, 40 s for the portal system, and 50–100 s for liver parenchyma.

With the spiral technique, a single noninvasive procedure can be used to diagnose the tumor and to stage its extension to surrounding organs and to the major vessels as well as to recognize metastatic lesions in the whole upper abdomen with the highest sensitivity.

In today's health care environment, a cost-effective strategy for the work-up of suspected pancreatic carinoma is needed. With recent advances in helical CT and the possibility of CT angiography, high resolution CT may be the sole imaging modality in staging pancreatic carcinoma.

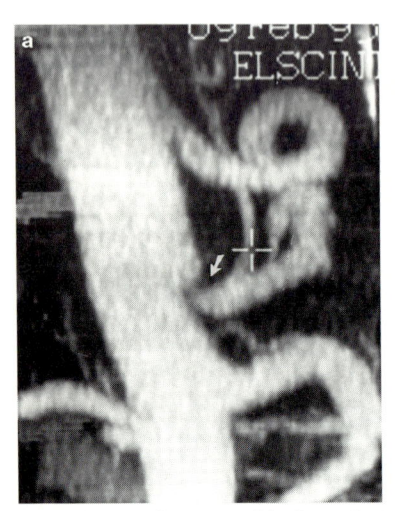

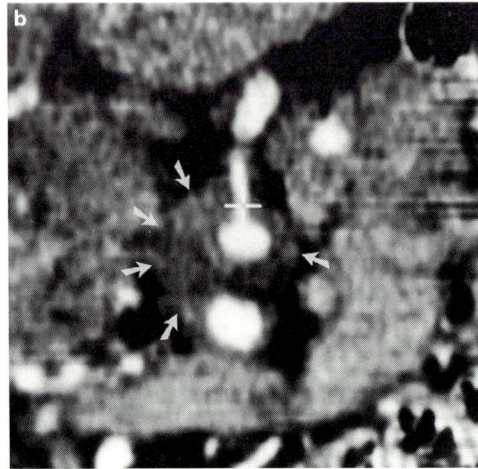

Fig. 3a, b. Two-dimensional high resolution reformation demonstrating encasement at the origin of the coeliac artery (*arrow* a). Reconstruction in coronal plane verifies perivascular tumor infiltration (*arrow*) with high contrast

Respiratory-related and motion artifacts do not favor abdominal imaging. Furthermore, bad contrast to surrounding intestinal structures and low sensitivity in detecting calcification may limit the role of **MRI in pancreatic disease.**

The introduction of ultrafast sequences and the phased array technique represent significant improvements in abdominal imaging [2].

Gradient echo sequences are the gold standard [9, 10]. They allow short acquisition in T1 and T2, because the TR and the TE are shortened, so that images of the pancreas can be obtained in one breathhold. We routinely use fat saturation techniques that decrease the signal intensity of fat and improve considerably imaging of the upper abdominal organs, especially the pancreas. Turbo spin echo techniques are not helpful in this context, as they do not allow data acquisition during one breathhold.

The spatial resolution is obtained with the use of phased array surface coil. Imaging planes include the transversal and coronal plane, and the slice thickness is between 5 and 8 mm. The usual contrast agent is gadolinium diethylenetriaminopentoacetic acid (Gd-DTPA) in concentrations of between 0.1 and 0.2 mmol/kg and shows an intestinal distribution like iodized contrast medium. Manganese dipyridoxyl diphosphate (Mn DPDP) shows parenchymal uptake, but has not yet been approved for clinical use.

Pancreatic Neoplasm

Pancreatic tumors are usually ductal adenocarcinomas, which are relatively difficult to diagnose by CT. These tumors metastasize early, which is why early diagnosis and better visualization of the adjacent structures of the pancreatic gland, especially the porta hepatis, are important. MRI offers an interesting approach to improve the diagnosis of pancretic carcinoma, as plenty of potential sequences are available. In the study by Steiner et al. [12], visualization of pancreatic tumors was better with MRI than with CT in 22 % of cases because the signal intensity was different from that in normal pancreas tissue; 63 % of pancreatic tumors had lower signal intensities than normal pancreas, whereas on T2-weighted sequences only 41 % had increased signal intensity.

Features of Pancreatic Tumor on Magnetic Resonance Imaging

Direct tumor signs include the following:

- Circumscript areas of decreased or (rarely) increased signal intensity
- Circumscript enlargement of pancreas
- Circumscript blurred margins of the pancreatic gland

Indirect tumor signs include the following:

- Dilatation of the pancreatic duct
- Dilatation of the extra and intrahepatic bile ducts
- Infiltration, compression, or occlusions of vessels

- Enlarged retroperitoneal lymph nodes
- Liver metastases

In our own study of 25 patients with suspected pancreatic tumors, we performed and compared different sequences. It was shown that breathhold images in 22 of 25 patients offered a better image quality than standard T1-weighted spin echo sequences. In all patients, a better delineation of the pancreas from the surrounding structures was achieved with fat suppression FLASH two-dimensional sequence. In two patients with no contrast between the tumor and the pancreatic parenchyma, even the T1-weighted breathhold images did not give additional information by improved image quality. The smallest depicted tumor measured 1.5 cm and showed a central area of low perfusion which was surrounded by a ring of high signal intensity. We usually had good contrast on the native T1-weighted images, which could be improved by application of Gd-DTPA in a few patients with hypovascularized lesions. The additional performance of fat suppression techniques, did not improve the contrast between the tumor and the surrounding parenchyma. On the other hand, fat suppression allows better delineation of the pancreas from surrounding structures. Especially after contrast injection, the otherwise masked pancreas is better shown using fat suppression sequences. The quantitative evaluation of the signal to noise ratio shows better tumor detection in 50 % after i.v. administration of Gd-DTPA. However, in 50 % tumor delineation was more difficult to achieve after contrast enhancement than on the native images. The complementary use of Gd-DTPA and fat suppression offered improved tumor contrast in 38 %. The use of fat suppression alone improved the signal to noise ratio between tumor and parenchyma in 25 %, and using additional contrast enhancement improved the signal to noise ratio in 44 %. Application of Gd-DTPA considerably worsened delineation of the pancreas on T1-weighted images, which means that there was usually no signal difference between pancreas parenchyma and surrounding fat tissue after Gd-DTPA application. This improved in 44 % after performing fat suppression.

Semelka et al. [9, 10] recommends FLASH sequences for stationary dynamic imaging, although the practical significance of this approach has not yet been proved. The best contrast between tumor and parenchyma is exptected on early images. All authors agree that the best contrast is obtained by using Gd-DTPA-enhanced fat suppression techniques (Fig. 4).

In Zollinger-Ellison syndrome, MRI was able to demonstrate gastrinomas with increased relative signal intensity on T2-weighted images, with the exception of calcified tumors [13].

In 12 patients with cystic neoplasm, Minami et al. [7] demonstrated that the cystic content was differentiated more easily with MRI than with CT. It was homogeneous in four of the five microcystic adenomas, which all had lobulated borders, best seen on T2-weighted images. The mucinous cystadenomas where all composed of multiple compartments that varied in signal intensity (Fig. 5a, b). Nevertheless, MRI showed only a limited ability to demonstrate calcifications of the tumor wall and septa.

Fig. 4. Fat suppressed and Gadolinium enhanced FLASH two-dimensional sequence (breath-hold). There is excellent contrast between the pancreas and the peripancreatic structures. Small carcinoma of the head of the pancreas with marked low signal intensity (*arrow*)

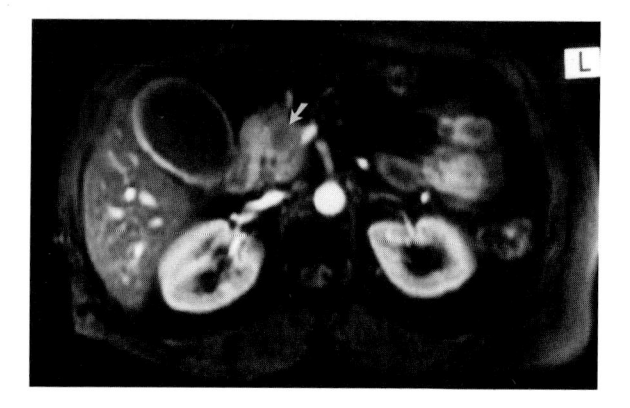

Further, liver and lymph node metastases had a low signal intensity on T1-weighted and an increased intensity on T2-weighted images. The signal intensity of primary and metastatic tumors is independent of size.

Insulinomas as small as 5 mm can be detected on T2-weighted images because these structures usually have a high signal intensity. However, not all

Fig. 5a, b. Partially cystic tumor of the head of the pancreas with occlusion of the main bile duct. CT features are strongly suspicious of malignancy. **b** Fat suppressed Gadolinium enhanced two-dimensional FLASH delimits the tumor much better, with evidence of an encapsulated process (cystadenoma) (*arrow*)

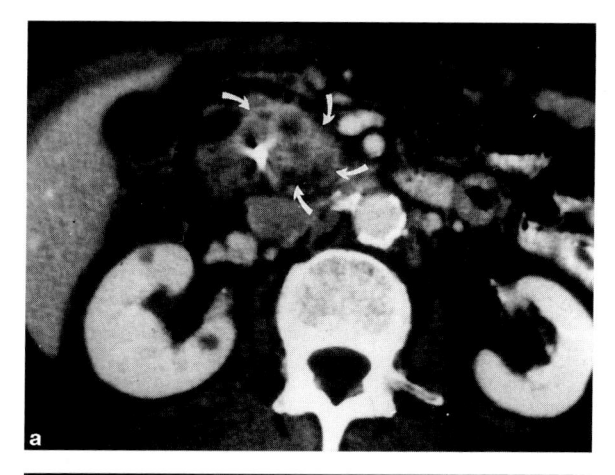

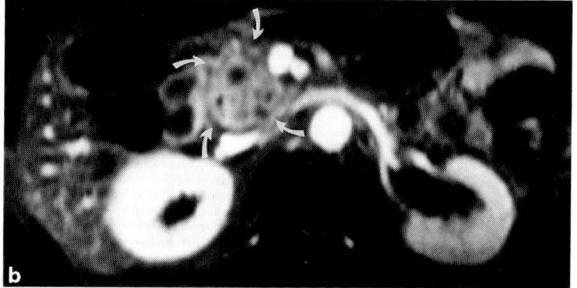

Fig. 6. MR cholangiopancreatography (HASTE) demonstrating proximal occlusion of the pancreatic duct (*double arrow*) in extended pancreatic carcinoma. Metastatic extension to the liver hilus with compression of the main bile duct (*arrow*)

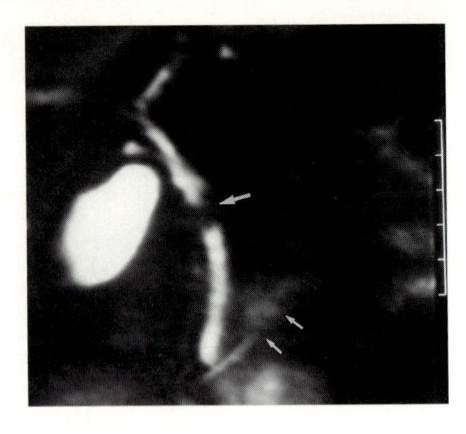

insulinomas have such a high T2 signal intensity, which renders detection of these small tumors very difficult. In contrast to adenocarcinomas, insulinomas are often hypervascularized, which results in good contrast after the application of Gd-DTPA.

Magnetic Resonance Angiography

In clinical use, two-dimensional FLASH and three-dimensional FISP/time of flight sequences are used. Sequence parameters may be adapted in order to depict slow or fast flow. Stenoses cause a turbulent flow, which may lead to a local signal loss, so that the exact extent of the stenoses may be exaggerated. Low-grade stenoses may be difficult to diagnose. Small vessels (diameter, < 2 mm) are not visualized. MR angiography provides the best overview of mesenteric and portal venous system, including the collateral circulation. Furthermore, with this technique, the flow direction (hepatopetal/hepatofugal) may be determined with certainty.

Magnetic Resonance Cholangiography

A heavily T2-weighted gradient echo sequence may be used for the biliary system [14]. With the newly introduced ultrafast echo planar techniques (HASTE/rapid acquisition relation-enhanced imaging, RARE), excellent imaging of the hepatic duct is becoming routine. The technique is particularly valuable in patients in whom endoscopic retrograde cholangiopancreatography (ERCP) is not possible. Further studies will need to compare the two methods in order to assess their viability (Fig. 6).

References

1. Claussen CD, Duda SH, Bautz WA (1990) Computertomographie des Pankreas. Röntgenpraxis 43(11): 397–402
2. Cohen MS, Weisskopf RM (1991) Ultra-fast-imaging. Magnetic Resonance Imaging, Vol. 9: 1–37
3. Freeny PC, Marks WM, Ryan JA, Traverso LW (1988) Pancreatic ductal adenocarcinoma: diagnosis and staging with dynamic CT. Radiology 166: 125–133
4. Friedrich JM, Tomczak R, Goldmann A (1996) Computed tomography in pancreatic cancer. In: Cancer of pancreas, HG Beger, M Büchler, Universitätsverlag Ulm, 225–262
5. Honda H, Kusumoto S, Nishikawa K (1991) Limitation of CT in diagnosis of pancreatic cancer. Radiation Medicine: Vol. 9 No. 2. 61–67
6. Johnson CD, Stephens DH, Charboneau JW, Carpenter HA, Welch TJ (1988) Cystic pancreatic tumors: CT and sonography assessment. AJR, 151 (6) 1133–1138
7. Minami M, Itaj Y, Ohtomo K, et al (1989) Cystic neoplasm of the pancreas: comparison of MR imaging with CT. Radiology 171: 53–56
8. Mori H, Miyake H, Aikawa H (1991) Dilated posterior superior pancreaticoduodenal vein: recognition with CT and clinical significance in patients with pancraeticobiliary carcinomas. Radiology 181: 793
9. Semelka RC, Chew W, Hricak H, et al (1990) Fat-saturation MR imaging of the upper abdomen. AJR 155, 1111–1116
10. Semelka RC, Simm FC, Recht MP, et al (1991) MR imaging of the pancreas at high field strength: comparison of six sequences. J. Comput Assist Tomogr 15(6) 966–971
11. Shimamoto K, Ishiguchi T, Sakuma S (1987) CT evaluation of pancreatic cancer. Europ. J Radiol 37
12. Steiner E, Stark DD, Hahn PF, et al (1989) Imaging of pancreatic neoplasm: comparison of MR and CT, AJR 152: 487–491
13. Tjon A, Tham RTO, Falke THM, Jansen JBMJ, et al (1989) CT and MR imaging of advanced Zollinger-Ellison-syndrome. J Comput Assist Tomogr 13(5) 821–828
14. Wallner B, Schumacher KA, Weidenmaier W, Friedrich JM (1991) Dilated biliary tract: evaluation with MR cholangiopgraphy with a T2-weighted contrast-enhanced fast sequence. Radiology 181: 805–808
15. Ward EM, Stephens DH, Sheedy PF II (1983) Computed tomographic characteristics of pancreatic carcinoma: an analysis of 100 cases. RadioGraphics 3: 547–565

Endoscopic Retrograde Cholangiopancreatography in the Diagnosis of Pancreatic Tumors

A. Hackelsberger · G. Manes

Introduction

A decade ago, a retrospective evaluation of the impact that the introduction of endoscopic retrograde cholangiopancreatography (ERCP), ultrasound (US), and computed tomography (CT) scan had on the diagnosis of pancreatic cancer was undertaken [1]. It stated that these imaging methods had failed in diagnosing pancreatic carcinoma at a resectable stage. Even now, a pancreatic tumor can only be suspected on the basis of the patient's history, clinical signs, laboratory tests, and tumor markers, with diagnosis relying on imaging procedures and confirmed by histology or cytology. As most exocrine tumors of the pancreas are of ductular origin [2], ductal alterations are the earliest visible changes caused by the tumor [3]. Therefore, the visualization of the pancreatic ductal system in great detail without surgical intervention by ERCP became the most important diagnostic tool soon after the introduction of this method in 1968 by McCune et al [4]. This chapter reviews the role of ERCP in the diagnosis of pancreatic tumors and updates the progress of the past decade. A focus is set on the following topics:

1. Typical findings, sensitivity, and specificity of ERCP in pancreatic cancer
2. Differential diagnosis
3. ERCP-associated methods for confirming malignancy and their value in clinical practice
4. ERCP in the diagnosis of pancreatic tumors other than adenocarcinoma

Typical Findings, Sensitivity, and Specificity of ERCP in Pancreatic Cancer

According to some of the earlier studies on ERCP in adenocarcinoma of the pancreas, the pathologic changes seen in pancreatography can be classified in the typical lesions [5–8] (Fig. 1). A malignant stenosis of variable length in the main duct can be found. It is frequently accompanied by a prestenotic (upstream) dilation. Alternatively obstruction of the main duct with cutoff is often seen. It may be abrupt with irregular contour, or of the tapering type with a cone shape (Fig. 2). Obstruction might be simulated by an underfilled duct. The clear visualization of downstream side branches and exclusion of a

Fig. 1a–f. Ductal patterns in pancreatic carcinoma. **a** Main duct stenosis with loss of side branches, upstream dilation, and normal downstream appearance. **b** Main duct obstruction, irregular, blunt contour. **c** Tapering type obstruction. **d** Extravasation of contrast into necrotic cavity from obstructed main duct. **e** Abnormal branching, circumscript loss of branches, main duct appears regular. **f** Diffuse narrowing of main duct

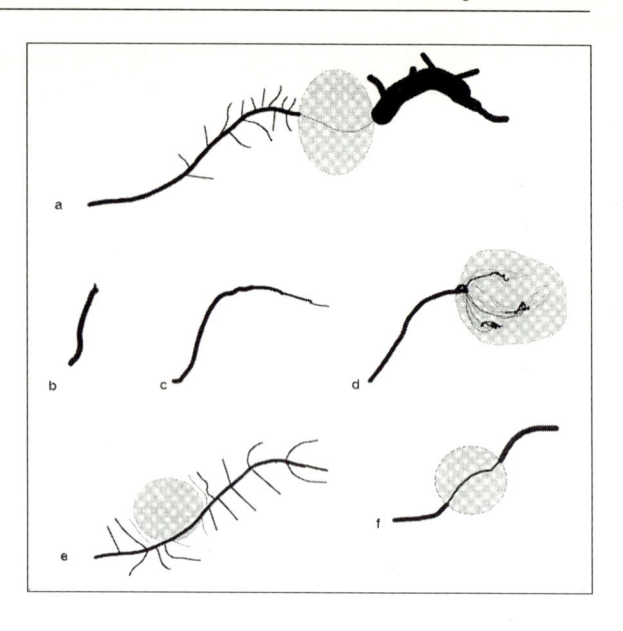

pancreas divisum by injecting a sufficient amount of contrast medium are therefore important before obstruction can be diagnosed. A further malignancy-derived pattern is extravasation of contrast medium from an obstructed main duct or side branch, which may fill a necrotic cavity. This type of lesion must be carefully differentiated from pseudocysts. Two other types of malignant lesions are rarely found and may be overlooked if only minor changes occur: Abnormal branching, mostly loss of branches in a circumscript area, may be found without alterations of the main duct. Only slight, or diffuse, narrowing of the main duct can occur in combination with altered branching. Two groups carried out a morphological analysis of pancreatic ductograms in larger samples of patients with pancreatic cancer [9, 10]. Obstruction and stenosis of the main duct were found to be the most common lesions, detectable in 89.3% of all patients. The tapering-type obstruction was rare (4%); it may occur with large carcinoma, usually in the body of the gland. Necrotic cyst formation and extraductal extravasation occurred in up to 15% of patients.

Secondary changes of the intrapancreatic bile duct occur typically in cancers of the pancreatic head. Encasement, stenosis, and obstruction are commonly found, resulting in the classic "double duct sign" [11], which may increase diagnostic accuracy of ERCP. Attempts at bile duct cannulation should therefore always be made if cancer of the pancreatic head is suspected [12], especially if only the ventral anlage has been opacified in patients with pancreas divisum [13]. The appearance of the malignancy-derived "double duct sign" – the two abruptly stenoted ducts in close proximity with upstream dilation – must, however, be carefully evaluated against bile duct involvement in chronic pancreatitis [14]. If ERCP is successful in patients with pancreatic cancer, conspicuous findings are the rule, as only 2.8%–3% of ductograms were normal [9, 15]. Special

Fig. 2. Endoscopic retrograde pancreatography (ERP) showing completely filled duct system with gradual tapering of duct caliber before cutoff in the pancreatic body; 58-year-old male patient with pancreatic carcinoma

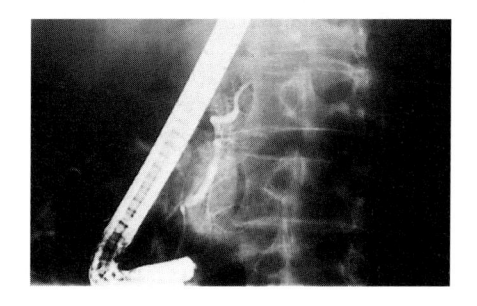

attention to ductal visualization in the uncinate portion is required if a small tumor is suspected here. As small cancer is often asymptomatic, diagnosis may occur by mere coincidence. If patients with early pancreatic cancer (tumor diameter < 2 cm, limited to pancreas without extension to adjacent structures, T1a, N0, M0) undergo a diagnostic evaluation, the lesion may be diagnosed by ERCP only while alterations on US and CT may be missed [16, 17]. Small tumors that arise in branch ducts far from the main duct are seldom found. For better visualization of such lesions, endoscopic retrograde parenchymography of the pancreas by overfilling the ducts and adding a surfactant to the contrast medium has been evaluated [18]. Routine use of this technique, however, is not recommended, as it bears a risk of pancreatitis and no minute carcinoma was detected in the series.

Until this day, ERCP with a complete pancreatic ductogram is the most reliable single method of excluding pancreatic carcinoma. In the diagnosis of this tumor, high diagnostic accuracy, sensitivity of up to 92%, and specificity of up to 95% were calculated for ERCP, clearly exceeding that of US and CT-scan [19–23]. However, ductal changes correlate poorly with actual tumor size. Therefore, ERCP is not a staging procedure in pancreatic cancer.

Differential Diagnosis

Although ERCP is diagnostic in a high portion of patients with pancreatic carcinoma, problems sometimes arise in differentiating malignancy-derived ductular changes from chronic pancreatitis [24]. On the one hand, there is a well-documented association of pancreatic cancer with preexisting chronic inflammation [25–28], and a chronically destructed duct system may mask a supervening malignant lesion. On the other hand, chronic inflammatory changes particularly in focal pancreatitis are able to mimic all the ductal patterns usually displayed by carcinoma to some extent [29]. In advanced stages of chronic inflammation, stricturing and stenosis of the main duct may occur [30]. The spectrum of ductal changes in chronic pancreatitis is depicted in the corresponding chapter of this book. Background clinical information and if possible comparison with previous ductograms are therefore indispensable when evaluating pancreatic duct strictures of unknown cause. Nevertheless, the differen-

Table 1. Ductal patterns in chronic pancreatitis and pancreatic carcinoma

Pancreatic duct	Chronic pancreatitis	Pancreatic carcinoma
Obstruction		
Contour	Smooth, hemispheric	Irregular, serrated, blunt, pointed, or tapered
Stricture, stenosis		
Number	Sometimes multiple	Singular
Contour	Smooth transition of caliber, flat, rod- or spindle-like	Abrupt change of caliber, irregular, serrated, eccentric
Length	Short < 5 mm	Usually > 10 mm [33]
Pancreatic main duct		
Upstream of stricture	Tortuosity, irregular dilation	Regular dilation
Downstream	Tortuosity, irregular dilation, "chain of lakes"	Normal aspect
Side branches		
At level of stricture	Ectatic, irregular	Lost, or destructed, not ectatic
Downstream	Ectatic, irregular	Normal aspect
Upstream	Ectatic, irregular	Regular dilation
Calcifications	Frequent	Rare
Extravasation pattern	Regular contour, cystic pseudocyst	Irregular necrotic cavity, diffuse extravasation
Common bile duct[a]		"Double duct sign"
Stenosis	Medium to high grade	Mostly high grade
Contour	Smooth, tube-like, symmetric	Irregular, abrupt, asymmetric
Length	Mostly > 10 mm	Mostly short

[a] Only if carcinoma/inflammation is present in the pancreatic head.

tiation of altered duct patterns is difficult even for the expert in some cases. It is estimated that diagnostic problems arise in some 10% of patients suspected of pancreatic cancer [31, 32]. Table 1 gives a comparative summary of typical duct patterns in malignancy and chronic inflammation of the gland. As a rule, an isolated stricture with a normal duct morphology downstream to the papilla and upstream dilation suggests malignancy. If the prestenotic downstream segment also shows tortuosity, dilation, and abnormal branching, chronic pancreatitis is proven, but coexisting malignancy must still be ruled out. A long (> 10 mm) strictured or stenotic duct segment almost invariably speaks for carcinoma (Fig. 3), while shorter strictures (up to 5 mm) are found in chronic pancreatitis [33]. The shape of malignant strictures is irregular and serrated, while inflammatory lesions are mostly smooth. A loss of side branches is frequently found in the duct segment occupied by cancer, but not in chronic pancreatitis. Although very rare in ordinary adenocarcinoma [34], the presence of pancreatic calcification cannot be considered a clear criterion for chronic inflammation since this may also be present in mucinous adenocarcinoma and cystic neoplasms [35]. Ductal disruption without cyst formation is not found in chronic pancreatitis, but diffuse extravasation of contrast medium into a necrotic irregular cavity may occur in carcinoma. If the head of the gland is involved, characteristic changes in bile duct morphology are found: The irregular abrupt high grade stenosis of carcinoma in most cases is easily distinguished from the long, smooth, and tube-like intrapancreatic narrowing in chronic pancreatitis (Fig. 4).

Fig. 3. Endoscopic retrograde cholangiopancreaticography (ERCP) showing 12-mm-long stenosis with near total loss of side branches and (incompletely filled) upstream dilation. Regular branch at downstream stenosis margin. Tumor has not reached the bile duct. 80-years-old patient (male). Malignancy confirmed by fine needle puncture

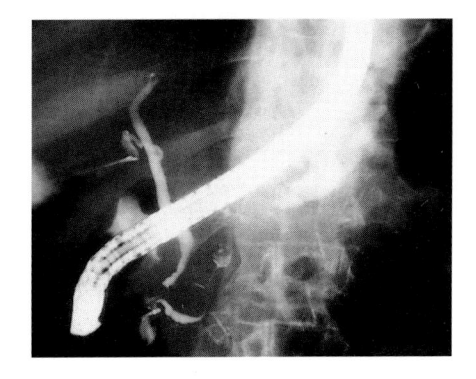

A rare differential diagnosis in isolated short strictures of the pancreatic body segment crossing the spine may represent previous blunt pancreatic trauma [36].

With all this in mind, however, there are some patients in whom ERCP allows no straightforward diagnosis. To these we must add the patients (< 5%) in whom ERCP is not successful. Theoretically, the best method to overcome these problems would be endosonography. It requires no access to the ductal system, can examine the whole parenchyma, and has high resolution. Yet even with EUS it may be difficult to differentiate chronic pancreatitis and carcinoma [37].

ERCP-Associated Methods for Conforming Malignancy – Value in Clinical Practice

Pancreatic Juice Cytology

If cancer cannot be ruled out, further diagnostic steps must obtain tissue, cytology, or other markers of malignant disease to confirm or reject this diagnosis. In an attempt to obviate explorative laparotomy, further ERCP-associated diagnostic methods have been evaluated. Endoscopic retrograde pancreatography

Fig. 4. Endoscopic retrograde choliangography (ERC) showing long, smooth contoured medium-grade stenosis of common bile duct with extrapancreatic dilation. Endoscopic retrograde pancreatography (ERP) showing the ventral anlage of pancreas divisum with irregular main duct and completely preserved ectatic, deformed side branches; 42-year-old male patient with long standing alcohol abuse. Findings compatible with chronic pancreatitis confirmed by identical ductograms 3 months later

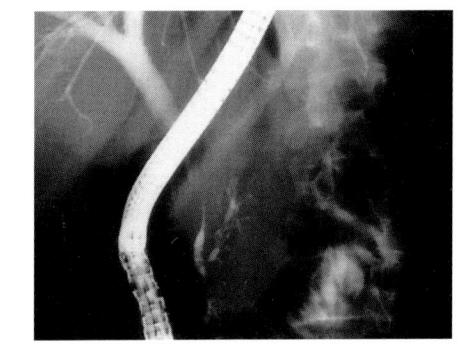

(ERP) provides access to the pancreas and thus allows the collection of pancreatic juice for cytology usually after IV administration of secretin [38-41]. Although highly specific (close to 100%), this method yielded a marked variation in sensitivity, from 50% to 84%. It has therefore not gained widespread acceptance. As exfoliated cells in juice may undergo rapid degeneration in contrast medium, intraductal brushing of accessible biliopancreatic strictures with a specially designed cytology brush has been evaluated [42-47]. In the case of pancreatic strictures, it may be difficult to move the brush (5F OD) far enough into the lesion when the duct is narrow and tortuous. In addition, this procedure carries a small risk of inducing pancreatitis. Brushing the distal common bile duct as well may be useful if malignant invasion has taken place [45]. The reported sensitivity of brush cytology in pancreatic cancer is 30%-60%, clearly less than in cholangiocarcinoma. In search of a further marker of malignant diseases besides brush cytology, additional flow cytometric analysis of DNA content was performed [48]. This combined approach yielded 63% sensitivity at a high rate of false-positive flow cytometric results (specificity, 69%). Both methods produce insufficient results and therefore are not recommended.

ERCP-Guided Puncture of Suspicious Lesions

Endoscopic fine needle aspiration has been studied with a shielded retractable needle catheter in the common bile duct and reached 61% sensitivity for malignancy [49]. After the performance of a satisfactory ERP, another group performed a percutaneous fine needle puncture of the lesion using biplanar fluoroscopic monitoring as guidance. This approach revealed 90% sensitivity in a small group of patients [50]. A confirmatory study would be welcome. Considerable time, effort, and skill are necessary to perform these procedures, which therefore will probably not gain widespread acceptance.

Tumor Antigens in Pancreatic Juice

To enhance their diagnostic potential, tumor markers such as CEA and CA 19-9 have been studied in pancreatic juice of patients with pancreatic carcinoma and chronic pancreatitis. The broad availability of these assays could make this approach particularly attractive for clinical practice. By now the results are somewhat conflicting: An earlier study showed equally elevated levels of CA 19-9 in patients with carcinoma and chronic pancreatitis [51]. In another study, determination of this tumor-associated antigen discriminated all patients with operable pancreatic carcinoma including small tumors from chronic pancreatitis [52]. A third group reported that this marker in pancreatic juice did not provide better diagnostic information than the serum assay [53]. Combining carcinoembryonic antigen (CEA) measurement and cytology in pancreatic juice yielded 93% diagnostic accuracy in a small group of patients, while low sensitivity was found for CA 19-9 in pancreatic juice [54]. Further studies in larger patient groups are necessary, but at the time there is no recommendation for this method in clinical routine.

Ki-*ras* Mutations in Pancreatic Juice

Ki-*ras* mutations are the most common genetic change in human pancreatic cancer, found in at least 85%–90% of cases by polymerase chain reaction (PCR)-based methods [55, 56]. The first report on this subject was published in 1988 [57]. Several recent studies in patients with diagnosed adenocarcinoma, or equivocal findings by ERP, investigated the diagnostic yield of Ki-*ras* mutations detected in cells from pancreatic juice and duct brushings [58, 59], or from duodenal juice obtained during a secretin test [60]. The detection of Ki-*ras* mutations in pancreatic juice or brushed cells showed a high sensitivity (77%–83%) and specificity (100%) for pancreatic carcinoma, even in cases with small carcinoma [58]. All patients with chronic pancreatitis had a negative *ras* test [58, 59]. Interestingly, the latter study found a positive result in two patients, in whom a pancreatic tumor was only evident at 18 and 40 months follow-up, respectively. This indicates a possible potential for detecting even small cancers not yet accessible to imaging methods. In the duodenal juice of 19 patients with pancreatic carcinoma, the *ras* test achieved 63% sensitivity, and one of 41 patients with benign pancreatic disorders showed a mutation [60]. Although very promising, the *ras* test is not feasible in clinical routine yet, due to restricted availability and cost. Even today, it is only performed in some highly specialized centers. Without being prophetic, in the near future widespread use of this test in conjunction with ERCP for diagnosing pancreatic carcinoma can be predicted.

The diagnostic potential of ERCP is presently being further enlarged by the development of new miniscopes for pancreatoscopy. A review on this exciting topic is given in the corresponding chapter of this book.

ERCP in the Diagnosis of Pancreatic Tumors Other Than Adenocarcinoma

Ductal adenocarcinoma accounts for more than 90% of pancreatic tumors [61]. The remaining ones are represented by a number of tumors that originate from different structures of the gland and show different biologic behavior: Endocrine neoplasms of the gland, sarcomas, and lymphomas are rare, metastatic disease from another primary site being more frequent. ERP in these tumors is generally not diagnostic as they have extraductal growth. Dislocation or compression of the duct may sometimes be detected by ERP, but the method is not diagnostic.

ERP may contribute ot the diagnosis of two further tumor types of the pancreas, which both belong to the spectrum of mucinous adenocarcinoma.

Mucinous Ductal Ectasia

ERCP led to description of this entity in 1986 [62], the clinical picture and pathology are well described at present [63–65]. Patients present with recurrent pain, US detects small cyst-like lesions in the pancreatic head, and on ERCP thick mucus extrudes from a patulous papilla. The pancreatic ductogram confirms the diagnosis: Dilation of smoothly outlined main duct and branches mostly in the head of the gland and an uncinate process with filling defects are demonstrated. Mucinous ductal ectasia is recognized as a premalignant lesion, and pancreatic resection is presently being advocated [66].

Mucinous Cystadenoma and Cystadenocarcinoma

If a larger (mostly > 5 cm diameter) cystic mass of the pancreatic body or tail is detected by US or CT in a younger person, often under 50 years old and generally female with epigastric pain and weight loss, then chronic pancreatitis with pseudocyst formation is the first differential diagnosis. If this is ruled out, however, a cystadenoma or cystadenocarcinoma may be suspected [67]. Most tumors do not communicate with the pancreatic duct, which may appear dislocated on ERP. Very rarely, communication of the cystic neoplasia with the otherwise inconspicuous duct system may nevertheless be demonstrated (Fig. 5). Although some patients show a longlasting benign course, resection of the tumor is advised as malignancy may be present already or develop later on.

Periampullary tumors are not of pancreatic origin. They are readily diagnosed by duodenoscopy and proven by biopsy. ERCP will demonstrate typical dilation of biliary and pancreatic ducts at the level of the papilla. This allows differential diagnosis of pancreatic carcinoma invading the duodenal wall.

Conclusion

At present ERCP and EUS in expert hands are the methods with the highest diagnostic accuracy for the diagnosis of pancreatic cancer. If carried out early in the course of the disease, ERCP has the potential to diagnose even small resectable pancreatic cancer. We hopefully predict that an improvement in diagnostic accuracy will be achieved in the near future by adding Ki-*ras* testing in cells from pancreatic juice or duct brushings. The development of pancreatoscopy may further enhance the diagnostic potential of ERCP. Regarding the role of ERCP in daily clinical practice, an important development must be consid-

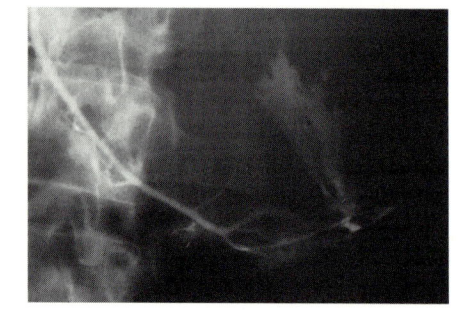

Fig. 5. Detailed endoscopic retrograde pancreatography (ERP) in the region of pancreatic tail ultrasound (US) had revealed a large cystic tumor in the region of pancreatic tail. ERP shows tumor cavity communicating with terminal branches of the otherwise regular pancreatic duct; 46-year-old emale patient with epigastric pain, diagnostic workup without signs of chronic pancreatitis. Resection specimen revealed mucinous cystadenoma without malignancy

ered, which until today has not been investigated systematically. In earlier years, ERCP was carried out in large centers with a high caseload by specialized endoscopists. The past decade in Germany, as probably in other countries, has seen a continuing spread of ERCP currently being performed by less trained endoscopists even in small hospitals. For these operators seeing fewer patients with pancreatic disease, there is an increasing need for training facilities to maintain the potential that ERCP has to offer.

References

1. Savarino V, Mansi C, Bistolfi L, et al. (1983) Failure of new diagnostic aids in improving detection of pancreatic cancer at a resectable stage. Dig Dis Sci 28: 1078–1082
2. Chen J, Baithun SI (1985) Morphological study of 391 cases of exocrine pancreatic tumours with special reference to the classification of exocrine pancreatic carcinoma. J Pathol 146: 17–29
3. Freeny PC, Ball TJ (1981) Endoscopic retrograde cholangiopancreaticography (ERCP) and percutaneous cholangiography (PTC) in the evaluation of pancreatic carcinoma: Diagnostic limitations and contemporary roles. Cancer 47 (suppl 1): 1666–1678
4. McCune WS, Shorb PE, Moscovitz H (1968) Endoscopic cannulation of the ampulla of Vater: a preliminary report. Ann Surg 167: 752–756
5. Ogoshi K, Hara Y (1972) Retrograde pancreatocholedochography. Jap J Clin Radiol 17: 455–461
6. Fukumoto K, Nakajima N, Murakami K, et al (1974) Diagnosis of pancreatic cancer by endoscopic pancreaticocholangiography. Am J Gastroenterol 62: 210–213
7. Nakajima M, Yamagichi Y, Akasaka Y (1979) Endoscopic retrograde cholangiopancreatography (ERCP) in the diagnosis of pancreatic cancer. In: Early Diagnosis of Pancreatic Cancer, Kawai K, ed. Iguaku Shoin, Tokyo, New York 140–145
8. Stadelmann O, Safrany L, Löffler A, et al (1974) Endoscopic retrograde cholangiopancreatography in the diagnosis of pancreatic cancer. Experiences with 54 cases. Endoscopy 6: 84–93
9. Kawai K, Yasuda K, Nakajima M (1987) Endoscopic diagnosis of cancer of the pancreas. In: Gastroenterologic endoscopy. M. Sivak ed. W.B. Saunders, Philadelphia, 821–838
10. Bilbao MK, Katon RM (1977) Neoplasms of the pancreas. In: Atlas of endoscopic retrograde cholangiopancreatography, Stewart ET, Vennes JA, Geenen JE, eds. Mosby, Saint Louis, 181–235
11. Freeny PC, Bilbao MK, Katon RM (1976) Blind evaluation of endoscopic retrograde cholangiopancreatography (ERCP) in the diagnosis of pancreatic carcinoma: the double duct and other signs. Radiology 119: 271–274
12. Malfertheiner P, Freeny PC (1991) Pankreas. In: Gastroenterologische Endoskopie, Lehrbuch und Atlas. R. Ottenjann, M. Classen eds. Enke, Stuttgart (2nd ed.), 202–221
13. Morris JB, Zollinger RM, Stellato TA, et al (1990) The pseudo-double duct sign: an ERCP finding in pancreatic carcinoma. Gastroint Endosc 36: 408–409
14. Schlauch D, Kohler B, Riemann RF (1993) Double duct sign – is it always cancer? Endoscopy 25: 489–490
15. Freeny PC (1989) Radiologic diagnosis and staging of pancreatic ductal adenocarcinoma. Radiol Clin North Am 27: 121–128
16. Gall FP, Kessler H (1987) Early cancer of the exocrine pancreas: diagnosis and prognosis. Chirurg 58: 78–83
17. Yoshimori M, Tajiri H, Nakamura K, et al (1984) Diagnosis of small carcinoma of the pancreas: importance of ultrasound scanning and endoscopic retrograde cholangiopancreatography (ERCP). Jpn J Clin Oncol 14: 359–367
18. Akasaka Y, Nakajima M, Yamaguchi K, et al (1979) Diagnosis of pancreatic cancer by endoscopic retrograde parenchymography of the pancreas (ERPP). In: Early diagnosis of pancreatic cancer. Kawai K, ed. Iguaku Shoin, Tokyo, New York 155–163
19. Nix GA, Schmitz PI, Wilson JH, et al (1984) Carcinoma of the head of the pancreas. Therapeutic implications of endoscopic retrograde cholangiopancreatography findings. Gastroenterology 87: 37–43

20. Gilinsky NH, Bornman PC, Girdwood AH, et al (1986) Diagnostic yield of endoscopic retrograde cholangiopancreatography in carcinoma of the pancreas. Br J Surg 73: 539–543
21. Meyer J, Sulkowski U, Kautz G, et al (1987) Die Wertigkeit diagnostischer Verfahren beim Pankreaskarzinom. Zentralbl Chir 112: 12–19
22. Nix GA, Van Overbeeke IC, Wilson JH, et al (1988) ERCP diagnosis of tumors in the region of the head of the pancreas. Analysis of criteria and computer-aided diagnosis. Dig Dis Sci 33: 577–586
23. Niederau C, Grendell JH (1992) Diagnosis of pancreatic carcinoma. Imaging techniques and tumor markers. Pancreas 7: 66–86
24. Neff CC, Simeone JF, Wittenberg J, et al (1984) Inflammatory pancreatic masses. Radiology 150: 35–38
25. Lowenfels AB, Maisonneuve P, Cavallini G, et al and the International Pancreatitis Study Group (1993) Pancreatitis and the risk of pancreatic cancer. N Engl J Med 328: 1433–1437
26. Lankisch PG, Lohr-Happe A, Otto J, et al (1993) Natural course in chronic pancreatitis. Pain, exocrine and endocrine pancreatic insufficiency and prognosis of the disease. Digestion 54: 148–155
27. Fernandez E, La Vecchia C, Porta M, et al (1995) Pancreatitis and the risk of pancreatic cancer. Pancreas 11: 185–189
28. Chari ST, Mohan V, Pitchumoni CS, et al (1994) Risk of pancreatic carcinoma in tropical calcifying pancreatitis: an epidemiologic study. Pancreas 9: 62–66
29. Jowell PS (1995) Assessment of pancreatic duct strictures. Gastrointest Endosc Clin Am 5: 125–143
30. Axon ATR (1989) Endoscopic retrograde cholangiopancreatography in chronic pancreatitis. Cambridge classification. Radiol Clin N Am 27: 39–50
31. Caletti G, Brocchi E, Agostini D, et al (1982) Sensitivity of endoscopic retrograde pancreatography in chronic pancreatitis. Br J Surg 69: 507–509
32. Rohrmann CA, Silvis SE, Vennes JA (1976) The significance of pancreatic ductal obstruction in differential diagnosis of the abnormal endoscopic retrograde pancreatogram. Radiology 121: 311–314
33. Shemesh E, Czerniak A, Nass S, Klein E (1990) Role of endoscopic retrograde cholangiopancreatography in differentiating pancreatic cancer coexisting with chronic pancreatitis. Cancer 65: 893–896
34. Furukawa H, Takayasu K, Mukai K, et al (1995) Ductal adenocarcinoma of the pancreas associated with intratumoral calcification. Int J Pancreatol 17: 291–296
35. Warshaw AL, Compton CC, Lewandrowski K, et al (1990) Cystic tumors of the pancreas. New clinical, radiological and pathologic observations in 67 patients. Ann Surg 212: 432–445
36. Carr ND, Cairns SJ, Lees WR, et al (1989) Late complications of pancreatic trauma. Br J Surg 76: 1244–1248
37. Grimm H, Maydeo A, Soehendra N (1990) Endoluminal ultrasound for the diagnosis an staging of pancreatic cancer. Baillieres Clin Gastroenterol 4: 869–888
38. Hatfield ARW, Smithies A, Wilkins R, Levi AJ (1976) Assessment of endoscopic retrograde cholangio-pancreatography (ERCP) and pure pancreatic juice cytology in patients with pancreatic disease. Gut 17: 14–21
39. Nakaizumi A, Tatsuta M, Vehara H, et al (1992) Cytologic examination of pure pancreatic juice in the diagnosis of pancreatic carcinoma. Cancer 70: 2610–2614
40. Endo Y, Morii J, Tanura N, Okuda S (1974) Cytodiagnosis of pancreatic malignant tumors by aspiration, under direct vision, using a duodenal fiberscope. Gastroenterology 67: 944–951
41. Del Favero G, Fabris C, Angonese C, et al (1988) Cytology in the diagnosis of pancreatic cancer. Int J Pancreatol 3 (suppl 1): 137–141
42. Venu RP, Geenen JE, Kin M, et al (1990) Endoscopic retrograde brush cytology: a new technique. Gastroenterology 99: 1474–1479
43. Sawada Y, Gonda H, Hayashida Y (1989) Combined use of brushing cytology and endoscopic retrograde pancreatography for the early detection of pancreatic cancer. Acta Cytol 33: 870–874
44. Ryan ME (1991) Cytological brushings of ductal lesions during ERCP. Gastrointest Endosc 37: 139–142
45. Scudera PL, Koizumi J, Jacobson IM (1990) Brush cytology evaluation of lesions encountered during ERCP. Gastrointest Endosc 36: 281–284
46. Foutch PG, Kerr DM, Harlan JR, et al (1990) Endoscopic retrograde wire guided brush cytology for diagnosis of patients with malignant obstruction of the bile duct. Am J Gastroenterol 36: 281–286

47. Ferrari Jr AP, Lichtenstein DR, Slivka A, et al (1994) Brush cytology during ERCP for the diagnosis of biliary and pancreatic malignancies. Gastrointest Endosc 40: 140–145
48. Ryan ME, Baldauf MC (1994) Comparison of flow cytometry for DNA content and brush cytology for detection of malignancy in pancreatobiliary strictures. Gastrointest Endosc 40: 133–139
49. Howell DA, Beveridge RP, Bosco J et al (1992) Endoscopic needle aspiration biopsy at ERCP in the diagnosis of biliary strictures. Gastrointest Endosc 38: 531
50. Gagnon P, Boustiere C, Ponchon T, et al (1991) Percutaneous fine-needle aspiration cytologic study of main pancreatic duct stenosis under pancreatographic guidance. Cancer 67: 2395–2400
51. Schmiegel W, Kreiker C, Eberl W, et al (1985) Monoclonal antibody defines CA 19-9 in pancreatic juices and sera. Gut 26: 456–460
52. Malesci A, Tommasini MA, Bonato C (1987) Determination of Ca 19-9 antigen in serum and pancreatic juice for differential diagnosis of pancreatic adenocarcinoma from chronic pancreatitis. Gastroenterology 92: 60–67
53. Hyoty M, Hyoty H, Aaran RK, et al (1992) Tumor antigens CA 195 and CA 19-9 in pancreatic juice and serum for the diagnosis of pancreatic carcinoma. Eur J Surg 158: 173–179
54. Matsumoto S, Harada H, Tanaka J, et al (1994) Evaluation of cytology and tumor markers of pure pancreatic juice for the diagnosis of pancreatic cancer at early stages. Pancreas 9: 741–747
55. Hruban RH, vanMansfeld ADM, Offenhaus GJA, et al (1993) K-*ras* oncogen activation in adenocarcinoma of the human pancreas. A study of 82 carcinomas using a combination of mutant-enriched polymerase chain reaction analysis and allele specific oligonucleotide hybridization. Am J Pathol 143: 545–554
56. Caldas C, Kern SE (1995) K-ras mutation and pancreatic adenocarcinoma. Int J Pancreatol 18: 1–6
57. Almoguera C, Shibata D, Forrester K, et al (1988) Most human carcinomas of the exocrine pancreas contain mutant c-K-ras genes. Cell 53: 549–554
58. Van Laethem JL, Vertongen P, Deviere J, et al (1995) Detection of c-Ki-*ras* gene codon 12 mutations from pancreatic duct brushings in the diagnosis of pancreatic tumors. Gut 36: 781–787
59. Berthelemy P, Bouisson M, Escorrou J, et al (1995) Identification of K-*ras* mutations in pancreatic juice in the early diagnosis of pancreatic cancer. Ann Intern Med 123: 188–191
60. Iguchi H, Sugano K, Fukayama N, et al (1996) Analysis of the K-ras codon 12 mutations in the duodenal juice of patients with pancreatic cancer. Gastroenterology 110: 211–226
61. Cubilla A, Fitzgerald PJ (1978) Pancreatic cancer. I. Duct adenocarcinoma. A clinical-pathologic study of 380 patients. Pathol Annu 1: 241–289
62. Itai Y, Ohhashi K, Nagai H, et al (1986) Ductectatic mucinous cystadenoma and cystadenocarcinoma of the pancreas. Radiology 161: 697–700
63. Bastid C, Bernard JP, Sarles H, et al (1991) Mucinous ductal ectasia of the pancreas: a premalignant disease and a cause of obstructive pancreatitis. Pancreas 6: 15–22
64. Raijman I, Kortan P, Walden D, et al (1994) Mucinous ductal ectasia: cholangiopancreatographic and endoscopic findings. Endoscopy 26: 303–307
65. Procacci C, Graziani R, Bicego E, et al (1996) Intraductal mucin-producing tumors of the pancreas: imaging findings. Radiology 198: 249–257
66. Fernandez-del-Castillo C, Rattner DW, Warshaw AL (1995) Standards for pancreatic resection in the 1990s. Arch Surg 130: 295–299
67. Compagno J, Oertel JE (1978) Mucinous cystic neoplasms of the pancreas with overt and latent malignancy (cystadenocarcinoma and cystadenoma): A clinical-pathological study of 41 cases. Am J Clin Pathol 69: 573–580

Role of Laparoscopy and Laparoscopic Ultrasound in Pancreatic Cancer

A. Klingler · M. Möschel · J. Tschmelitsch · K. S. Glaser

Introduction

The accurate diagnosis and staging of intra-abdominal neoplasms is still a challenge for the clinician's diagnostic abilities and methods. This is especially true for pancreatic cancer, where the anatomical position of pancreas, duodenum, hepatic and mesenteric vessels as well as peripancreatic lymph nodes aggravate the correct assessment of tumor stage, local resectability, and existence of extrapancreatic tumor spread. Moreover, precise preoperative staging is indispensable in the surgeon's decision between radical and extensive curative treatment with hope of better prognosis on the one side and palliation of symptoms with maximization of quality of life for the limited remaining life span on the other side. The availability of new palliative procedures (e.g. laparoscopic cholecystojejunostomy [1] and gastrojejunostomy [2], endoscopic stenting [3]) as well as neoadjuvant approaches in radical therapy [4, 5] will make exact preoperative tumor assessment even more important.

Laparoscopy has been advocated as a staging tool for pancreatic and other gastrointestinal neoplasm for several years [6–13]. Nevertheless, clinicians have been rather reluctant to employ this method in daily routine. The most important reasons may probably be found in the former lack of nonsurgical treatment options, prolonged hospital stay, increased costs, and possible complications of laparoscopy as well as in the simplicity and assumed accuracy of noninvasive diagnostic methods (computed tomography and percutaneous ultrasound) – although the superiority of laparaoscopy in comparison to these methods has been well documented:

1. The existence of metastatic tumor in the liver is a frequent contraindication for curative surgery. Computed tomography scan (CT) and percutaneous ultrasound fail to detect this condition in 20%–30% of patients with pancreatic cancer [10, 11], especially if the lesions are small (< 2 cm). Laparoscopy is valuable in detecting lesions on the surface of the liver, with a sensitivity of 96% in these cases [11] and therefore helps avoid unnecessary laparotomy.
2. Laparoscopy – possibly in combination with peritoneal cytology – is able to disclose peritoneal tumor spread in 24%–73% of patients in whom such lesions had previously been excluded by CT [6–15]; again, these lesions are chiefly very small (1–2 mm). Positive peritoneal cytology is associated with low survival probability [8, 15] and with a high proportion of unresectable

disease [14]. Histologic evaluation is attainable through laparoscopic biopsies.
3. The incidence of complications during or after diagnostic laparosopy is very low. There are major complications including hemorrhage, gas embolism, cardiovascular arrest, pneumothorax, or perforation of viscera with an incidence of 0.6%-2.49% [16, 17]. Minor complications (hematoma, pain, transient ileus, emphysema, etc.) occur with a frequency of 1.07%-5.1%. The frequency of these complications is evidently related to the investigator's experience of laparoscopic techniques, which today increases steeply. There are a few reports of port-site metastases [18, 19] and the dissemination of tumor cells in the abdominal cavitiy [20] after laparoscopic surgery, but the mechanism and clinical significance of these findings still remain to be evaluated.

The application of intraoperative ultrasound (IOUS) has been investigated mainly in the setting of liver metastases of colorectal cancer [21, 22]. The sensitivity of IOUS in the detection of liver metastases is in the range of that of palpation (80%-90% [13, 22]). Even modern methods of radiologic diagnostics (delayed CT, CT during arterial portography, bolus contrast-enhanced dynamic CT, etc.) do not seem to reach this high level of precision [13, 22], although these methods still have to be evaluated. IOUS differs from laparoscopy in that IOUS primarily detects deeply situated small metastases, whereas palpation and laparoscopic exploration are preferable for the diagnosis of surface lesions. The combination of laparoscopy and IOUS seems to be the logical consequence, reaching the highest sensitivity by revealing both surface and subsurface liver metastases.

Several authors investigated laparoscopic ultrasound (LUS) in the context of pancreatic cancer [23-28]. Despite the preliminary nature of these results, LUS in combination with laparoscopy seems to provide complete und exact tumor staging within one preoperative diagnostic step:

1. Due to the high resolution capacity, small (< 0.5 cm) intrahepatic lesions are appropriately identified with LUS [23, 25, 26]. Cytological evaluation of these lesions was obtained by means of ultrasound-guided aspiration biopsy [29, 30]. Special probes for LUS with a working channel for biopsies are not as yet commercially available, but prototypes are currently being developed. Together with the visualization of retroperitoneal lymph nodes, LUS completes laparoscopy with respect to the assessment of lymph node and liver metastases.
2. LUS is very reliable in the judgment of local resectability of pancreatic cancer [23, 24, 26, 31]. The relationship between tumor and adjacent vessels or organs is probably visualized better than by any other diagnostic method (Fig. 1) – with the exception of endoscopic ultrasound (EUS). EUS, however, is limited to pancreatic head tumors and insufficient in the visualization of the uncinate process, celiac axis, and adjacent lymph nodes [32].

We established laparoscopic ultrasound at the Second Surgical Department of the University Hospital of Innsbruck in 1990, and it was first used experimentally during laparoscopic cholecystectomy. Today, laparoscopy and LUS are regularly performed in the staging of pancreatic cancer with the aim of investigating the diagnostic value of these methods.

Methods

Several prototypes of ultrasound probes were used when dedicated probes were not available – including the application of EUS probes [27, 33]. We used a 7-MHz Picker intraoperative finger-tip probe (EUP-F334, curved array, frequency shifts between 7.5 and 10 MHz), which was attached to a 30-cm-long metal tube (diameter 12 mm). In four cases, LUS was performed with an Aloka US probe (Aloka Ltd., Tokyo, Japan). At present, we use a new, flexible LUS probe (5.0–7.5 MHz, Brüel & Kjaer 8555, B&K Medical, Gentofte, Denmark).

After creation of the pneumoperitoneum (12 mm Hg) and insertion of the umbilical trocar, a 10-mm port was introduced under direct visualization into the upper gastrointestinal region. The video camera was then put into the epigastric port, and insertion of the ultrasonic probe through the umbilical incision under visual supervision could begin. Maintenance of the pneumoperitoneum during LUS was technically difficult until the dedicated B&K LUS probe was available, which can be inserted through a standard trocar (11 mm).

It is not necessary to fill the abdominal cavity with water in order to improve visibility of the upper gastrointestinal (GI) organs during LUS. Filling the stomach with water via a gastric tube can improve visibility of the pancreatic corpus and tail. During LUS the liver, pancreas, biliary tract, stomach, and kidneys are investigated routinely.

Fig. 1. Cross-section of the pancreatic neck (*P*) at the confluence of the superior mesenteric vein (*SMV*) and splenic vein

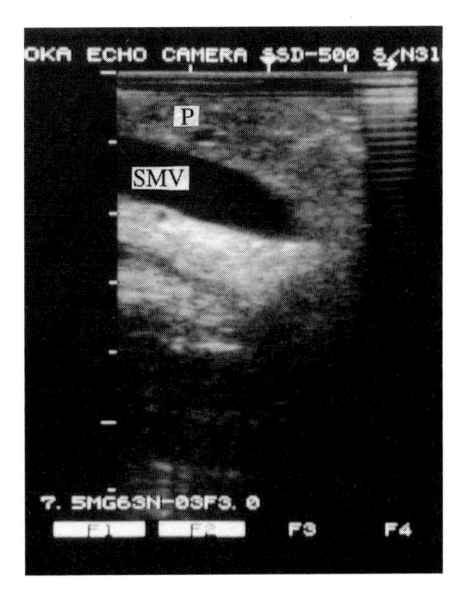

Results

From 1984 to 1990, 45 patients with cancer of the pancreatoduodenal region were included in a study at our institution to investigate the advantages and pitfalls of laparoscopy [34]. Results of preoperative screening for liver or peritoneal metastases by CT and percutaneous US were negative in all cases. In two patients, laparoscopy was abandoned due to intra-abdominal adhesions which made the investigation impossible. In 16 patients (37%), metastatic spread to liver and/or peritoneum could be disclosed either macroscopically (11 cases, Fig. 2), cytologically (three cases), or by means of biopsy (one case), which was obtained during laparoscopy. In all but two cases with only positive cytologic findings, these lesions were confirmed during subsequent surgery for palliation. In seven of 27 cases, laparoscopy gave false-negative results, and peritoneal carcinosis or liver metastases were disclosed during the surgical procedure.

Since 1990, laparoscopy in combination with LUS was performed in 32 patients with gastrointestinal neoplasms, among them 13 patients with suspected pancreatic disease. We had severe technical and organizational problems with our initial US prototype and could only accomplish a few investigations for a period of two years. Thus, LUS was impossible in the majority of patients with pancreatic disease.

Although pancreatic neoplasm were suspected preoperatively, chronic pancreatitis with postpancreatitic calcifications was stated by LUS in two cases. In a further case, retroperitoneal lymph node metastases from a gynecological malignancy were disclosed as the cause of biliary obstruction. These cases were treated conservatively. In the remaining nine cases, pancreatic neoplasms were confirmed by LUS. In one patient with hyperinsulinism, a well-delineated, partly calcified tumor of the pancreatic tail was identified and judged as operable. One case presented with a multifocal endocrine tumor (MEN II syndrome)

Fig. 2. Small liver metastases not detectable by percutaneous ultrasound or computed tomography

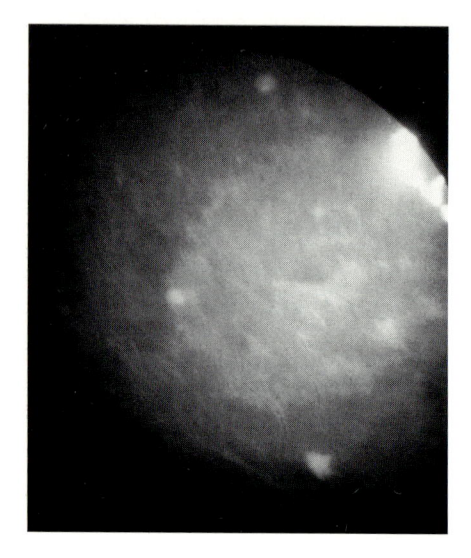

Fig. 3. Small tumor (*TU*) originating from the common bile duct (*CBD*)

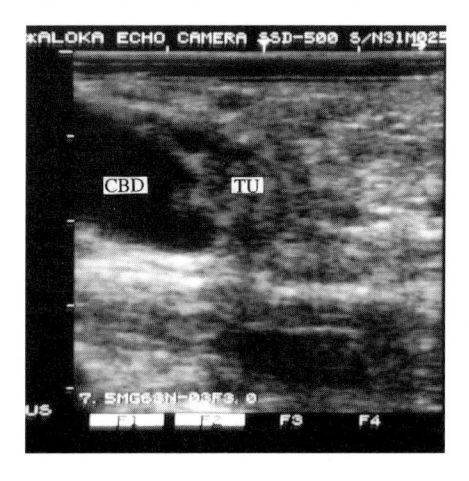

which was not operated on due to endocrinological considerations. In three of the remaining seven pancreatic malignancies, local resectability was established by LUS (Figs. 3, 4) and confirmed by intraoperative findings. The remaining four patients were judged unresectable, three of them presenting with liver and/or peritoneal metastases and two with clear infiltration of the portal vein. These patients were treated by palliative surgical procedures, and the diagnosis of LUS was confirmed.

There were no intraoperative mishaps or complications that could have been attributed to laparoscopy or LUS. All patients had an uneventful postoperative course and were discharged on the third postoperative day.

Fig. 4. Periampullary carcinoma (*TU*) with infiltration of the common bile duct (*CBD*), but a clear resectional margin towards the superior mesenteric vein (*SMV*) and duodenal wall (*DW*)

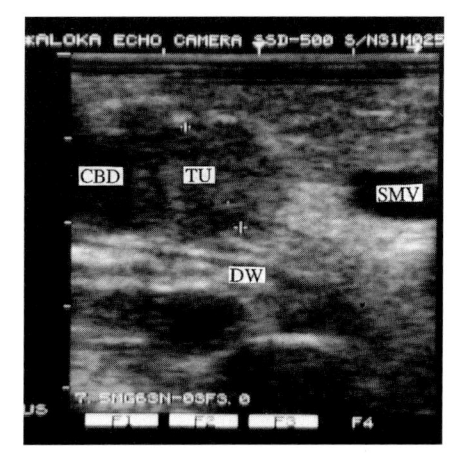

Discussion

The necessity of exact preoperative staging of pancreatic cancer is still discussed controversially: Operations with radical intention can be converted to palliative procedures should the intraoperative macroscopic findings disclose metastatic spread or local unresectability. Additionally, pancreaticoduodenectomy is increasingly considered to be a reasonable palliative approach due to its low postoperative mortality, at least in specialized centers. Furthermore, postoperative mortality of palliative surgery is also decreasing [35, 36], and nonsurgical palliative treatments are not yet widely accepted. On the basis of these arguments, the necessity of exact preoperative distinction between cases with a chance of surgical cure and a dominating need for relief of symptoms is often doubted.

In contrast, we think that there are several developments in the management of pancreatic cancer that make preoperative staging increasingly important: the improvement in endoscopic stenting procedures [3] and laparoscopic palliative measures [1, 2], consideration of costs and quality of life in cases with metastatic spread or local unresectability, referral of selected patients to specialized centers with excellent operative results [35], and the advent of neoadjuvant modalities (including genetic modulations of tumor cells [4, 5]) with the promising opportunity of downstaging and subsequent radical surgery.

According to our experience, laparoscopy alone is a valuable, yet insufficient method for complete and exact staging of pancreatic cancer: In 43 cases without suspicion of metastatic disease, tumor spread to liver and/or peritoneum was disclosed with a sensitivity of 67% and specificity of 91%. Assessment of local resectability and existence of intrahepatic metastases is impossible by means of laparoscopy alone. Moreover, there are pitfalls that have to be kept in mind: In seven of 27 cases (26%) with negative laparoscopy, tumor spread was later found intraoperatively. In these cases, laparoscopy could not visualize some distant sites of metastatic spread, especially the dorsal surface of the liver, serosa of the mesenteric root, Douglas' pouch, and bursa omentalis.

In two of 16 cases (13%) with positive findings, subsequent surgery gave negative results. There was one case in which peritoneal spread was not seen macroscopically, but indicated by peritoneal lavage cytology. The misinterpretation of mesothelial proliferation was the reason for this false-positive result. In another case, a cytologic smear was obtained for a single, small peritoneal lesion of unclear status. The pathologist was not sufficiently informed about the investigational site and therefore misdiagnosed peritoneal spread. Although positive findings of peritoneal cytology could be an independent predictor of poor prognosis [6, 8, 15], we are convinced that positive findings of peritoneal lavage cytology alone can not be regarded as an indicator of noncurative surgery.

The application of LUS allows assessment of local resectability and intrahepatic as well as lymph node metastases, therefore compensating the majority of the disadvantages of laparoscopy mentioned above. Nevertheless, one must take into consideration that LUS is generally not applicable to the diagnosis of peritoneal tumor spread. The combination of laparoscopy and LUS thus still leaves a group of patients (albeit small) with peritoneal spread to the sites mentioned above in whom diagnosis has to be established intraoperatively.

Although we have demonstrated that LUS yields good results with our self-constructed prototype, the acceptance of LUS as a routine procedure in preoperative staging of gastrointestinal neoplasm depends on the availability of technically reliable and flexible ultrasonic probes. There are several dedicated LUS probes that are obtainable or currently under construction, and they remain to be investigated with regard to their aptitude in daily routine. According to our experience, a linear or curved array is best suited for LUS due to the large coupling area and easier interpretation of anatomical structures. The probe itself has to be flexible, so convex organ surfaces and vessels serving as landmarks during ultrasound investigations can be followed. It is necessary to be able to fixate the position of the probe after deflection so that pressure can be applied to the underlying anatomical structures. Thus, the probe can be completely coupled with the surface, and gases in hollow viscera can be pushed aside for the clear visualization of wall layers and underlying organs (especially pancreas). Finally, a separate working channel for laparoscopic aspiration cytology would facilitate the confirmation of macroscopic results and therefore minimize the risk of false-positive findings.

Prospective studies that compare the diagnostic value of LUS with modern radiological methods are rare. At our institution, we prospectively investigate the additive value of LUS in comparison to percutaneous US, angiography, and CT during arterial portography in an ongoing trial. Our results so far are encouraging, and we are confident that LUS will play a major role in the future of preoperative staging and therapeutic decision-making in pancreatic cancer.

References

1. Shimi S, Banting S, Cuschieri A (1992) Laparoscopy in the management of pancreatic cancer: endoscopic cholecystojejunostomy for advanced disease. Br J Surg 79: 317–319
2. Mouiel J, Katkhouda N, White S, Dumas R (1992) Endolaparoscopic palliation of pancreatic cancer. Surg Laparosc Endosc 2: 241–243
3. Ballinger AB, McHugh M, Catnach SM, Alstead EM, Clark ML (1994) Symptom relief and quality of life after stenting for malignant bile duct obstruction. Gut 35: 467–470
4. Hoffman JP, Weese JL, Solin LJ, Engstrom P, Agarwal P, Barber LW, Guttman MC, Litwin S, Salazar H, Eisenberg BL (1995) A pilot study of preoperative chemoradiation for patients with localized adenocarcinoma of the pancreas. Am J Surg 169: 71–78
5. Ishikawa O, Ohigashi H, Imaoka S, Teshima T, Inoue T, Sasaki Y, Iwanaga T, Nakaizumi A (1991) Concomitant benefit of preoperative irradiation in preventing pancreas fistula formation after pancreatoduodenectomy. Arch Surg 126: 885–889
6. Warshaw AL, Tepper JE, Shipley WU (1986) Laparoscopy in the staging and planning of therapy for pancreatic cancer. Am J Surg 151: 76–80
7. Cuschieri A (1988) Laparoscopy for pancreatic cancer: does it benefit the patient? Eur J Surg Oncol 14: 41–44
8. Castillo CF, Warshaw L (1993) Peritoneal metastases in pancreatic carcinoma. Hepatogastroenterology 40: 430–432
9. Sackier JM, Berci G, Paz-Partlow M (1991) Elective diagnostic laparoscopy. Am J Surg 161: 326–331
10. Warshaw AL, Gu ZY, Wittenberg J, Waltman AC (1990) Preoperative staging and assessment of resectability of pancreatic cancer. Arch Surg 125: 230–233
11. Cuschieri A, Hall AW, Clark J (1978) Value of laparoscopy in the diagnosis and management of pancreatic carcinoma. Gut 19: 672–677

12. Cuesta MA, Meijer S, Borgstein PJ (1992) Laparoscopy and assessment of digestive tract cancer. Br J Surg 79: 486–487
13. Soyer P, Levesque M, Elias D, Zeitoun G, Roche A (1992) Detection of liver metastases from colorectal cancer: comparison of intraoperative US and CT during arterial portography. Radiology 183: 541–544
14. Castillo CF, Rattner DW, Warshaw AL (1995) Further experience with laparoscopy and peritoneal cytology in the staging of pancreatic cancer. Br J Surg 82: 1127–1129
15. Warshaw AL (1991) Implications of peritoneal cytology for staging of early pancreatic cancer. Am J Surg 161: 26–30
16. Evans RM, Hulbert JC, Reddy PK (1992) Complications of laparoscopy. Sem Urology 10: 164–168
17. Shifren JL, Adlestein L, Finkler NJ (1992) Asystolic cardiac arrest: a rare complication of laparoscopy. Obstet Gynecol 79: 840–841
18. Carmichael AR, Jackson BT (1995) Diagnostic laparoscopy combined with laparoscopic ultrasonography in staging of cancer of the pancreatic head region (letter). Br J Surg 82: 1703–1704
19. Jorgensen JO, McCall JL, Morris DL (1995) Port side seeding after laparoscopic ultrasonographic staging of pancreatic carcinoma. Surgery 117: 118–119
20. Bouvy ND, Marquet RL, Jeekel J, Bonjer HJ (1995) Gasless versus CO_2 pneumoperitoneum in relation to the development of abdominal wall metastases. Eur Surg Res (Suppl I) 27: 4
21. Stone MD, Kane R, Bothe A, Jessup M, Cady B, Steele GD (1994) Intraoperative ultrasound imaging of the liver at the time of colorectal cancer resection. Arch Surg 129: 431–436
22. Knol JA, Marn CS, Francis IR, Rubin JM, Bromberg J, Chang AE (1993) Comparisons of dynamic infusion and delayed computed tomography, intraoperative ultrasound, and palpation in the diagnosis of liver metastases. Am J Surg 165: 81–88
23. Bemelman WA, Wit LT, Delden OM, Smits NJ, Obertop H, Rauws EJA, Gouma DJ (1995) Diagnostic laparoscopy combined with laparoscopic ultrasonography in staging of cancer of the pancreatic head region. Br J Surg 82: 820–824
24. Glaser KS, Tschmelitsch, J, Klingler A, Klingler P, Bodner E (1995) Is there a role for laparaoscopic ultrasonography (LUS)? Surg Laparosc Endosc 5: 370–375
25. Cuesta MA, Meijer S, Borgstein PJ, Mulder LS, Sikkenk AC (1993) Laparoscopic ultrasonography for hepatobiliary and pancreatic malignancy. Br J Surg 80: 1571–1574
26. Murugiah M, Paterson-Brown S, Windsor JA, Miles WFA, Garden OJ (1993) Early experience of laparoscopic ultrasonography in the management of pancreatic carcinoma. Surg Endosc 7: 177–181
27. Miles WFA, Paterson-Brown S, Garden OJ (1992) Laparoscopic contact hepatic ultrasonography. Br J Surg 79: 419–420
28. Frank K, Bliesze H, Bönhof JA, Beck K, Hammes P, Linhart P (1985) Laparoscopic sonography: a new approach to intraabdominal disease. J Clin Ultrasound 13: 60–65
29. Bönhof JA, Linhart P, Bettendorf U, Holper H (1984) Liver biopsy guided by laparoscopic sonography. A case report demonstrating as new technique. Endoscopy 16: 237–239
30. Rau B, Hünerbein M, Schlag PM (1994) Laparoskopische Sonographie mit einem Ultraschallendoskop. Chirurg 65: 400–402
31. John TG, Garden OJ (1994) Laparoscopic ultrasonography: extending the scope of diagnostic laparoscopy. Br J Surg 81: 5–6
32. Rösch T, Braig C, Gain T, Feuerbach S, Siewert JR, Schusdziarra V, Classen M (1992) Staging of pancreatic and ampullary carcinoma by endoscopic ultrasonography. Gastroenterology 102: 188–199
33. Röthlin M, Schlumpf R, Largiadèr F (1991) Die Technik der intraoperativen Sonographie bei der laparoskopischen Cholezystektomie. Chirurg 62: 899–901
34. Glaser K, Judmaier G, Prior G, Vogel W, Tschmelitsch J, Bodner E (1991) The value of laparoscopy in the management of IORT for pancreatic cancer. In: Abe M, Takahashi M (eds.) Intraoperative Radiation Therapy. Pergamon Press Inc., pp 263–264
35. Janes RH, Niederhuber JE, Chmiel JS, Winchester DP, Ocwieja KC, Karnell LH, Clive RE, Menck HR (1996) National patterns of care for pancreatic cancer. Results of a survey by the commission on cancer. Ann Surg 223: 261–272
36. Cameron JL (1995) The current management of carcinoma of the head of the pancreas. Annu Rev Med 46: 361–370

Intraportal Ultrasonography for Evaluation of Resectability in Pancreatic Cancer

Å. Andrén-Sandberg · C. Lundstedt · P. Hannesson · H. Stridbeck · I. Ihse

Introduction

A wide variety of radiographic techniques are available for evaluation of patients with pancreatic carcinoma. When the accurate diagnosis has been provided, a second goal is to define the extent of disease and establish if the tumor is resectable or not.

The most commonly used radiological methods have been ultrasonography (US), computed tomography (CT), angiography, and magnetic resonance imaging (MRI). US and CT are both accurate methods in detecting unresectable tumors; the positive predictive values (PPV) approach 100% in both methods [1]. Angiography and MRI can hardly add anything to this. However, it is much more difficult to correctly identify the patients with resectable tumors radiologically, for whom PPV obtained by CT varies between 35% and 80%. In controlled studies, US has fared no better than CT in this group of patients [1].

In patients in whom the tumor seems to be confined to the pancreatic parenchyma without distant spread, possible involvement of the portal vein is one of the most important factors to consider when evaluating the possibility or resection. The frequency of venous involvement is related to the size of the pancreatic tumor, but even large cancers in the pancreatic head may occasionally grow in such a way that the portal vein is respected and a radical operation is possible. In one series, tumor involvement of the large extrapancreatic veins (portal, superior mesenteric, and splenic) was found in 67% of 341 cases with pancreatic cancer [2].

The portal venous system may be studied by arterial portography or by direct portal venography. In arterial portography, the portal venous system is opacified by injecting a large amount of contrast medium into the superior mesenteric or splenic artery [3]. Transhepatic portal venography was first described in 1952 [4]. However, it was not until 1974, when Lunderquist described the first cases of transhepatic obliteration of gastroesophageal varices, that the procedure gained wider acceptance [5]. Subsequently, a number of investigators have used this technique for direct portal venography and selective pancreatic venography [6, 7].

Transabdominal US and CT have about the same accuracy as angiography in evaluating vascular involvement in pancreatic adenocarcinoma [1]. The most difficult area to evaluate properly is the portal vein adjacent to the uncinate process, an area where tumor overgrowth is not uncommon. Improved resolution can be obtained with helical CT using thinner slices, and in US resolution will increase with increasing US frequency. However, with increasing frequency penetration of US will decrease, and the frequencies used in transabdominal US examinations are a compromise between resolution and penetration. This problem can be partially ovecome by using endoluminal (gastric or duodenal) [8] or translaparoscopic US.

A more direct option is to use intravascular US, with a probe placed in the portal vein itself. Intravascular ultrasound (IVUS) is a relatively new technique in which a high-frequency US probe is mounted inside a vascular catheter. The technique has until now most commonly been used in the evaluation of atherosclerosis [9]. We have used this technique in the evaluation of patients with potentially resectable pancreatic cancer.

Preoperative Approach: Normal Anatomy

Normal peripancreatic anatomy, as demonstrated by IVUS, has been described by us [10] in a series of ten patients investigated during surgery for colorectal carcinoma. Prior to surgery, gross abnormalities in the liver and hepatoduodenal ligament were excluded by transabdominal US. In all cases, surgical evaluation of the hepatoduodenal ligament was normal.

The IVUS catheters used were 2.0 mm in diameter with a 20-MHz transducer (Boston Scientific Corp., Watertown, MA, USA). The intravascular imaging system was a Sonos M2400A (Hewlett Packard Co., Andover, MA, USA). This system gives a 360° cross-sectional, high-resolution real-time image perpendicular to the catheter. The field of view was 30 mm. During laparotomy, a mesenteric vein was punctured with a 1.4-mm sheathed needle (Viggo-Spectramed, Helsingborg, Sweden), and a 0.64-mm guidewire (Meadox, Helsingborg, Sweden) was introduced. The guidewire was blindly advanced into the portal vein and up into the liver. Subsequently, the IVUS catheter was advanced over the guidewire into the right or left main branch of the portal vein. The entire portal vein was evaluated down to below the confluence between the splenic and superior mesenteric vein and recorded on a super VHS video recorder. No complications to the procedure were seen.

The appearance of the portal vein and its surroundings was consistent. The vein had a variable diameter (8–16 mm) and in some patients it was partially collapsed at the confluence. The wall of the portal vein appeared as a single hyperechoic layer 0.5–0.8 mm thick. Its echogenicity was often similar to that of the surrounding fat tissue. At times, the venous wall could not be clearly separated from the fatty tissue. The wall was often slightly thicker in the juxtahepatic than in the distal part of the vein. The parenchyma of the pancreas had an intermediate echogenicity, mostly clearly separable from the portal venous wall. Normal structures adjacent to the vein, such as the common bile duct, the hepatic artery, and small lymph nodes, were clearly separated from the lumen of the portal vein and surrounding fatty tissue.

Fig. 1. 55-year-old male with a short history of jaundice. Transabdominal ultrasound shows an expanding, hypoechoic lesion in the head of the pancreas (arrow). The common bile duct is dieated, measures almost 15 mm in diameter. The dilatation can be followed down to the lesion in the pancreatic head

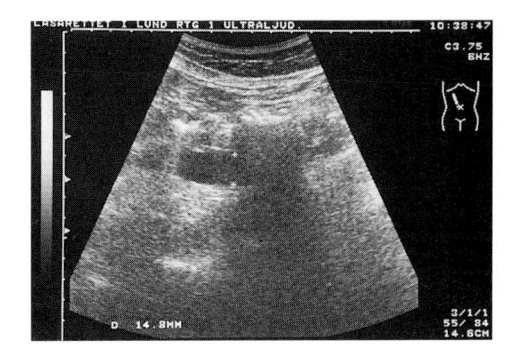

Preoperative Approach:
Patients with Pancreatic Adenocarcinoma

Using the same technique as described above, eight patients with exocrine pancreatic cancers were examined preoperatively. No evidence of irresectability could be found prior to operation in any of the cases, and laparotomy was performed in all cases with the intention of radical surgery.

Of the eight cases, one case showed infiltration of the portal vein as seen in IVUS and confirmed by laparotomy. No resection was performed. In the remaining seven cases, preoperative radiological and routine preoperative surgical evaluation on the whole showed a resectable tumor, and resection was performed. However, in all of these patients IVUS suggested portal vein involvement of the tumor. This was confirmed by the histopathological evaluation of the resected specimens.

Preoperative Approach:
Transhepatic Approach

After completion of the second series of eight patients described above, two further patients have been examined with IVUS prior to surgery, using the transhepatic route.

Both patients were male, 52 and 55 years old, respectively, and had been jaundiced only for a short period of time before surgery. In both patients, preoperative US and CT showed a pancreatic tumor (Figs. 1, 2). Percutaneous transhepatic portography (PTP) was performed using a right lateral intercostal puncture site in the midaxillary line. Using fluoroscopic control, the patient was asked to hold his breath and a 25-cm-long, 5 F (outer diameter 1.6 mm) sheathed needle was advanced into the liver towards Th 12. The stylet was removed and the patient instructed to breath normally. The catheter was

Fig. 2. CT of the same patient shows a slightly expanded head of the pancreas. Biliary decompression has been performed by PTC insertion. The superior mesenteric vein (arrow) is well delineated towards the pancreatic head

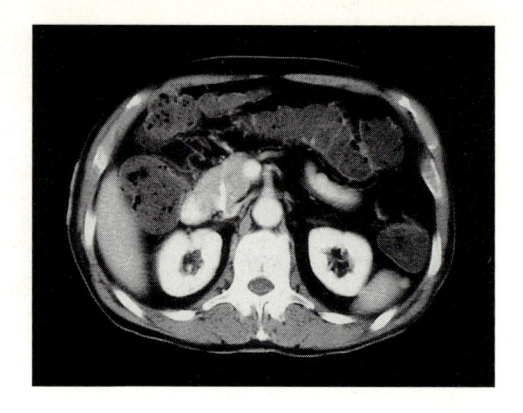

retracted under continuous aspiration, and when blood was obtained, the position of the catheter was checked by contrast medium injection. When the tip was in the portal vein, a 0.97-mm guidewire was inserted into the main portal vein and the catheter advanced to a suitable location. The catheter was then replaced with an 8 F (2.7 mm) vascular sheath, and through this sheath the IVUS catheter was later advanced into the portal vein.

A portal venogram obtained before the IVUS examination showed an impression of the venous wall (Fig. 3). In IVUS, a discontinuous portal venous wall was seen in both patients, suggesting tumoral involvement of the vessel wall (Fig. 4).

In one of the patients, portal venous pressure was noted to be higher than normal during PTP (blood drained freely from the portal vein through the catheter). In that patient, about 1000 ml of clotted blood in the upper right quadrant of the abdomen, most of it between the liver and the diaphragm, were found by laparotomy. There was no ongoing bleeding at that time (24 h after PTP). The second patient showed no evidence of portal hypertension during

Fig. 3. Transhepatic portogram shows as smooth impression in the portal venous wall (arrow heads). This could be due to pancreatitis or to tumor. The PTC catheter is also well seen (arrow)

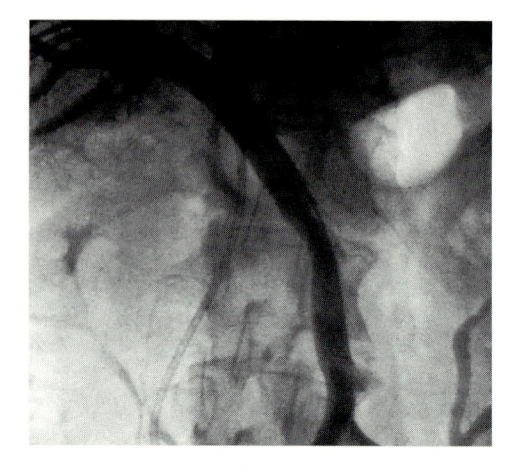

Fig. 4. At portal ultrasonograph the venous wall is discontinuous (arrows). This suggests tumorous involvement of the portal venous wall

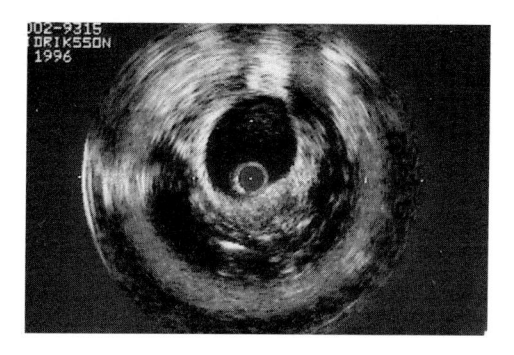

PTP, and only about 100 ml of blood were noted in the abdomen during surgery. The first of the patients had an irresectable adenocarcinoma of the head of the pancreas at laparotomy, whereas most of the duodenum was normal. However, the well-circumscribed tumor was larger than expected, $4 \times 5 \times 6$ cm^3, encasing the portal vein at least from the right side. There was no spread of the tumor outside the pancreas. The second patient had a well-defined tumor in the head of the pancreas. A radical subtotal pancreaticodenectomy was performed. The surgical specimen showed a superficial adenocarcinoma in the common bile duct and fibrous and lipomatous infiltration in the pancreas adjacent to the portal vein.

Discussion

Pancreatic and other periampullary carcinomas are liable to invade the major vessels, particularly the portal vein. It is well documented [11] that local recurrence is a major problem after radical pancreatic cancer resection, making more aggressive operation techniques, i.e., including portal vein resection, an option [12, 13]. Regional pancreatectomy, i.e., removal en bloc of the pancreas, regional lymph nodes, duodenum, gastric antrum, and intrapancreatic portal vein, has as yet not been shown to be superior to less extensive surgical procedures in terms of either operative mortality, morbidity, or long-term survival [14]. However, patients selected for these extensive operations usually had advanced disease, making the results obtained difficult to compare to those of pancreaticoduodenectomy without portal vein resection. If it were known preoperatively that there was local tumor overgrowth on the portal vein, the decision to perform a radically intended operation could be based on more solid ground. Some patients should then probably be offered palliative procedures instead, and in those cases in which there was limited involvement of the portal vein, local resection ot that part could be planned in advance, or in selected cases regional pancreatectomy could be discussed. Therefore, in patients with pancreatic cancer confined to the pancreatic bed, preoperative information on portal vein involvement by the tumor, and even invasive preoperative examination techniques, can be accepted, given that the information on this matter is reliable.

It seems as if our results and those of others [15-17] regarding evaluation of the portal venous wall by IVUS strongly favor the view that this examination is is capable of detecting subtle signs of tumoral venous wall invasion in pancreatic carcinoma. It is possible to introduce the catheter transhepatically, and an IVUS examination can thus be performed prior to surgery to detect tumoral involvement of the venous structures not detectable by other methods. If the accuracy of a preoperative IVUS performed transhepatically can be shown in a larger series to be sufficiently high, this could lead to a decision not perform an unnecessary laparotomy, or it could give a better basis for preoperative planning of a portal vein resection in a pancreaticoduodenectomy. However, as seen in one of our transhepatically examined patients, fibrotic and fatty changes in the pancreatic tissue might cause false-positive results in an IVUS examination.

It seems, however, that IVUS has great potential for improving preoperative staging of pancreatic carcinoma, and also might become a valuable tool in the preoperative tailoring of the surgical procedure – both to the patient and to the tumor – regardless if a portal vein resection is contemplated or not.

References

1. Reznek RH, Stephens DH (1993) Review: the staging of pancreatic adenocarcinoma. Clin Radiol 47: 373-381
2. Freeny PC, Lawson TL (1982) Radiology of the pancreas. New York: Springer-Verlag 466
3. Nebesar RA, Pollard JJ (1966) Portal venography by selective arterial catheterization. Am J Roentg 97: 477-487
4. Bierman HR, Steinbach HL, White LP, et al. (1952) Portal venipuncture. A percutaneous transhepatic approach. Proc Soc Exper Biol Med 79: 550-552
5. Lunderquist A, Vang J (1974) Transhepatic catherization and obliteration of the coronary vein in patients with portal hypertension. N Eng J Med 291: 646-649
6. Göthlin J, Lunderquist A, Tylén U (1974) Selective phlebography of the pancreas. Acta Rad Diag 15: 474-480
7. Reichard W (1979) Phlebography of the pancreas: anatomy, technique and clinical applications. Lund University: Department of Radiology, (thesis)
8. Grimm H, Maydeo A, Soehendra N (1990) Endoluminal ultrasound for the diagnosis and staging of pancreatic cancer. Clin Gastroenterol 4: 869-888
9. Nissen SE, Gurley JC (1991) Application of intravascular ultrasound for detection and quantification of coronary atherosclerosis. Int J Card Imaging 6: 165-170
10. Hannesson PH, Stridbeck H, Lundstedt C, Andrén-Sandberg Å, Ihse I (1996) Intravascular ultrasound of the portal vein – normal anatomy. Acta Radiol 36: 388-392
11. Westerdahl J, Andrén-Sandberg Å, Ihse I (1993) Recurrence of exocrine pancreatic cancer – local or hepatic? Hepatogastroenterol 40: 384-387
12. Sindelar WF (1989) Clinical experience with regional pancreatectomy for adenocarcinoma of the pancreas. Arch Surg 124: 127-132
13. Nakao A, Nonami T, Harada A, Kasuga T, Takagi H (1990) Portal vein resection with a new antithrombogenic catheter. Surgery 108: 913-918
14. Hiraoka T (1990) Extended radical resection of cancer of the pancreas with intraoperative radiotherapy. Clin Gastroenterol 4: 985-993
15. Kaneko T, Nakao A, Harada A, Toshiaki N, Takagi H (1994) Intraportal endovascular ultrasonography in pancreatic cancer – a new technique for the diagnosis of portal vein invasion: a preliminary report. Surgery 115: 438-444

16. Kaneko T, Nakao A, Inoue S, Nomoto S, Hosono J, Harada A, Nonami T, Takagi H (1995) Intraportal endovascular ultrasonography as a new diagnostic procedure in pancreatic surgery. Hepatogastroenterology 42: 711–716
17. Hannesson PH, Stridbeck H, Lundstedt C, Dawiskiba S, Andrén-Sandberg Å, Ihse I (1996) Intravascular ultrasound for evaluation of portal venous involvement in pancreatic cancer. Europ Radiol, in press

II
Other Diagnostic Procedures

Serological Diagnosis of Pancreatic Cancer

M. Ebert · P. Malfertheiner

Introduction

Pancreatic cancer is a devastating malignancy characterized by increasing incidence, poor prognosis, and limited therapeutic opportunities [1–3]. Overall, 5-year survival for these patients is less than 1% [1], and the vast majority of these patients present with advanced disease. Thus there have been multiple approaches in order to find effective serological markers for this disease. These markers should be specific for this kind of tumor, and give clinicians a tool to screen, diagnose, and monitor patients with pancreatic cancer (Table 1). Furthermore, these serum markers should ideally help identify patients with a more favorable prognosis, as well as detect recurrent disease. Finally, the determination of these markers should be standardized, reproducible, and cost-effective. However, to date none of the presently known markers fulfills these criteria. Nonetheless, new molecular approaches have been helpful in identifying patients with this malignancy. This review will give a brief overview of currently used serum markers and will also focus on the role of molecular markers.

Conventional Serum Markers

In the past, three groups of serum markers have been studied extensively. Analysis of the sensitivity and specificity of enzyme measurement, such as galactosyltransferase II [4], ribonuclease, or elastase [5], for the diagnosis of pancreatic

Table 1. Mandatory features of serum tumor markers in pancreatic cancer

Feature type	Feature
Diagnostic features	Specific for pancreatic ancer Diagnosis Differential diagnosis Screening Follow-up Prognosis Recurrent disease
Technical features	Standardized and reproducible determination Cost-effective

cancer have led to disappointing results. Generally, sensitivity of these markers varies between 60% and 90%, and false-positive results occur in benign gastrointestinal disease and nonpancreatic tumors at a rate of approximately 10%–60% and 15%–70%, respectively [3–5]. Furthermore, the measurement of the ratio of testosterone to dihydrotestosterone, which is below 5 in 70% of patients with pancreatic cancer, represents the second group of potential serum markers for pancreatic cancer. However, this is again not a sensitive marker for pancreatic cancer and thus has no clinical relevance [6].

A third group of intensively studied serum markers are tumor-associated antigens. A wide variety of these markers has been studied. Today's most common and best studied tumor marker is Ca 19-9. Ca 19-9 is defined by monoclonal antibodies 1116 NS 19-9 which react with sialylated Lewis A blood group antigen [7]. Overall sensitivity of Ca 19-9 for the diagnosis of pancreatic cancers is 70%–90% and specificity is close to 90% [8, 9]. Furthermore, the diagnostic accuracy of Ca 19-9 is superior to other tumor-associated antigens, which serve as potential alternative markers for pancreatic cancer, such as CA 50, TPA, and Dupan-2 [9–11]. Combining the determination of Ca 19-9 with other serum markers does not improve diagnostic accuracy [9–11]. Tumor resection is associated with decreased Ca 19-9 values, and recurrent or progressive disease leads to increased Ca 19-9 values [8, 12, 13]. A study by the Japan Pancreatic Cancer Study Group in 1994 [14] evaluated the effectivity of Ca 19-9 as part of a screening program for the detection of early pancreatic cancers. In symptomatic patients presenting with jaundice, diabetes, or gastrointestinal complaints versus asymptomatic patients, the combined determination of Ca 19-9 and elastase-1 coupled with an ultrasound proved to be effective in the detection of early, resectable pancreatic cancers (Table 2). However, Ca 19-9 measurement, is often false-positively elevated in benign disease, such as chronic pancreatitis, an important differential diagnosis of pancreatic cancer. Furthermore, false-negative results occur in patients with localized cancers and in patients with a Lewis-negative phenotype. In conclusion, Ca 19-9 is a widely used serum marker with reasonably high sensitivity and specificity and, based on its diagnostic accuracy, is superior to all other currently known and used serum markers. Nonetheless, it is not suitable for the identification of small cancers and cannot be used for screening purposes (Table 3) [8, 15, 16].

Ca 242 is a new serum marker based on the monoclonal antibody c242 obtained after immunization of mice with a human colorectal adenocarcinoma cell line [17]. The structure of the antigenic determinant is a sialylated carbo-

Table 2. Results of the Japan Pancreatic Cancer Study Group Screening Program 1994 [14]

	Asymptomatic (n)	Symptomatic (n)
Total cases	12800	8700
Pancreatic cancers	4	141
Resectable cancers	1:4	47:141

Screening program: Ca 19-9, elastase-1, ultrasound in patients over 40 years of age.

Table 3. Role of Ca 19-9 in the diagnosis of pancreatic cancer

Pro
Satisfactory sensitivity and specificity
Follow-up
Prognosis
Low cost and rapid result
Contra
Screening
False-negative in localized pancreatic cancer
False-positive results in benign disease (obstructive jaundice)
False-negative in Lewis negative phenotype

hydrate structure and is related, but not identical to, Ca 19-9 and Ca 50. Haglund et al. studied the diagnostic value of this marker in pancreatic cancer [11]. Using serum samples from 179 patients with pancreatic cancer, overall sensitivity of the Ca 242 assay was 74% and specificity was 91%. In conclusion, CA 242 might have similar sensitivity and specificity as Ca 19-9; however, false-positive results also occur in benign obstructive jaundice, and the CA 242 assay is also dependent on the Lewis blood group status [17, 18].

New Molecular Markers

Molecular analysis of pancreatic carcinoma has revealed a number of molecular and genetic alterations associated with pancreatic carcinogenesis. Thus pancreatic cancers exhibit a high frequency of K-*ras* mutations [19, 20] and mutations of the p53 tumor suppressor gene [20–22]. Furthermore, pancreatic cancers express and overexpress a wide variety of growth factors and their receptors [23–25]. Based on these findings, there have been multiple attempts to develop new assays leading to serological detection of molecular alterations that occur in pancreatic carcinoma.

Mutations of the p53 tumor suppressor gene lead to a mutant protein with an increased half-life which can be detected by immunohistochemistry, and further studies have shown that the immunohistochemically detected mutant p53 protein correlates well with the presence of p53 gene mutation [21]. Serological detection of p53 antibodies has been reported for breast cancers, lung cancer, and other human malignancies [26, 27]. Again, the presence of these antibodies correlates well with the presence of mutant p53 and p53 gene mutation. Laurent-Piug et al. [28] analyzed the presence of antibodies against p53 in the serum of 29 patients with pancreatic cancer, 33 with biliary tract cancer, and 33 patients with benign biliary or pancreatic disease. p53 antibodies were detected in 8/29 (28%) pancreatic cancer patients, in five of 33 biliary tract cancer patients, and in one patient with stones of the common bile duct. Overall sensitivity and specificity in distinguishing between malignant and benign pancreatic or biliary diseases was 21% and 96% for p53, respectively (Table 4). The combination of elevated Ca 19-9 levels and the presence of p53 antibodies was associated with a specificity of 97%. Though the authors did not study the pres-

Table 4. Molecular markers for pancreatic cancer

Author	Reference	Type	Sensitivity	Specificity
Laurent-Puig	[28]	p53 antibodies	8/29 (28%)	32/33 (96%)
Tada	[29]	K-*ras* mutations	2/6 (33%)	2/2 (100%)

ence and type of p53 mutation present in the primary tumor, this study is the first to use genetic alterations in pancreatic cancer as a novel marker for pancreatic cancer.

In a different approach, Tada et al. [29] used a modified polymerase chain reaction (PCR) technique and peripheral blood from eight patients, two of whom were suffering from insulinoma and six from pancreatic ductal adenocarcinoma, in order to detect K-*ras* mutations in the peripheral blood of these patients. K-*ras* mutations occur at a frequency of approximately 90% in pancreatic cancers. Tada et al. detected two GTT mutations in the peripheral blood in two of the six pancreatic cancer patients, of whom one patient was diagnosed with metastatic disease (Table 4). In contrast, none of the patients with insulinoma exhibited K-*ras* mutations in the DNA extracted from the peripheral blood. Again, the presence and type of K-*ras* mutation in the primary tumor was not determined; nonetheless, further studies will have to correlate the presence or absence of K-*ras* mutations detected in peripheral blood with the presence and type of K-*ras* mutations in the primary tumor.

Conclusion

Ca 19-9 is the most widely used and best studied serum marker currently available. It is useful in the diagnosis of advanced pancreatic cancer and has a role in its follow-up. However, its diagnostic accuracy is limited by false-positive elevation in benign obstructive jaundice and low sensitivity in early stages of pancreatic cancer.

p53 antibodies and K-*ras* mutations detected in peripheral blood of patients with pancreatic cancer are novel and interesting approaches based on the recently revealed molecular and genetic alterations in pancreatic cancer.

References

1. Gudjonsson B (1987) Cancer of the pancreas. 50 years of surgery. Cancer 60: 2284–2303
2. Hermanek P, Scheibe O, Spiessl, Wagner G (1987) TNM Klassifikation maligner Tumoren. Berlin, Heidelberg, New York: Springer
3. Warshaw AL, Castillo C (1992) Pancreatic carcinoma. New Engl J Med 326: 455–465
4. Podolsky DK, McPhee MS, Alpert E, Warshaw AL, Isselbacher KJ (1981) Galactosyltransferase isoenzyme II in the detection of pancreatic cancer. comparison with radiologic, endoscopic, and serologic tests. N Engl J Med 304: 1313–1318
5. Hamano H, Hayakawa T, Kondo T (1987) Serum immunoreactive elastase in diagnosis of pancreatic diseases: a sensitive marker for pancreatic cancer Dig Dis Sci 32: 50–56

6. Robles-Diaz G, Diaz-Sanchez V, Mendez JP, Altamirano A, Wolpert E (1987) Low serum testosterone/dihydrotestosterone ratio in patients with pancreatic carcinoma. Pancreas 2: 684–687
7. Koprowski H, Steplewski Z, Mitchell K, Herlyn M, Herlyn D, Fuhrer P (1979) Colorectal carcinoma antigens detected by hybridoma antibodies. Som Cell Gen 5: 957–972
8. Safi F, Beger HG, Bittner R, Büchler M, Krautzberger W (1985) Ca 19-9 and pancreatic adenocarcinoma. Cancer 57: 779–783
9. Steinberg WM, Gelfand R, Anderson KK, et al (1986) Comparison of the sensitivity and specificity of the Ca 19-9 and carcinoembryonic antigen assays in detecting cancer of the pancreas. Gastroenterology 90: 343–349
10. Panucci A, Fabris C, Del Favero G, et al (1985) Tissue polypeptide antigen in pancreatic cancer diagnosis. Br J Cancer 52: 801–803
11. Haglund C, Lundin J, Kuusela P, Roberts PJ (1994) Ca 242, a new tumor marker for pancreatic cancers: a comparison with Ca 19-9, Ca 50 and CEA. Br J Cancer 70: 487–492
12. Forsmark CE, Lambiase L, Vogel SB (1994) Diagnosis of pancreatic cancer and prediction of unresectability using the tumor-associated antigen Ca 19-9. Pancreas 9: 731–734
13. Serti C, Pasquali C, Catalini S, et al (1993) Ca 19-9 as a prognostic index after resection for pancreatic cancer. J Surg Oncol 52: 137–141
14. Satake K, Takeuchi T, Homma T, Ozaki H (1994) Ca 19-9 as a screening and diagnostic tool in symptomatic patients: the japanese experience. Pancreas 9: 703–706
15. Frebourg T, Bercoff E, Manchon N, Senant J, Basuyau JP, Breton P, Janvresse A, Brunelle P, Bourreille J (1988) The evaluation of Ca 19-9 antigen level in the early detection of pancreatic cancer. Cancer 62: 2287–2290
16. Malesci A, Tommasini MA, Bonato C et al (1987) Determination of Ca 19-9 antigen in serum and pancreatic juice for differential diagnosis of pancreatic carcinoma from chronic pancreatitis. Gastroenterology 92: 60–67
17. Nilsson O, Jansson EL, Johansson C, Lindholm L (1988) CA 242, a novel tumor-associated carbohydrate antigen with increased tumor specificity and sensitivity. J Tumor Marker Oncol 3: 314–319
18. Röthlin MA, Joller H, Largiader F (1992) Ca 242 is a new tumor marker for pancreatic cancer. Cancer 71: 701–707
19. Almoguera C, Shibata D, Forrester K, Matin J, Arnheim N, Perucho M (1988) Most human carcinomas of the exocrine pancreas contain mutant c-K-ras genes. Cell 53: 549–554
20. Kalthoff H, Schmiegel W, Roeder C, Kasche D, Schmidt A, Lauer G, Thiele HG, Honold G, Pantel K, Riethmüller G, Scherer E, Maurer HG, Deppert W (1993) p53 and K-ras alterations in pancreatic epithelial lesions. Oncogene 8: 289–298
21. Casey G, Yamanaka Y, Friess H, Kobrin MS, Lopez ME, Büchler MW, Beger HG, Korc M (1993) p53 mutations are common in pancreatic cancer and absent in chronic pancreatitis. Cancer Lett 69: 151–160
22. Levine AJ, Momand J, Finlay CA (1991) The p53 tumor suppressor gene. Nature 351: 453–456
23. Ebert M, Yokoyama M, Kobrin MS, Friess H, Lopez ME, Büchler MW, Johnson GR, Korc M (1994) Induction and expression of amphiregulin in human pancreatic cancer. Cancer Res 54: 3959–3962
24. Ebert M, Yokoyama M, Friess H, Büchler MW, Korc M (1994) Coexpression of the c-met protooncogene and hepatocyte growth factor in human pancreatic cancer. Cancer Res 54: 5775–5778
25. Ebert M, Yokoyama M, Friess H, Kobrin MS, Büchler MW, Korc M (1995) Induction of platelet-derived growth factors (PDGF) and overexpression of their receptors in human pancreatic cancer. Int J Cancer 62: 529–535
26. Crawford LV, Pim DC, Bulbrook RD (1992) Detection of antibodies against the cellular protein p53 in sera from patients with breast cancer. Int J Cancer 30: 403–408
27. Schlichtholz B, Tredaniel J, Lubin R, Zalcman G, Hirsch A, Soussi T (1994) Analysis of p53 antibodies in sera of patients with lung carcinoma define immunodominant regions in the p53 protein. Br J Cancer 69: 809–816
28. Laurent-Puig P, Lubin R, Semhoun-Ducloux S, Pelletier G, Fourre C, Ducreux M, Briantais MJ, Bufet C, Soussi T (1995) Antibodies against p53 protein in serum of patients with benign or malignant and biliary diseases. Gut 36: 455–458
29. Tada M, Omata M, Kawai S, Saisho H, Ohto M, Saiki RK, Sninsky JJ (1993) Detection of ras gene mutations in pancreatic juice and peripheral blood of patients with pancreatic adenocarcinoma. Cancer Res 53: 2472–2474

Role of Cytology in the Diagnosis of Pancreatic Tumors

H. U. Kasper · A. Roessner

Introduction

Prior to the establishment of modern imaging procedures such as computer tomography and sonography, the cytologic diagnosis of pancreatic diseases was usually limited to cells obtained by exfoliative methods. Cells were collected from the pancreatic duct through a tube located in the duodenum, mostly after stimulation of pancreatic secretion. This method consumed time and money and, furthermore, was not very successful.

Fine needle aspiration cytology, now well established in the management of patients with suspicious pancreatic lesions, improved the validity of pancreatic cytology. The aspirates can be obtained directly during explorative laparoscopy (peri- or intraoperative fine-needle aspiration cytology) or via a percutaneous approach (preoperative fine needle aspiration cytology).

The perioperative cytology technique of pancreas allows taking of defined samples of suspect areas of the organ. This improves the accuracy of the procedure, leading to a higher validity. No serious complications are reported. However, intraoperative aspiration cytology competes with rapid section diagnostics, a method for analyzing tissue samples in cryostate sections. The latter is characterized by a higher risk of complication, and, due to fibrosis, it is less likely to obtain tumor cells. However, either method is faced with the difficulty of distinguishing between a highly differentiated carcinoma and chronic pancreatitis.

Preoperative aspiration cytology is becoming increasingly important. It is performed under computer tomographic or ultrasonographic guidance under vizualization and can even be performed as an outpatient procedure. The accuracy of this procedure is high, even in small tumors. Complications including transient pancreatitis or small hematoma and, in some cases, fatal pancreatitis, significant hemorrhage, or tumor cell seeding into the puncture channel occur very rarely [3, 13].

Cytologic Observations

Normal Pancreas

Aspiration samples of the normal pancreas contain cells from the acinar and the ductal epithelium. Acinar cells are cuboidal, show a finely vacuolated, finely granulated, and well-demarcated cytoplasm, and possess a small, round, often eccentric nucleus with a dispersed chromatin pattern and no or only one very small nucleolus. These cells almost always form clusters. Sometimes, it is also possible to observe single naked nuclei that can be assigned to acinar cells.

The amount of ductal cells is always smaller. They are larger than the acinar cells mentioned above and have a cuboidal or columnar shape, depending on the caliber of the original structure. These cells have distinct, eosinophilic cytoplasm with defined borders. Ciliae are not visible. The round to oval eccentric nucleus shows finely distributed chromatin, a distinct nuclear membrane, and contains one or, in very rare cases, more than one small nucleus. The cells form flat cluster in a honeycombed arrangement (Fig. 1) or, when located on the side, they resemble palisades.

The islet cells, which theoretically account for approximately 2 % of the aspirate, are extremely rarely encountered in routinely obtained material. Sometimes, such material is interspessed with blood components or occasionally contains hepatocytes. Occurrence of inflammatory cells is extremely rare. Mesothelial cells may be present und must be differentiated from atypical cells.

Pancreatitis

The dominant feature in aspirates from pancreatitis is the debris, forming a dirty background and containing a variable number of epithelial and inflammatory cells. Within the first group, ductal cells are more common than acinar cells. They often exhibit features of regeneration with hyperchromatic, enlarged nuclei. The nuclear contour is regular. In general, nucleoli are inconspicuous, but sometimes they are prominent, making differential diagnosis of carcinoma more difficult (Fig. 2).

Among the inflammatory cells, polymorphic leukocytes and macrophages, often presenting with foamy cytoplasm, are the most common types. Giant cells

Fig. 1. Normal ductal epithelium with honeycombed arrangement of uniform cells. Mai-Grünwald-Giemsa

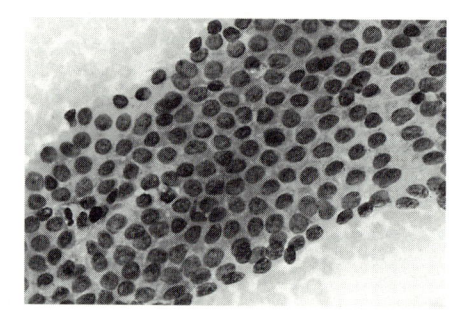

Fig. 2. Cells from chronic pancreatitis showing reactive changes. Mai-Grünwald-Giemsa

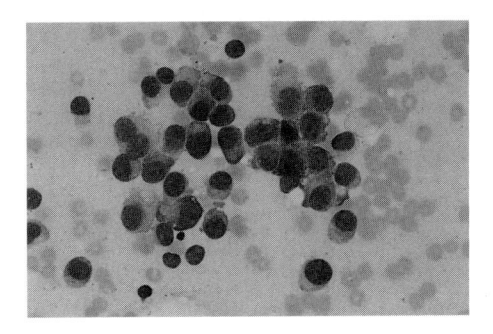

are also visible. Fragments of granulation tissue and degenerated fatty tissue can be observed. Some cases of subacute and chronic pancreatitis also include calcifications.

Pancreatic pseudocysts can develop as complications of pancretitis. Along with a few inflammatory cells, the aspirates show activated fibrocytes and macrophages as well as amorphous debris and calcifications. Theoretically, they do not have an epithelial component, but cells from adjacent pancreatic tissue may be intermingled, thus complicating differentiation from cystic neoplasm.

Ductal Adenocarcinoma

More than 90% of all pancreatic cancers are made up of adenocarcinomas of duct origin with different grading. Among them, the well-differentiated ones are particularly difficult to evaluate cytologically.

The cells of well-differentiated adenocarcinoma have a cuboidal to polygonal shape. The cytoplasm is granular, and the nuclei are oval to round and show a chromatin pattern similar to reactive atypia. However, nuclear crowding occurs. The nuclear membranes are irregular and mitotic figures can be seen. The cells are mostly organized in sheets, but cellular dyshesion can be observed. The background, often containing mucus, is clearer than in chronic inflammation, but the coexistence of tumor and inflammation should always be considered (Table 1).

The moderately and poorly differentiated variants show the common criteria of malignancy and are much more easily detectable in the aspirate. The cells are pleomorphic and have granulated cytoplasm. The nuclei are enlarged, differ in size and shape, and possess prominent macronuclei within clumped chromatin (Fig 3). Architectural disorganization can be observed. Tumor diathesis is subject to alterations. Anaplastic carcinoma can also exhibit a dominance of spindle-shaped and multinucleated cells (giant cell carcinoma of the pancreas). In such cases, differential diagnosis of retroperitoneal sarcoma can be performed. However, smears from pancreatic carcinoma show carcinoma cells of a more obvious appearance, often with intracellular mucus.

Table 1. Criteria for differentiation of benign cells (normal and reactive ductal cells) from pancreatic carcinoma cells

Criterium	Benign	Malignant
Cell size	Uniform	Pleomorphic
Nucleus		
Size	Small	Enlarged
Chromatin pattern	Fine	Coarse
Nucleolus	Absent or tiny, sometimes prominent	Prominent, multiple, macronucleoli
Nuclear membrane	Smooth	Irregular, foldings
Cell clusters	Cohesive, only a few single cells, orderly	Dissociated, many single cells, loose and discorderly, microacini
Mitosis	Few	Increased
Smear composition	Mixed	One dominant cell type

Neuroendocrine Tumors of the Pancreas

These tumors, predominantly located in the body and the tail of the pancreas, are cytologically characterized by a monotonous picture of small cells with an abundance of granular cytoplasm and small eccentric nuclei of regular shape and equal size. The cromatin is dispersed, and an unsuspicious central nucleolus often occurs. The cells tend to appear singly, but small clusters and even rosette-like structures are sometimes seen. Increased nuclear pleomorphism, nuclear molding, and a dirty necrotic background are signs of increased malignancy.

Rare Tumors

Acinar cell carcinoma, originating from acinar cells, is an uncommon variant of pancreatic cancer. The aspirates contain polygonal cells, which are smaller than ductal cancer ones. The cytoplasm is abundant in granules, and the nuclei are round and dark with a rather uniform appearance. The nuclear membrane may exhibit foldings with the cells building up solid nests.

Fig. 3. A cluster of atypical cells from a moderately differentiated ductal carcinoma with cellular and nuclear pleomorphism and architectural disorganization. Mai-Grünwald-Giemsa

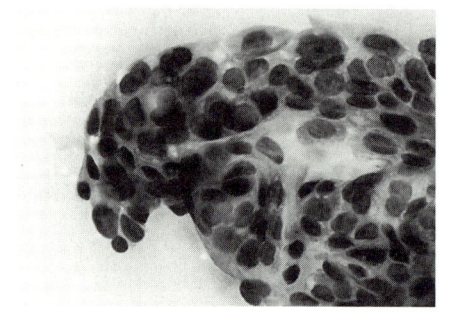

The cystic neoplasm of pancreas is also very uncommon. Aspirates from microcystic tumors contain small groups of cuboidal cells, presenting a uniform picture. The cells have a fine pale cytoplasm, and the nuclei are round and oval, displaying a dark and regular contour. Mucin is not detectable intracytoplasmatically, nor can it be found in the background. In contrast, mucinous cystic neoplasms show an abundance of mucin. The cellular morphology varies from bland in cystadenoma to malignant in cystadenocarcinoma.

Papillary cystic neoplasm occurs mostly in adolescents and young women. The cells are monomorphous and contain round nuclei with a regular membrane as well as finely dispersed chromatin but rather conspicuous nucleoli. They are organized in clusters and sometimes pseudorosettes are found.

Metastatic neoplasm with primary sites in organs such as stomach, breast lung, and kidney may also occur in the pancreas.

Further Developments

Mutations in the ras genes are genetic aberrations very often involved in the oncogenesis of human cancer. In pancreatic carcinoma, the majority of cells (65%–100%) also harbor activated K ras genes with a mutation at codon 12. Other known gene abnormalities occur less frequently.

Molecular detection of such a frequent genetic change could be used to overcome the limits of traditional cytomorphologic cancer detection, particularly regarding the differentiation of reactive atypia in chronic pancreatitis and well-differentiated cancer. Particularly the first studies performed on the basis of polymerase chain reaction (PCR) [1, 12] yielded encouraging results. A combination of cytologic and molecular biologic tests leads to higher sensitivity. Cytologic smears would not require any special handling. In a reference center, the procedure could be completed within 2 days. However, additional confirmatory studies must be performed in the future before such developments can influence routine diagnostics.

Conclusion

In fine-needle aspiration of pancreas, sensitivity and specifity is very high, ranging from 70% to 96% [2, 4, 9] and can be increased by using recently developed molecular biologic procedures.

The percutaneous technique with radiologic detection of the lesion is rather simple, but accuracy depends on the experience of radiologist performing the aspiration. The major advantage of this procedure is to be able to obtain a preoperative diagnosis to help the surgeon to plan the therapeutical strategy. Total pancreatectomy can be performed on resectable tumors in case of positive cytology. Patients with resectable tumors in whom preoperative cytology is negative, but who have a high suspicion index of pancreatic malignancy due to clinical findings and imaging procedures can benefit from intraoperative cytology, thus avoiding any delay. In patients deemed to be unresectable due to the large size of the tumor or because of metastasization, fine needle aspiration cytology can establish the presence of a tumor, thus paving the way for palliative measures.

In summary, fine needle aspiration cytology of pancreas is a safe and economical technique that can be performed percutaneously under computed tomography (CT) or ultrasonographic guidance or intraoperatively to provide an accurate preoperative or intraoperative diagnosis.

References

1. Apple SK, Hecht R, Novak JM, Nieberg RK, Rosenthal DL, Grody WW (1996) Polymerase chain reaction-based K-ras mutation detection of pancreatic adenocarcinoma in routine cytology smears. Anal Pathol 105: 321-326
2. Edoute Y, Lemberg S, Malberger E (1991) Preoperative and intraoperative fine-needle aspiration cytology of pancreatic lesions. Am J Gastroenterol 86: 1015-1019
3. Ferrucci JT, Wittenberg J, Margolies MN, Carey RW (1979) Malignant seeding of the tract after thin-needle aspiration biopsy. Radiol 130: 345-346
4. Hyoty MK, Mattila JJ, Salo K (1991) Intraoperative fine-needle aspiration cytology examination of pancreatic lesions. Surg Gynecol Obstet 173: 193-197
5. Koss LG (1992) Diagnostic Cytology and its Histopathologic Bases. 4th Edition. J. B. Lippincott, Philadelphia
6. Koss LG, Woyke S, Olszewski W (1992) Aspiration Biopsy. Cytologic Interpretation and Histologic Bases. New York, Igaku-Shoin, Ed. 2
7. Lindholm (1995) Punktionszytologie im Abdominalbereich. In: Schenck U, Schenk UB, Eberhard HD (eds.) 13. Fortbildungstagung für Klinische Zytologie. Referate, München
8. Nakamura R, Machado R, Amikura K, Ruebner B, Frey CF (1994) Role of fine needle aspiration cytology and endoscopic biopsy in the preoperative assessment of pancreatic and peripancreatic malignancies. Int J Pancreatol 16: 17-21
9. Schadt ME, Kline TS, Neal HS, Scoma RS, Naryshkin S (1991) Intraoperative pancreatic fine needle aspiration biopsy: Results in 166 patients. Am Surg 57: 73-75
10. Stormby N (1992) Aspiration cytology of the pancreas. In: Wied GL, Keebler CM, Koss GL, Patten SF, Rosenthal DL (ed) Compendium on diagnostic cytology. Tutorials of cytology. Chicago, Ill.
11. Urrutia R, Dimango EP (1996) Genetic markers. The key to early diagnosis and improved survival in pancreatic cancer? Gastroenterology 110: 306-310
12. Villanueva A, Reyes G, Cuatrecasas M, Martinez A, Erill N, Lerma E, Farre A, Lluis F, Capella G (1996) Diagnostic utility of K-ras mutation in fine-needle aspirates of pancreatic masses. Gastroenterol 110: 1587-1594
13. Weiss H, Düntsch U, Weiss A (1988) Risiken der Feinnadelpunktion - Ergebnisse einer Umfrage in der BRD (DEGUM-Umfrage). Ultraschall 9: 121-127

Scintigraphic Procedures in the Detection of Pancreatic Tumors: The Role of FDG PET

J. Mester · K. H. Bohuslavizki · W. Beyer · M. Clausen · E. Henze

The Clinical Problem

One of the current challenges in diagnostic radiology is the early and accurate detection of pancreatic carcinoma and its differentiation from mass-forming pancreatitis using noninvasive imaging methods [1, 2]. The diagnostic accuracy of morphologically oriented imaging techniques is presently suboptimal. Ultrasonography is hampered by the dorsal position of the pancreas in the abdomen and the location of the bowel in front of it. Computed tomography (CT) and magnetic resonance imaging (MRI) have excellent geometric resolution, but the differentiation between malignant and benign lesions remains difficult even with these leading technologies. Conversely, functionally oriented nuclear medicine procedures enable imaging of organ metabolism using appropriate radiolabelled tracers. At the beginning, the aim of radioisotope studies was merely the visualization of pancreatic tissue. To this purpose selenium-75-selen methionine and ^{123}I-N,N,N'-trimethyl-N'-(2-hydroxy-3-methyl-5-iodobenzyl)-1,3-propanediamine ([^{123}I] HIPDM) were tested. Both tracers accumulate in normal pancreatic tissue, but they cannot differentiate between malignant tumors and benign lesions [3, 4]. Thus, in the era of high resolution radiological methods, they are of a more historical interest. Recently, the introduction of several new types of tracers opened exciting perspectives. In this chapter the possibilities of these radiopharmaceuticals will be discussed.

Immunoscintigraphy

Since the mid 1980s high hopes have been set on the introduction of radiolabeled monoclonar antibodies against tumor-associated antigens to oncologic nuclear medicine. The characteristic feature of these antibodies is their extremely high specificity. Using chemical procedures, they can be broken either into Fc and F(ab')$_2$ fragments or into Fc and Fab fragments. The F(ab')$_2$ and Fab fragments are responsible for the antigen specificity of the antibodies. These antibodies can be labelled with ^{123}I, ^{131}I, ^{111}In, or, more recently, with Tc-99m.

For detection of pancreatic cancer, different types of monoclonal antibodies have been tested. A cocktail of ^{131}I-labelled F(ab')$_2$ fragments of antibodies directed against the tumor-associated antigens CA 19-9 and carcinoembryonic antigen (CEA) was used by Montz [5]. Despite detection of some large tumors without elevated level of tumor markers in the peripheral blood, they considered this tracer of only limited diagnostic value due to its relatively poor sensitivity. Using ^{111}In for labeling and SPECT acquisition at least 3 days after tracer injection, a moderate increase in diagnostic accuracy due to elimination of unspecific early tracer accumulation was reported by Bares in various gastrointestinal carcinomas [6]. As a further attempt at detection of pancreatic cancer, preliminary results have been reported with the ^{131}I-labeled murine monoclonal antibody AR-3-IgG1 directd against the mucin-like antigen CAR-3 [7].

Investigations with the ^{111}In- and ^{131}I-labeled F(ab')$_2$ fragments of the monoclonal antibody BW 494/32, the corresponding antigene of which is often expressed by pancreatic carcinomas, failed as well in presenting a breakthrough in immunoscintigraphy [8]. Nevertheless, in a study with only three patients, Abdel Nabi and coworkers presented favorable images of primary tumors as well as of their metastases using ^{111}In-labeled monoclonal anti-CEA antibody ZCE 025 [9]. In conclusion, at present there is no radiolabeled monoclonal antibody available with clearly documented high clinical performance necessary for routine patient management. Despite this, immunoscintigraphy can be considered as a possible investigative method in diagnostically difficult cases.

Receptor Scintigraphy

New possibilities in tumor imaging have opened up recently by the introduction of small receptor-analogue molecules. A subgroup of these compounds, the radiolabeled somatostatine analogues, can be used for imaging of endocrine tumors, i.e., tumors derived from so-called APUD cells. Somatostatine analogues have primarily been used for imaging of carcinoids and islet cell tumors of the pancreas. Bakker and coworkers reported the successful localization of pancreatic tumors in rats using ^{123}I-Tyr-3-octreotride [10]. However, the main disadvantage of this radiopharmaceutical is its predominantly hepatic clearance and, therefore, its high accumulation in the liver, which may mask pancreatic tracer uptake.

When labeling octreotide with [^{111}In] DTPA, the longer half-life of ^{111}In can be combined with the facilitated renal clearance of the DTPA-containing compound. These features offer the advantage of 24-h imaging when interfering background activity is already minimized by renal clearance. Bakker and coworkers reported successful investigations of pancreatic tumors in a rat model using (^{111}In-DTPA-D-Phe1)-octreotride [11]. They documented an increase in tracer uptake with time within the tumor tissue, which could be clearly visualized by gamma camera scintigraphy in somatostatin-receptor-positive rat pancreatic carcinoma [11]. As an attempt at supporting surgical interventions, Ohrvall and coworkers introduced a nonimaging method for the intraoperative detection of tumors and their metastases by using a hand-held gamma probe. However, the feasibility of this interesting method is limited by relatively high background activity [12].

Nonspecific Perfusion Tracers

Thallium-201 uptake is considered to reflect the regional perfusion as well as the viability of tumor cells [13]. The theoretical background of this feature of ^{201}Tl is the correlation of the growth of malignant transformed cells with the activity of Na/K-ATPase [14].

In 1993 Suga and coworkers demonstrated the possibility of monitoring the efficacy of antineoplastic treatment using quantified ^{201}Tl uptake in pancreatic cancer. In three patients, ^{201}Tl uptake by the tumor correlated well with the serum level of the tumor marker CA 19-9 [15]. In a subsequent publication of this group, results obtained by subtraction scintigraphy were presented [16]. When the boundary between abnormal ^{201}Tl uptake and adjacent liver activity was unclear on the ^{201}Tl SPECT image, a SPECT image of the liver using Tc-99m-phytate was acquired and subtracted from the ^{201}Tl image in order to separate hepatic and pancreatic ^{201}Tl uptake. Using this technique, a favorable sensitivity of 91 % was demonstrated. However, in the same study, four of 16 patients with benign pancreatic disorders exhibited abnormal, increased ^{201}Tl uptake. Based on these data, ^{201}Tl scintigraphy is a nuclear medicine method with relatively low cost and acceptabe clinical performance in detecting pancreatic cancer and can be recommended, especially when positron emission tomography (PET) facilities are not available.

Positron Emission Tomography Investigations Using Fluorodeoxyglucose

The rationale of using radiolabeled glucose analogues for tumor imaging is the increased metabolic activity of tumor tissue. The accelerated rate of glycolysis in aggressive malignantly transformed tumors was first described by Warburg in 1956 [17].

Fluorodeoxyglucose (FDG), a glucose analogue, is supposed to enter cells by the same transport mechanisms as used by native glucose. After phosphorylation, however, FDG phosphate is trapped intracellularly due to its extremely slow dephosporylation as compared to native glucose. This feature enables imaging of FDG distribution by PET. Experimental and human studies have demonstrated an increase in FDG uptake in various malignant tumors [18–20]. All of these studies have confirmed that increased FDG uptake is a reliable indicator of the presence of viable malignant tumor tissue. In contrast, benign processes or metabolically less active neoplasms generally have lower or even normal levels of glucose uptake [21]. The mechanism of FDG accumulation in tumors is probably multifactorial. First, it is induced by activation of glucose transporter proteins and elevated glucose consumption, which are both considered to be early and prominent features of an oncogene-mediated malignant transformation in cell culture systems [22]. Second, tumor-associated tissue inflammation produces increased FDG uptake as well [23]. The value of [^{18}F] FDG for the detection of malignant pancreatic processes was first documented in patients by Zanzi and coworkers in 1990 [24]. Based on the results of [^{18}F] FDG PET, Lever and coworkers reported clear differentiation of pancreatic carcinoma and chronic pancreatitis [25] (see Figs. 1, 2). Bares and coworkers [26] found focally increased FDG accumulation in 12 out of 13 patients with histologically proven pancreatic adenocarcinoma. Eight of nine known lymph nodes and four of five known liver metastases were detected in their study. In contrast, in two patients with chronic pancreatitis, no FDG uptake was documented. One patient suffering from an adenocarcinoma and lacking FDG uptake had diabetes, probably because the fasting state could not be established sufficiently prior to the study. In a second study with 40 patients investigated by the same group [27], PET helped to correctly classify 25 of 27 malignant pancreatic tumors and 11 of 13 benign disorders of the pancreas. False-negative findings were again obtained in two patients with insulin-dependent diabetes. False-positive findings were associated either with retroperitoneal fibrosis or, in one patient, with pancreas divisum accompanied by chronic pancreatitis. However, FDG PET was shown to be superior to both CT and ultrasound in the detection of lymph node metastases. These results have been confirmed by Friess and coworkers [28].

Forty-one of 42 patients with pancreatic cancer and four of six patients with a periampullary carcinoma presented focally increased FDG uptake. In contrast, in 28 of 32 patients with chronic pancreatitis, no FDG accumulation occured.

In a comparative study of 46 patients suspected of having pancreatic cancer, the diagnostic performance of FDG PET was superior to CT as well as transabdominal and endoscopic ultrasound [29]. This superiority of FDG PET over CT was also demonstrated by Stollfuss and coworkers [30]. Based on the result of a recent comparative study with FDG PET and ^{201}Tl SPECT in patients with histologically proven pancreatic cancer, it can be concluded that FDG PET is presently the nuclear medicine method of choice if PET facilities are available [31].

An exciting and widely discussed possibility of increasing the performance of PET studies is the use of quantitative methods to obtain numerical values of the phosphorylation rate of deoxyglucose. To this purpose, several methods have been suggested. Most of them are based on the three-compartmental model introduced by Sokoloff [32]. However, there are some practical and theoretical difficulties connected to the application of the three-compartmental model of FDG metabolism, especially to the determination of the velocity constants of the biochemical reactions and to determination of the lumped constant [33-35]. Therfore, most investigators simply use ratios of FDG uptake in tumors compared to those in normal tissues. A further method of quantification is the estimation of net uptake of FDG in the tumor tissue standardized to the body surface or body weight.

The most widely used quantitative method of estimation of FDG uptake in tissue is the determination of standardized uptake values (SUV). The main advantage of the SUV method is its methodologic simplicity. The main disadvantage is the fact that SUV itself is time-dependent and, therefore, potentially subject to error if images are not obtained at the same time after tracer injection [36, 37].

The impact of quantification of FDG uptake by SUV was shown in patients with pancreatic cancer. The tumor region exhibited significantly higher values than pancreatic regions in patients with pancreatitis [28]. Using ROC analysis,

Fig. 1. F-18-fluorodeoxyglucose PET in a patient with pancreatic carcinoma. Four consecutive transverse slices. Note the intense accumulation of the tracer in the pancreas. (Courtesy of M. Schwaiger, Nuklearmedizinische Klinik, Technische Universität, Munich)

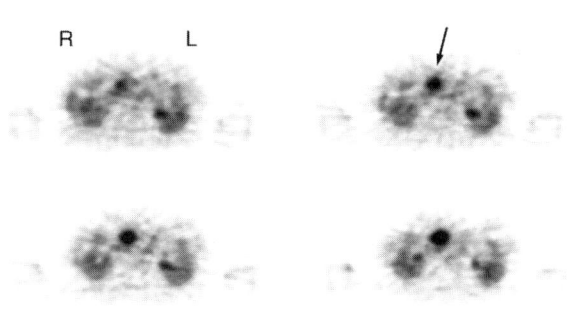

it was demonstrated that an SUV of approximately 1.5 optimally separates malignant and benign pancreatic processes [30].

However, very recent investigations in clinical patients report lower accuracy than in the early studies [38, 39]. Dohmen and coworkers found an accuracy of approximately 80% regarding the differentiation of pancreatic cancer from chronic pancreatitis. Furthermore, they could not demonstrate any advantage of using quantitative parameters as compared to simple visual analysis [38]. The limited performance of SUV was also reported by Vomocil and coworkers [39].

Position Emission Tomography Tracers for Endocrine Pancreatic Tumors

Recently, results obtained using ^{11}C-labeled L-dihydroxyphenylalanine (L-DOPA) and hydroxytryptophan (HTP) have been reported in pancreatic endocrine tumors with promising results, particularly regarding glucagonomas [40]. These findings, based on the investigation of 22 patients, suggest further possibilities in metabolic characterization of tumors. However, the role of FDG in this type of tumors has not yet been explored.

Fig. 2. Pancreatic cyst in a patient with chronic pancreatitis. Note the cold area within the pancreas. No pathologic accumulation of F-18-fluorodeoxyglucose in the pancreatic region. (Courtesy of M. Schwaiger, Nuklearmedizinische Klinik, Technische Universität, Munich)

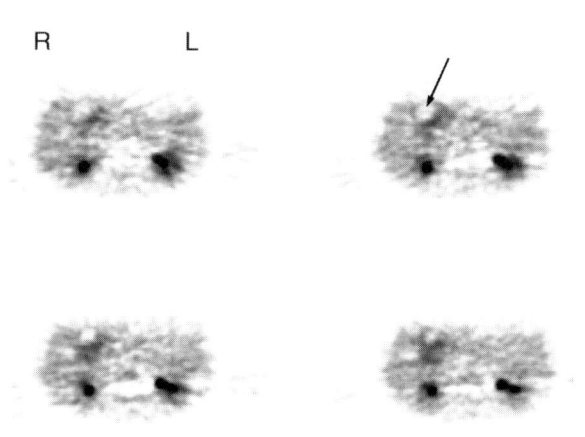

Multimodality Imaging

The combination of morphologic and functional information is a very new and exciting trend in diagnostic imaging. It is especially helpful in the exact anatomic localization of functional disorders. Detailed morphologic information presented by the excellent geometric resolution of CT or MRI can be combined with the visualization of metabolic parameters and presented in a single image. However, the coregistration of tomographic images from different modalities requires sophisticated external or anatomical markers. The first successful fusion of [^{18}F] FDG PET and MR images using a system of surface markers in patients with pancreatic adenocarcinoma was demonstrated by Benyounes and coworkers [41]. The combined images impressively delineated the tumor exactly on the high quality slices of the MR study. Thus, multimodality imaging might be of increasing interest in future studies.

Conclusion

One of the main challenges in diagnostic radiology is the early and accurate detection of pancreatic carcinoma, which is indeed difficult by morphologically oriented methods, i.e., ultrasonography, CT, and MRI.

Therefore, functionally oriented nuclear medicine procedures may be useful. In patients with suspected pancreatic cancer, several imaging procedures have been investigated, i.e., immunoscintigraphy, receptor scintigraphy, and unspecific perfusion scintigraphy. However, none of them were convincing in routine patient management. Best diagnostic results were obtained using [^{18}F] FDG PET. However, critical analysis of the literature presented so far show overall accuracy tending to be below than above 80%. Due to inherent technical limitations, PET probably cannot depict lesions smaller than 15 mm in size even when a high-resolution PET scanner is used. Thus it is probably not suitable for early detection of pancreatic carcinoma. It is not yet clear whether the performance of FDG PET is efficient enough to reduce the current number of diagnostic laparotomies. Prospectively performed comparative studies with CT, ultrasonography, endoscopic retrograde cholangiopancreatography (ERCP), and MRI using state-of-the-art equipment are still needed to establish an optimal diagnostic strategy. Apart from lesion detection, FDG PET may offer valid data on both the prognosis of pancreatic masses and the effectiveness of therapeutic procedures. However, further effort is still necessary to define the exact position of nuclear medicine in the management of pancreatic cancer.

References

1. Megibow AJ (1992) Pancreatic adenocarcinoma: designing the examination to evaluate the clinical question. Radiology 183: 297–303
2. Steiner E, Stark DD, Hahn, Haini S, Simeone JF, Mueller PR, Wittenberg J, Ferrucci JT (1989) Imaging of pancreatic neoplasms: comparison of MR and CT. AJR 152: 487–491
3. Yamamoto K, Shibata, T, Saji H, Kubo S, Aoki E, Fujita T, Yonekura Y, Konishi J, Yokoyama A (1990) Human pancreas scintigraphy using iodine-123-labelled HIPDM and SPECT. J Nucl Med 31: 1015–1019
4. Antunez AR (1964) Pancreatic scanning with selenium-75-methionine, utilizing morphine to enhance contrast: a preliminary report. Cleveland Clin Quart 31: 213–218
5. Montz R, Klapdor R, Kremer B, Rothe B (1985) Immunoszintigraphie und SPECT bei Patienten mit Pankreaskarzinom. Nuklearmedizin 24: 232–237
6. Bares R, Fass J, Truong S, Büll U, Schumpelick V (1987) Radioimmunszintigraphie mit SPECT: Methodik, Probleme und klinische Erfahrungen. Nuklearmedizin 26: 202–205
7. Mariani-G, Molen N, Bacciardi D, Boggi U, Bonino C, Costa A, Viacava P, Castagna M, Bodei L, Tarditi L (1994) Biodistribution and pharmacokinetic screening in humans of monoclonal antibody AR-3 as a possible immunoscintigraphy agent in patients with pancreatic cancer. J Nucl Biol Med 38(4 Suppl 1): 145–150
8. Montz R, Klapdor R, Rothe B, Heller M (1986) Immunoscintigraphy and radioimmunotherapy in patients with pancreatic carcinoma. Nuklearmedizin 25: 239–244
9. Abdel-Nabi HH, Schwartz AN, Wechter DG, Higano CS, Ortman-Nabi JA, Unger MW (1991) Scintigraphic detection of gastric and pancreatic carcinomas with In-111 ZCE 025 monoclonal antibody. World J Surg 15: 122–127
10. Bakker WH, Krenning EP, Breeman WA, Koper JW, Kooij PP, Reubi JC, Klinjn JG, Visser TJ, Docter R, Lamberts SW (1990) Receptor scintigraphy with a radioiodinated somatostatin analogue: radiolabeling, purification, biologic activity, and in vivo application in animals. J Nucl Med 31: 1501–1509
11. Bakker WH, Krenning EP, Reubi JC, Breeman WA, Setyono HB, de Jong M, Kooij PP, Bruns C, van Hagen PM, Marbach P (1991) In vivo application of (111In-DTPA-D-Phe1)-octreotride for detection of somatostatin receptor-positive tumours in rats. Life-Sci 49: 1593–1601
12. Ohrvall U, Westlin JE, Nilsson S, Wilander E, Juhlin C, Rastad J, Akerstrom G (1995) Human biodistribution of (111In)diethylenetriaminepentaacetic acid-(DTPA)-D-(Phe1)-octreotide and perioperative detection of endocrine tumours. Cancer Res 55(23 Suppl): 5794s–5800s
13. Ito Y, Muranka A, Harada T, Matsudo A, Yokobayashi T, Terashima H (1978) Experimental study on tumour affinity of Tl-201 chloride. Eur J Nucl Med 3: 81–86
14. Elligsen JD, Thomson JE, Frey HE, Kruuv J (1974) Correlation of Na-K ATPase activity with growth of normal and transformed cells. Exp Cell Res 87: 233–240
15. Suga K, Fujita T, Nakada T, Yoneshiro S, Uchisako H, Nishigauchi K, Nakanishi T, Hamada Y (1993) Preliminary Tl-201 SPECT for assessment of treatment efficacy in three patients with pancreatic cancer. Clin Nucl Med 18: 771–775
16. Suga K, Nishigauchi K, Kume N, Fujita T, Nakanishi T, Hamasaki T, Suzuki T (1995) Thallium-201 SPECT and technetium-99m-phytate subtraction liver imaging in the evaluation of pancreatic cancer. J Nucl Med 36: 762–770
17. Warburg O (1956) On the origin of cancer cells. Science 123: 309–314
18. Som P, Atkins AD, Bandoypadhyay D, Fowler JS, MacGregor RR, Matsui K, Oster ZH, Sacker DF, Shiue CY, Turner H, Wan CN, Wolf AP, Zabinski SV (1980) A fluorinated glucose analogue, 2-fluoro-2-deoxy-D-glucose (F18): nontoxic tracer rapid tumour detection. J Nucl Med 21: 670–675
19. Strauss LG, Conti PS (1991) The application of PET in clinical oncology. J Nucl Med 32: 623–648
20. Hawkins RA, Hoh C, Dahlbom M, Choi Y, Glaspy J, Tse N, Slamon D, Chen B, Messa C, Maddahi J, Phelps M (1991) PET cancer evaluation with FDG. J Nucl Med 32: 1555–1558
21. Hawkins RA (1995) Pancreatic Tumours: Imaging with PET (editorial). Radiology 195: 320–322
22. Flier JS, Mueckler MM, Usher P, Lodish HF (1987) Elevated levels of glucose transport and transporter messenger RNA are induced ras or src oncogenes. Science 235: 1492–1495
23. Kubota R, Yamada S, Kubota K, Ishiwata K, Tamahashi N, Ido T (1992) Intratumoural distribution of fluorine-18-fluorodeoxyglucose in vivo: high accumulation in macrophages and granulation tissues studied by microautoradiography. J Nucl Med 33: 1972–1980

24. Zanzi I, Robeson W, Vinciguerra V (1990) Positron tomography (PET) imaging in patients with carcinoma of the pancreas (abstr.). Proc. ASCO 9: A434
25. Klever P, Bares R, Fass J, Büll U, Schumpelick V (1992) PET with fluorine-18 deoxyglucose for pancreatic disease. Lancet 340: 1158–1159
26. Bares R, Klever P, Hellwig D, Hauptmann S, Fass J, Hambuechen U, Zopp L, Mueller B, Buell U, Schumpelick V (1993) Pancreatic cancer detected by positron emission tomography with 18F-labelled deoxyglucose: method and first result. Nucl Med Commun 14: 596–601
27. Bares R, Klever P, Hauptmann S, Hellwig D, Fass J, Cremerius U, Schumpelick V, Mittermayer C, Büll U (1994) F-18 fluorodeoxyglucose PET in vivo evaluation of pancreatic glucose metabolism for detection of pancreatic cancer. Radiology 192: 79–86
28. Friess H, Langhans J, Ebert M, Beger HG, Stollfuss J, Reske SN, Buchler MW (1995) Diagnosis of pancreatic cancer by 2(18F)-fluoro-2-deoxy-D-glucose positron emission tomography. Gut 36: 771–777
29. Inokuma T, Tamaki N, Torizuka T, Magata Y, Fujii M, Yonekura Y, Kajiyama T, Ohshio G, Imamura M, Konishi J (1995) Evaluation of pancreatic tumours with positron emission tomography and F-18 fluorodeoxyglucose: comparison with CT and US. Radiology 195: 345–352
30. Stollfuss JC, Glatting G, Friess H, Kocher F, Berger HG, Reske SN (1995) 2-(fluorine-18)-fluoro-2-deoxy-D-glucose PET in detection of pancreatic cancer: value of quantitative image interpretation. Radiology 195: 339–344
31. Inokuma T, Tamaki N, Torizuka T, Fujita T, Magata Y, Yonekura Y, Ohshio G, Imamura M, Konishi J (1995) Value of Fluorine-18-Fluorodeoxyglucose and Thallium-201 in the detection of pancreatic cancer. J Nucl Med 36: 229–235
32. Sokoloff L, Reivich M, Kennedy C, Des Rosiers MH, Patlak CS, Pettigrew KD, Sakurada O, Shinohara M (1977) The (C-14)-deoxyglucose method for the measurement of local cerebral glucose utilization: theory, procedure and normal values in the conscious and anesthetized albino rat. J Neurochem 28: 897–916
33. Huang SC, Phelps ME, Hoffmann EJ, Sideris K, Selin CJ, Kuhl DE (1980) Noninvasive determination of local cerebral metabolic rate of glucose in normal human subjects with 18-F-Fluoro-2'-Deoxyglucose and emission computed tomography. Amer J Physiol 238: E69–E82
34. Blomquist G (1984) On the construction of functional maps in positron emission tomography. J Cerebr Blood Flow Metab 4: 629–632
35. Patlak CS, Blasberg RG, Fenstermacher JD (1983) Graphic evaluation of blood to brain transfer constants from multiple time uptake data. J Cerebr Blood Flow Metab 3: 1–7
36. Hawkins RA, Choi Y, Huang SC, Messa C, Hoh CK, Phelps ME (1992) Quantitating tumour glucose metabolism with FDG and PET (editorial). J Nucl Med 33: 339–344
37. Hamberg LM, Hunter GJ, Alpert NM, Choi NC, Babich JW, Fischman AJ (1994) The dose uptake ratio as an index of glucose metabolism: useful parameter or oversimplification? J Nucl Med 35: 1308–1312
38. Dohmen BM, Bares R, Teusch M, Buell U (1996) Classification of pancreatic tumours by FDG-PET: Comparison of visual and quantitative image interpretation by ROC analysis (abstr.). J Nucl Med 36: 140P
39. Vomocil B, Hübner KF, Adams LJ, Smith GT, Buonocore E (1995) The complimentary role of PET using C-11-aminocyclobutanecarboxylic acid (C-11-ACBC) and F-18-FDG in suspected pancreatic cancer (abstr.). J Nucl Med 36: 193P
40. Ahlström H, Eriksson B, Bergström M, Bjurling P, Langström B, Öberg K (1995) Pancreatic neuroendocrine tumours: diagnosis with PET. Radiology 195: 333–337
41. Benyounes H, Smith FW, Campbell C, Evans NT, Mikecz P, Heys SD, Bruce D, Eremin O, Sharp PF (1995) Superimposition of PET images using 18F-fluorodeoxyglucose with magnetic resonance images in patients with pancreatic carcinoma. Nucl Med Commun 16: 575–580

III
Molecular Biology

Clinical Applicability of Molecular Procedures in the Diagnosis of Pancreatic Cancer

H. Friess · J. Kleeff · P. Berberat · M. W. Büchler

Introduction

Pancreatic cancer is a devastating disease with a median survival of five months after diagnosis [24, 56]. The incidence of pancreatic carcinoma in Western industrialized countries has increased significantly as the median life expectancy has been prolonged and better diagnostic options have become available. At present, approximately 10/100 000 individuals die of pancreatic cancer every year, making it the fourth to fifth most common cause of cancer-related mortality [24, 56, 69, 77].

Complete surgical resection of pancreatic tumors presently offers the only effective treatment for this disease. However, between 75% and 85% of pancreatic cancer patients have unresectable tumors at the time of diagnosis, and therefore palliative treatment is the predominant therapy in this disease [24, 56, 69, 77]. Although the potential for cure in patients with pancreatic cancer is restricted to those who are able to undergo complete surgical resection, the 5-year survival rate following such operations is only about 10%–25%. Management of individuals with unresectable pancreatic cancer includes palliative surgical options, such as biliary or enteral bypass operations. Conservative oncological strategies such as chemotherapy and radiotherapy do not appear to prolong survival, although a sufficient reduction in tumor size may lead to palliation of pain [55, 57]. Antihormonal modalities using tamoxifen or buserelin [2, 22] or the systemic use of specific antipancreatic cancer cell monoclonal antibodies [8, 21] have also failed to lead to a significant improvement in prognosis. Furthermore, most patients deemed resectable at the time of diagnosis develop metastatic disease or local recurrence within the first two postoperative years, without any option of further effective treatment modalities.

The reasons for the aggressive growth and metastatic behavior of pancreatic cancer are poorly understood. However, studies on human pancreatic carcinoma cell lines [30, 40] have highlighted the important role of the expression and overexpression of growth factors and growth factor receptors in the pathogenesis of pancreatic cancer. These cell lines overexpress the epidermal growth factor (EGF) receptor and exhibit an increase in EGF-receptor mRNA [41]. In addition, these cells produce transforming growth factor (TGF)-α, a polypeptide that binds to the EGF receptor [30]. Following binding of EGF or TGF-α, both factors are internalized. EGF often gets recycled, whereas TGF-α is rapidly degraded [40]. The latter was found to be 10- to 100-fold more potent then EGF in enhancing the anchorage-independent growth of pancreatic cancer cell lines. Both EGF and TGF-α induce EGF receptor downregulation, indicating that the functions of this receptor/ligand system are at least in part under its own control. EGF is more efficient than TGF-α in this regard. These findings suggest that overexpression of the EGF receptor in conjunction with production of TGF-α and the recycling of EGF may give pancreatic cancer cells a growth advantage. Based on these experimental data, analysis of several growth factor and growth receptor families as well as gene mutations was started in human pancreatic cancer.

A better understanding of the pathobiology of pancreatic cancer is a precondition for the development of new diagnostic procedures and treatment strategies. In the following paper, we present part of the molecular work we have done during the past four years and the possibilities for using this knowledge in clinical practice in the diagnosis of cancer of the pancreas.

Growth Factor Receptors and Their Ligands in Pancreatic Cancer

EGF Receptor Family and Its Ligands in Pancreatic Cancer

The EGF receptor, also known as human EGF receptor-1 (HER-1), is probably the best-known and -studied growth factor receptor. Other members of this growth factor receptor family are c-erbB2 (HER-2) [14], c-erbB3 (HER-3) [43], and c-erbB4 (HER-4) [60]. These four growth factor receptors consist of an extracellular domain, a transmembrane domain, and an intracellular domain which possesses tyrosine kinase activity [60]. Binding of ligands to the extracellular receptor domain leads to the phosphorylization of various intracellular substrates such as phospholipase C-γ which stimulates cell growth [64].

EGF and TGF-α have been characterized as the prototypes of a growth factor family which binds and activates the EGF receptor. In addition, amphiregulin, betacellulin, and heparin-binding EGF (HB-EGF) belong to this growth factor family. All members share close structural homology with EGF [3, 13, 35, 61].

Early studies on cancer cells showed that overexpression of the EGF receptor leads to malignant transformation and that the presence of TGF-α additionally stimulates the proliferation of transformed cells [1, 50]. These in vitro studies provided the initial indication that alterations within the EGF receptor family and their ligands might be important for the course and prognosis of tumor diseases in vivo.

Research over the post 5 years has provided new insights into the role of the EGF receptor family and its ligands in pancreatic carcinomas. Immunohistochemical analysis, together with modern molecular biology techniques, demonstrated the overexpression of the EGF receptor, EGF, and TGF-α in human pancreatic cancers [42, 82]. Many cancer cells show concomitant overexpression of the EGF receptor and EGF and/or TGF-α, indicating that autocrine and paracrine mechanisms of this receptor-ligand system might play a crucial role in the pathogenesis of cancer of the pancreas [56]. This was confirmed by immunohistochemical studies in 87 human pancreatic cancer tissues showing

Table 1. Growth factors and growth factor receptors in human pancreatic cancer

Growth factor receptors	Growth factors
EGF receptor[a] [42, 82]	EGF[a] [42, 82]
	TGF-α[a] [42, 82]
	Amphiregulin[a] [16, 85]
c-erbB-2 receptor [83]	Betacellulin [86]
c-erbB-3 receptor[a] [27]	Heparin-binding EGF [87]
FGF receptor [39]	Acidic FGF [81]
	Basic FGF[a] [81]
TGF-β receptor type II and type III [25]	TGF-β[a] (all three isoforms) [26]

Patients whose tumors overexpress amphiregulin and/or epidermal growth factor (EGF) and/or transforming growth factor (TGF)-α concomitantly with the EGF receptor die significantly earlier than patients whose tumors express only the ligands, only the EGF receptor, or none of these.
FGF, fibroblast growth factor.
[a] Factors with a negative influence on patient survival.

that patients overexpressing the EGF receptor and EGF and/or TGF-α died earlier postoperatively than those who did not simultaneously overexpress the EGF receptor with one of its ligands (Table 1) [82]. The epidermal growth factor receptor is also activated by other EGF-like growth factors such as betacellulin, amphiregulin, and HB-EGF [28].

Betacellulin has 50% aminoacid sequence homology with TGF-α and 32% sequence homology with EGF [66]. Five of six human pancreatic cancer cell lines we investigated expressed betacellulin at increased levels in comparison with the levels observed in the normal pancreas. EGF and HB-EGF increased betacellulin mRNA levels, indicating that betacellulin expression can be induced in pancreatic cancer cells through ligands of the EGF family [86].

Another EGF-like growth factor is amphiregulin. Immunohistochemical analysis of 62 pancreatic cancers demonstrated the presence of cytoplasmatic amphiregulin immunoreactivity in 37% of the tumors. In 15 of 31 tumors (48%), cytoplasmic amphiregulin immunoreactivity was concomitantly present with the EGF receptor. Analysis of patient survival periods revealed that patients concomitantly overexpressing the EGF receptor and amphiregulin died earlier postoperatively than patients who did not simultaneously overexpress the EGF receptor and amphiregulin (Table 1) [16, 85].

In an additional study characterizing the biological actions of HB-EGF, immunohistochemical analysis of 47 pancreatic tissues revealed the presence of HB-EGF immunoreactivity in half of the tumors. However, neither the presence of HB-EGF in the pancreatic cancer cells nor the concomitant presence of the EGF receptor and HB-EGF was associated with shorter patient survival following tumor resection (Table 1) [87].

The potential role of c-erbB2 in tumor pathogenesis of pancreatic cancer has also been investigated [34, 83]. The c-erbB2 gene encodes a transmembrane receptor with a molecular weight of 185 kDa. This receptor is activated through binding of specific ligands such as neu differentiation factor (NDF), glial growth factors, and heregulin [37, 52, 64]. Overexpression of c-erbB2 leads to malignant cell transformation in vitro [64]. Immunohistochemical analysis of 76 pancreatic cancer samples showed that 34 (45%) exhibited increased c-erbB2 immunoreactivity in pancreatic cancer cells [83]. In situ hybridization and Northern blot analysis of these samples indicated that the increase in c-erbB2 immunoreactivity was associated with overexpression of the corresponding mRNA moiety [83]. Statistical analysis revealed that enhanced expression of c-erbB2 mRNA in pancreatic cancer cells was associated with better tumor differentiation [83]. In contrast to the EGF receptor, the presence of c-erbB2 was not associated with advanced tumor stage or shorter postoperative survival periods (Table 1). These findings suggest that the activation of c-erbB2 in human pancreatic cancer leads to better differentiation of the cancer cells, a theory that has already been described in studies with cultured cancer cell lines [58].

The third member of the EGF-receptor-related family of growth factor receptors is c-erbB3 [43]. In 1992, immunohistochemical studies demonstrated moderate to intense immunoreactivity of c-erbB3 in human pancreatic cancer cells [45]. Analysis of c-erbB3 mRNA expression indicated that pancreatic cancer cells also overexpress this growth factor receptor. In our own studies, we detected low levels of cerbB3 mRNA in the normal human pancreas [27]. Conversely, our quantitative mRNA analysis demonstratd a sixfold increase in c-erbB3 mRNA in pancreatic cancer tissues. With immunohistochemistry, 47% (27 of 58) of our pancreatic cancer samples exhibited positive immunoreactivity for c-erbB3. This was associated with advanced tumor stages and significantly shorter postoperative survival (Table 1) [27]. Although the ligand that activates c-erbB3 has not yet been identified, these findings suggest that overexpression of the EGF receptor and/or c-erbB3 seem to play an important role in pancreatic cancer progression and patient prognosis [27].

TGF-β and TGF-β-receptors in Pancreatic Cancer

Another important family of growth factors influencing cell growth is that of TGF-β and its homologues. In general, TGF-β inhibit growth in many epithelial cells, influence the structure of the extracellular matrix, stimulate angiogenesis, and have been described as immunosuppressive factors [53, 54, 62, 70]. However, cell proliferation is not inhibited in all pancreatic carcinoma cell lines by TGF-β1, which represents the prototype of this growth factor family. Meanwhile, it has been shown that the influence of TGF-β on growth of tumor cell lines is dependent on culture conditions [70, 71, 73]. Therefore, alterations in culture conditions can change the effect and function of TGF-β from an inhibitory to a stimulative agent.

The role of TGF-β in human pancreatic carcinomas has been characterized in a recent study [26]. This study demonstrated that all three mammalian TGF-β isoforms – TGF-β1, TGF-β2, and TGF-β3 – are overexpressed in many human pancreatic cancer cells in vivo [26]. Overexpression of the TGF-β as determined by in situ hybridization and northern blot analysis was associated with increased immunoreactivity of the corresponding peptides in pancreatic tumor cells [26].

Analysis of the survival data of 60 resected pancreatic cancer patients demonstrated that the presence of TGF-β1, TGF-β2, or TGF-β3 in pancreatic tumor cells was associated with more aggressive tumor growth and significantly reduced postoperative survival periods (Table 1) [26]. These findings indicate that TGF-β may act as growth stimulators in human pancreatic cancer in vivo.

TGF-β act through specific cell surface receptors. Three major TGF-β-binding receptors have been identified in the past years: TGF-β receptor I, TGF-β receptor II, and TGF-β receptor III [25, 51, 79]. Several biochemical studies indicate that TGF-β receptor II activates signal transmission by an intracellular serine-threonine-kinase [51, 79]. However, signaling is dependent on the presence of TGF-β receptor I. On the other hand, TGF-β receptor II is necessary for binding TGF-β to the TGF-β receptor I [51, 79]. TGF-β receptor III is a proteoglycan also known as betaglycan, and is not directly involved in signal transmission [25]. All three TGF-β receptors are present in the normal human pancreas [25]. Pancreatic cancer cells often overexpress TGF-β receptor II, but not TGF-β receptor III [25]. In situ hybridization showed that TGF-β receptor II mRNA expression was primarily located within pancreatic cancer cells and in the desmoplastic tissue adjacent to the tumor [25]. These findings suggest that TGF-β might contribute to the neoplastic process and thus enhance proliferation of tumor cells in human pancreatic carcinomas by autocrine and/or paracrine activation of the TGF-β receptor II [25, 26, 80].

Acidic and Basic Fibroblast Growth Factor in Pancreatic Cancer

Acidic fibroblast growth factor (aFGF) and basic fibroblast growth factor (bFGF) belong to a third family of growth factors capable of influencing various biological functions such as cell differentiation, cell migration, and angiogenesis [7, 20, 31, 32]. Other members of the fibroblast growth factor gene family are int-2 (FGF 3), the gene product of hst (Kaposi FGF, or FGF 4), FGF 5, FGF 6, keratinocyte growth factor (FGF 7), androgen-induced growth factor (FGF 8), and glia-activating growth factor FGF 9 [20, 31, 32, 38].

aFGF and bFGF are prototypes of this growth factor family. aFGF has been found in nerve tissue, heart, kidney, prostate, and liver, while bFGF seems to be more ubiquitous in human tissues. aFGF and bFGF bind to specific transmembrane receptors which stimulate intracellular tyrosine kinase activity, and which possess an extracellular domain consisting of two or three immunoglobulin-like regions [38, 39]. Binding of aFGF and bFGF to their receptors requires the presence of heparin sulfate proteoglycans, which are usually found on the cell surface or in the extracellular matrix [20, 31, 32, 38]. aFGF, bFGF, and four high-affinity FGF receptors have already been detected in the normal human pancreas [23]. In addition, studies with isolated rat pancreatic acini have shown that aFGF and bFGF stimulate amylase release, suggesting a physiological role for these factors in the regulation of the exocrine pancreas [12].

Recently, we have observed that aFGF and bFGF are overexpressed in a significant number of human pancreatic cancers [81]. In situ hybridization localized the overexpression of both mRNA moieties within the pancreatic cancer cells [81]. Tumor cells surrounding areas with chronic pancreatitis-like alterations also exhibited increased expression of aFGF and bFGF mRNA in the pancreatic acinar and ductal cells [81]. Enhanced expression of aFGF and bFGF mRNA was associated with increased levels of the corresponding proteins, as demonstrated by intense immunoreactivity for aFGF and bFGF in pancreatic cancer cells and in the desmoplastic tissue surrounding the cancer mass. Furthermore, Western blot analysis revealed an eightfold and an 11-fold increase, respectively, in aFGF and bFGF levels in the cancer samples compared with the corresponding levels in normal samples.

In the case of aFGF, the cancer samples exhibited the characteristic 16.5-kDa band and a faint 20-kDa band, as well as several small bands in the molecular weight range of 10–15 kDa. These low molecular weight forms could be degradation products of aFGF. Recently, it has also been reported that low molecular forms of FGF-4 have higher receptor affinity and biological activity than FGF-4 itself [5]. Therefore it is possible that the low molecular forms of aFGF are also biologically active in human pancreatic cancer tissues. In the case of bFGF, a major 18-kDa and a minor 24-kDa band were visible in pancreatic cancer. In addition, a 15-kDa minor band was visible in the cancer samples. The 24-kDa protein and other high molecular weight forms of bFGF have previously been described in cell extracts of mammary gland cells, neonatal fibroblasts, and hepatocellular tumor cells [29, 65]. It is thought that these high molecular forms of bFGF are transported directly into the nucleus after synthesis in the cytoplasm [9]. Also, in the case of the 18-kDa bFGF protein, transport into the nucleus is known to occur after binding to the cell surface and subsequent internalization into the cytoplasm [7]. The histological detection of nuclear bFGF immunoreactivity in pancreatic cancer cells could therefore be caused by nuclear bFGF accumulation from intracellular and/or extracellular sources [7, 9].

Keratinozyte growth factor (KGF) is also a member of the fibroblast growth factor group of heparin-binding polypeptides. It is an important mitogen for a variety of epithelial cells, and it is often expressed by stromal fibroblasts and other types of mesenchymal cells [19]. In contrast to aFGF and bFGF, the KGF precursor contains a signal sequence, allowing for its efficient secretion from its cell of origin. Following release, KGF stimulates epithelial cell growth in a paracrine manner, thereby contributing to epithelial-mesenchymal interactions [19]. In a recent study, it was demonstrated that pancreatic cancer samples often exhibit KGF mRNA levels that are approximately fivefold higher than levels in normal controls [67]. In pancreatic cancer, both the 2.4-kb and the 5.0-kb KGF RNA species which result from transcription of the same gene at two different initiation sites were overexpressed [67]. It is likely that KGF is expressed by the stromal elements within the tumor mass, and that it exerts paracrine effects on neighboring cancer cells. It is also possible that some pancreatic cancer cells express KGF, which can then act in a paracrine manner on stromal cells, thereby enhancing aberrant epithelial–mesenchymal interactions. In addition, cancer cell-derived KGF may act in an autocrine manner to directly enhance the growth of these cells. These observations suggest that KGF may participate together with a variety of other growth-promoting factors in the promotion of pancreatic cancer cell growth in vivo [19].

Platelet-Derived Growth Factors and Their Receptors in Pancreatic Cancer

Platelet-derived growth factors (PDGF) are dimerized proteins consisting of A and/or B chains linked via disulfide bonds, forming the three isoforms PDGF-AA, -AB, and -BB. These isoforms bind to two PDGF receptors which both possess tyrosine kinase activity. PDGF receptor-A binds all three PDGF isoforms with high affinity, whereas PDGF receptor-B binds only PDGF-BB with high affinity [78]. PDGFs are mitogenic and chemoattractant toward fibroblasts, monocytes, and endothelial cells, and play an important role in wound healing and tissue repair [68]. They also stimulate the production of stromal tissue in malignant tumors, thereby potentially contributing to tumor development and progression.

In a recent study, we demonstrated the presence of the PDGF A and B chains and PDGF receptor-B mRNA in the human pancreatic cancer cell lines PANC-1 and HPAF. However, these cells did not express PDGF receptor-A. Addition of PDGF-AA and PDGF-BB to the cell culture medium did not alter the growth of these cancer cell lines. These findings suggest that cultured pancreatic cancer cells do not have a PDGF-dependent mitogenic autocrine loop. However, in pancreatic cancer tissues, increased expression of the PDGF B chain and both PDGF receptors' mRNA were present in the cancer cells. It is conceivable, therefore, that pancreatic cancer cells derive a growth advantage in vivo as a result of a PDGF-dependent autocrine loop. In addition, PDGF receptors were present in the fibroblasts and endothelial cells in the surrounding desmoplastic tissue. These findings raise the possibility that PDGFs produced by pancreatic cancer cells may enhance the desmoplastic response in the surrounding tissue, which may contribute to chronic pancreatitis-like lesions surrounding the tumor mass [17].

Gene Mutations in Pancreatic Cancer

p53 Mutations in Pancreatic Cancer

p53 is a tumor suppressor gene that is located on the short arm of chromosome 17 and encodes a 53-kDa nuclear phosphoprotein [48, 75]. Mutations of the p53 gene are the most common somatic genetic alteration in human cancer [36, 47, 49], present in 40%–45% of all tumors. Various studies have found the prevalence of p53 mutations in pancreatic cancer to be between 40% and 60% [4, 11].

Normally, the p53 gene seems to be responsible for inhibition of oncogene-induced transformation, maintenance of genomic stability, modulation of the G_1 phase of the cell cycle, and expression of growth control genes [15]. Following p53 mutations, these regulatory functions are lost, which might contribute to malignant cell transformation. The most common change is a point mutation with amino acid substitution in the four evolutionary-conserved domains (exons 3, 4, 5, and 6). However, point mutations have also been reported at codons 35, 105, 133, 213, 258, and 299. Finally, a 3-bp inframe insertion has been identified between codons 261 and 262.

Mutant p53 proteins have a much longer half-life than wild-type protein. These accumulate in the transformed cells and can be detected by immunohistochemistry. Immunohistochemical studies have demonstrated a high correlation between nuclear p53 immunoreactivity and the presence of mutated p53 genes.

Although p53 mutations have been reported in pancreatic cancer, they have not been reported in chronic pancreatitis [11]. Therefore, it seems that the presence of p53 mutations is one of the major molecular differences between pancreatic cancer and chronic pancreatitis. p53 mutations are associated in pancreatic cancer with more advanced tumor stage, local lymph node involvement, and shorter survival periods, but not with a higher incidence of distant metastases or increased tumor size [84]. These findings confirm those of other studies suggesting that p53 mutations are a relatively late event in pancreatic carcinogenesis, and that mutations of p53 entail more rapid progression of the disease. In addition, the presence of p53 antibodies in the serum of patients seems to be very specific (90%) for malignant pancreatic and biliary diseases. However, the low sensitivity of the tests presently available reduces the clinical value of p53 as a new and highly accurate tumor marker [44].

K-ras Mutations in Pancreatic Cancer

Point mutations of the K-ras proto-oncogene are among the most frequent genetic changes in human pancreatic cancer. These have been identified in tumor needle biopsies and aspirations in 85%–95% of pancreatic adenocarcinomas, but not in chronic pancreatitis [33, 46]. K-ras mutations occur in pancreatic cancer almost exclusively on codon 12, which is located on the short arm of chromosome 21. A large majority of tumor samples have G-T transversions at the first or the second base of codon 12. These findings have been interpreted as tissue-, species-, and possibly mutagen-specific factors. In colorectal adenocarcinomas, a rather different mutation spectrum of the K-ras proto-oncogene has been described. In addition, in experimental pancreatic cancer models no K-ras mutations are present during carcinogenesis [63].

The product of the K-ras gene is a plasma-membrane-bound 21-kDa guanine nucleotide-binding protein with GTPase activity. After mutation the protein seems to lose GTPase activity and thereby affect the tumorgenic process by altering the signal transduction pathway across the membrane.

Studies of ductal pancreatic tumors with different degrees of anaplasia have reported that K-ras mutations occur early in pancreatic carcinogenesis – even in mucous cell hyperplasia appearing in association with chronic pancreatitis and in intraductal papillary neoplasms, which are considered as potentially precancerous lesions of ductal carcinomas [59]. However, K-ras mutations have not been found to be correlated with decreased patient survival, as is the case with p53 mutations [84]. Together, these data suggest that K-ras mutations are more involved in initiation of the tumorgenic process, and that p53 mutations might maintain progression of the disease. In contrast, some authors suggest that the mutations of the K-ras oncogenes have little effect on neoplastic transformation of epithelial cells [76]. They support the idea of a multistep concept involving oncogenes and tumor suppressor genes in combination, but they point out that total accumulation of changes is much more important than the order in which the changes appear [18].

Because K-ras mutations ostensibly occur early in pancreatic cell transformation, they are potential candidates for a gene-based diagnostic test. Searching for K-ras mutations might improve the diagnostic sensitivity of duct brushing or needle aspiration and could lead to the detection of curable early stages of pancreatic tumor genesis.

The development of highly sensitive polymerase chain reaction (PCR) procedures has allowed detection of K-ras mutations in pancreatic juice taken from patients with pancreatic cancer [72]. In two clinical trials, K-ras mutations were evaluated in 120 patients undergoing ERCP due to suspected pancreatic disease [6, 74]. In 37 of 46 patients (80%) with pancreatic malignancies, K-ras mutations were present in the pancreatic juice samples. In addition, K-ras mutations have been detected in stool samples of patients with pancreatic adenocacinomas [10]. Although only a limited number of patients have been studied, the first results of this work are promising. Stool samples can be collected easily, and therefore further development of a new diagnostic tool might improve early diagnosis in patients with pancreatic cancer. However, K-ras mutation analysis in pancreatic juice and stool samples is at present far from clinical practice, and further studies using these new diagnostic tools in pancreatic centers are needed to evaluate the sensitivity and specificity of K-ras mutations in the early detection of pancreatic cancer.

Clinical Impact of Molecular Findings in Pancreatic Cancer

Over the past 5 years, molecular studies in pancreatic cancer have increased our knowledge of the pathophysiology of this malignancy. We understand that enhanced expression of growth factors and growth factor receptors and the presence of mutations of protooncogenes and tumor suppressor genes give pancreatic cancer cells a major growth advantage, which may lead to tumor progression and may also be responsible for unresponsiveness to therapeutic modalities such as chemotherapy, radiotherapy, and hormonal therapies. Several studies have reported that the presence of some of these molecular alterations in pancreatic cancer is associated with tumor aggressiveness and shorter survival following tumor resection (Table 1). The use of molecular techniques allows us to select patients with poor prognosis who might benefit from more aggressive surgery and postoperative adjuvant treatment. A major clinical problem, however, is that we neither have effective drugs to cure patients or offer them prolongation of recurrence-free survival, nor drugs that have a palliative effect in patients with local recurrence or nonresectable disease. Therefore, molecular tumor analysis can already select patients who might profit from effective adjuvant therapy.

Another use of molecular techniques is to establish a diagnosis in patients for whom other procedures – such as contrast-enhanced computed tomography scanning and endoscopic retrograde cholangiopancreaticography (ERCP) – do not provide a conclusive answer. Molecular biology techniques are also providing the basis for new treatment concepts in pancreatic cancer. Initial results of gene therapy in other malignancies are promising, and indicate the possibility that gene therapy can also be established as a new treatment in pancreatic cancer. The identification of genetic changes that are specific and present in high frequency in pancreatic cancer cells is an important step toward designing gene therapy for this disorder.

Further molecular characterization of pancreatic cancer will contribute to a better understanding of its pathogenesis, making it possible to characterize the crucial steps in the malignant transformation of pancreatic cells in vivo.

Acknowledgements. This study was supported in part by the SNF Grant 32-39529 awarded by the Swiss National Funds to Helmut Friess.

References

1. Aaronson SA (1991) Growth factors and cancer. Science 254: 1146–1153
2. Andrén-Sandberg A (1990) Treatment with an LHRH analogue in patients with advanced pancreatic cancer. Acta Chir Scand 156: 549–551
3. Barton CM, Hall PA, Hughes CM, Gullick WJ, Lemoine NR (1991) Transforming growth factor alpha and epidermal growth factor in human pancreatic cancer. J Pathol 163: 111–116
4. Barton CM, Staddon SL, Hughes CM, Hall PA, O'Sullivan C, Klöppel G, Theis B, Russel RCG, Neoptolemos J, Willaimson RCN, Lane DP, Lemoine NR (1991) Abnormalities of the p53 tumor suppressor gene in human pancreatic cancer. Br J Cancer 64: 1076–1082
5. Bellosta P, Talarico D, Rogers D, Basilico C (1993) Cleavage of K-FGF produces a truncated molecule with increased biological activity and receptor binding affinity. J Cell Biol 121: 705–713
6. Bertheleny Ann Int Med (1995) 123: 188
7. Bouche G, Gas N, Prats H, Baldin V, Tauber JP, Teissie J, Amalric F (1987) Basic fibroblast growth factor enters the nucleus and stimulates the transcription and ribosomal genes in ABAE cells undergoing G0-G1 transition. Proc Natl Acad Sci USA 84: 6770–6774
8. Büchler M, Friess H, Schultheiss KH, Gebhardt Ch, Kübel R, Muhrer KH, Winkelmann M, Wagener T, Klapdor R, Kaul M, Müller G, Schulz G, Beger HG (1991) A randomized controlled trial of adjuvant immuno-therapy (murine monoclonal antibody 494/32) in resectable pancreatic cancer. Cancer 68: 1507–1512
9. Bugler B, Amalric F, Prats H (1991) Alternative initiation of translation determines cytoplasmic or nuclear localization of basic fibroblast growth factor. Mol Cell Biol 11: 573–577
10. Caldas C, Hahn SA, Hurban RH, Redston MS, Yeo CJ, Kern SE (1994) Detection of K-ras mutations in the stool of patients with pancreatic adenocarcinoma and pancreatic ductal hyperplasia. Cancer Research 54: 3568–3573
11. Casey G, Yamanaka Y, Friess H, Kobrin MS, Lopez ME, Büchler M, Beger HG, Korc M (1993) p53 mutations are common in pancreatic cancer and are absent in chronic pancreatitis. Cancer Letters, 69: 151–160
12. Chandrasekar B, Korc M (1992) Binding and biological actions of acidic and basic fibroblast growth factors in isolated rat pancreatic acini. Gastroenterology 102: A725, Abstract
13. Ciccodicola A, Dono R, Obici S, Simeone A, Zollo M, Persico MG (1989) Molecular characterization of a gene of the 'EGF family' expressed in undifferentiated human NTERA2 teratocarcinoma cells. EMBO J 8: 1987–1991

14. Coussens L, Yank-Feng TL, Liao YC, Chen E, Gray A, McGrath J, Seeburg PH, Libermann TA, Schlessinger J, Francke U (1985) Tyrosine kinase receptor with extensive homology to EGF receptor shares chromosomal location with neu oncogene. Science 230: 1132–1139
15. Diller L, Kassel J, Nelson CE, Gryka MA, Litwak G, Gebhardt M, et al (1990) p53 functions as a cell cycle control protein in osteosarcoma. Mol Cell Biol 10: 5772–5781
16. Ebert M, Yokoyama M, Kobrin MS, Friess H, Lopez M, Büchler MW, Johnson GR, Korc M (1994) Induction and expression of amphiregulin in human pancreatic cancer. Cancer Res 54: 3959–3962
17. Ebert M, Yokoyama M, Friess H, Kobrin MS, Büchler MW, Korc M (1995) Induction of platlet-derived growth factor A and B chains and over expression of their receptors in human pancreatic cancer. Int J Cancer 62: 529–535
18. Fearon ER, Vogelstein B (1990) A genetic model for colorectal tumorigenesis. Cell 61: 759–767
19. Finch P, Rubin J, Miki T, Ron D, Aaronson S (1989) Science 245: 752–755
20. Folkman J, Klagsbrun M (1987) Angiogenic factors. Science 235: 442–447
21. Friess H, Büchler M, Schulz G, Beger HG (1989) Therapie des Pankreaskarzinoms mit dem monoklonalen Antikörper BW 494/32: erste klinische Ergebnisse. Immun Infekt 17: 24–26
22. Friess H, Büchler M, Krüger M, Beger HG (1992) Treatment of duct carcinoma of the pancreas with the LH-RH analogue buserelin. Pancreas 7: 516–521
23. Friess H, Kobrin MS, Korc M (1992) Acidic and basic fibroblast growth factors and their receptors are expressed in the human pancreas. Pancreas 7: 737, Abstract
24. Friess H, Büchler M, Beglinger C, Krüger M, Beger HG (1993) Low-dose octreotide treatment is not effective in patients with advanced pancreatic cancer. Pancreas 8: 540–544
25. Friess H, Yamanaka Y, Büchler M, Beger HG, Kobrin MS, Baldwin RL, Korc M (1993) Enhanced expression of the type II transforming growth factor-beta receptor in human pancreatic cancer cells without alteration of type III receptor expression. Cancer Res 53: 2704–2707
26. Friess H, Yamanaka Y, Büchler M, Ebert M, Beger HG, Gold LI, Korc M (1993) Enhanced expression of transforming growth factor-beta isoforms in pancreatic cancer correlates with decreased survival. Gastroenterology 105: 1846–1856
27. Friess H, Yamanaka Y, Kobrin MS, Do AD, Büchler MW, Korc M (1995) Enhanced erbB-3 expression in human pancreatic cancer correlates with tumor progression. Clin Cancer Res 1: 1413–1420
28. Friess H, Berberat P, Schilling M, Kunz J, Korc M, Büchler MW (1996) Pancreatic cancer: the potential clinical relevance of alterations growth factors and their receptors. J Mol Med 74: 35–42
29. Fu Y-M, Spirito P, Yu Z-X, Biro S, Sasse J, Lei J, Ferrans VJ, Epstein SE, Casscells W (1991) Acidic fibroblast growth factor in the developing rat embryo. J Cell Biol 114: 1261–1273
30. Glinsmann-Gibson BJ, Korc M (1991) Regulation of transforming growth factor-alpha mRNA expression in T_3M_4 human pancreatic carcinoma cells. Pancreas 6: 142–149
31. Gospoderowicz D, Neufeld G, Schweigerer L (1986) Molecular and biological characterization of fibroblast growth factor, an angiogenic factor which also controls the proliferation and differentiation of mesoderm and neuroectoderm derived cells. Cell Diff 19: 1–17
32. Gospoderowicz D, Ferrara N, Schweigerer L, Neufeld G (1987) Structural characterization and biological functions of fibroblast growth factor. Endocrine Rev 8: 95–114
33. Grünewald K, Lyons J, Fröhlich A, Feichtinger H, Weger RA, Schwab G, Janssen JWG, Bartram CR (1989) High frequency of Ki-ras codon 12 mutations in pancreatic adenocarcinomas. Int J Cancer 43: 1037–1041
34. Hall PA, Hughes CM, Staddon SL, Richman PI, Gullick WJ, Lemoine NR (1990) The c-erbB-2 protooncogene in human pancreatic cancer. J Pathol 161: 1995–2000
35. Higashiyama S, Abraham JA, Miller J, Fiddes JC, Klagsbrun M (1991) A heparin-binding growth factor secreted by macrophage-like cells that as related to EGF. Science 251: 936–939
36. Hollenstein M, Sidransky D, Vogelstein B, Harris CC (1991) p53 mutations in human cancers. Science 253: 49–53
37. Holmes WE, Sliwkowski MX, Akita RW (1992) Identification of heregulin, a specific activator of p185erbB2. Science 256: 1205–1210
38. Klagsbrun M (1989) The fibroblast growth factor family: structural and biological properties. Progress in Growth Factor Res 1: 207–235
39. Kobrin MS, Yamanaka Y, Friess H, Lopez ME, Korc M (1993) Aberrant expression of the type I fibroblast growth factor receptor in human pancreatic adenocarcinomas. Cancer Res 53: 4741–4744

IV
Guidelines

Pancreatic Cancer: Diagnostic Guidelines for General Practitioners and Clinicians in Community Hospitals and Specialized Centers

L. Fernandez-Cruz · L. Sabater · S. Navarro · C. Parada

Pancreatic cancer is one of the most common neoplastic diseases, responsible for over 20% of deaths due to gastrointestinal malignancies. The prognosis of patients with pancreatic cancer is extremely poor with 5-year survival rates lower than 5% in large series.

The majority of pancreatic cancers arise in the exocrine pancreas, and ductal adenocarcinoma is the most common type, accounting for approximately 75%–80% of cases.

Surgical resection remains at present the only potentially curative possibility for these patients. However, in less than 25% of cases this curative treatment can be performed, since the majority of patients are diagnosed later, with metastatic spread or local invasion making resection of the tumor useless. Therefore, most patients will be treated on palliative basis by surgery or by any other therapeutic modality such as chemotherapy, external beam radiotherapy, brachytherapy, immunotherapy, or endocrine therapy. Nevertheless, these treatment options have not shown any clear advantages over supportive therapy alone, but as new protocols and trials are currently in progress, the future will clarify their role in the treatment of pancreatic cancer.

While these newly evolving therapy strategies develop, the best and probably only way to modify the prognosis in patients with pancreatic cancer is to diagnose the disease at an early stage and to perform immediate surgical treatment by an experienced surgeon.

How can this early diagnosis be achieved? Some risk factors have been related to cancer of the pancreas [1]: age over 40–50 years, male sex, cigarette smoking, coffee and alcohol consumption, high intake of fat or meat, previous peptic ulcer surgery, diabetes, organic solvents, and petroleum derivatives. However, no high-risk group of patients has been identified by epidemiologists, and therefore there is no role for screening programs in an asymptomatic population.

In the absence of screening possibilities, the suspicion of pancreatic cancer by the physician involved in the patient's care becomes the most important factor for the performance of a prompt diagnosis [2, 3].

Signs and symptoms of patients with cancer of the pancreas vary widely, especially depending on the location and extension of the tumor. In some instances, a high index of suspicion is easily derived from the clinical picture. The presence of weight loss, pain, and palpable gallbladder in a jaundiced patient is clearly suggestive of pancreatic malignancy. However, there is a high percentage of patients with insidious and nonspecific symptomatology normally attributed by the general practitioner to other disorders of the gastrointestinal tract such as gallstones, peptic ulcer disease, or gastroesophageal reflux. Awareness should be, therefore, the first rule for an early diagnosis.

Pain is a common symptom in pancreatic cancer patients, and often this symptom leads to seeking medical attention. Pain is usually of progressive intensity and diffuse localization. If the tumor is located at the head or at the uncinate process, pain may be the result of obstruction of the pancreatic duct and is not necessarily associated with neural plexus involvement. If the tumor is located at the body and tail, pain normally results from perineural and retroperitoneal invasion since in these areas the tumor has a silent growth and clinical manifestations are derived from its large size. In patients with a clinical presentation of pain localized to the lower thoracic or upper lumbar area, the differential diagnosis process must include pancreatic cancer, even in the absence of any other symptom.

Weight loss is present in approximately 90 % of patients at the time of diagnosis. Its etiology remains unknown, but a combination of decreased caloric intake, maldigestion, and increased resting energy expenditure [4] as well as abdominal discomfort have been related.

Jaundice and the associated signs of dark urine and pale stools are frequent features that require careful evaluation. Classically, a picture of painless jaundice was almost pathognomonic of pancreatic cancer. This description is not reliable at present, since the vast majority of patients have some sort of pain. The presence of a really painless jaundice must induce the suspicion of carcinoma of the bile duct or Vater's papilla more than pancreatic cancer. When the tumor is located at the head of the pancreas (60 % of cases), jaundice can be considered either an early or late symptom since the obstruction of the common bile duct can be produced by tumors of small size. However, if the tumor is located at the body and tail (25 % and 10 % of cases, respectively), jaundice is not observed until the disease has developed liver metastases or invaded the nodes around the porta hepatis. In fact, in the experience of Moossa [1], in approximately 45 % of patients with jaundice and pancreatic cancer the lesion was resectable, while resectability was performed only in 10 % of nonjaundiced patients.

The obstruction of the distal bile duct causes enlargement of the gallbladder. This fact is clinically relevant in 30 % of patients in whom palpation of the gallbladder (Courvoisier's sign) is possible by exploration. This sign is not generally associated with a dismal prognosis. However, the presence of duodenal obstruction with nausea and vomiting, venous thrombosis, splenomegaly, and migratory thrombophlebitis (Trousseau's sign) usually represent late and ominous manifestations of the disease.

New onset of diabetes mellitus is observed in 20 %–60 % of patients with pancreatic cancer. Destruction of islet cells secondary to associated pancreatitis and fibrosis has been suggested as an explanation of this glucose intolerance. The occasional association of pancreatitis and pancreatic cancer has resulted in confusion over the relationship between the two entities. Only the exceptional form of hereditary pancreatitis seems to be clearly related to the development of pancreatic malignancy. However, any patient suffering from pancreatic cancer may present an acute episode or recurrent acute episodes of pancreatitis. Therefore, neither acute nor chronic pancreatitis constitute a risk factor by themselves.

Depression has frequently been described especially in the past in patients with pancreatic cancer. This reactive state, probably secondary to several months of abdominal discomfort, weight loss, anorexia, weakness, and absence of an established diagnosis, can occasionally be the initial symptom in the diagnostic workup.

Since clinical features of pancreatic cancer vary widely, the diagnosis at an early stage has to be based on a high index of suspicion by the physician. Several studies illustrate how difficult it is to achiev this goal. In the prospective study by DiMagno et al. [5], the tumor was confirmed only in 30 out of 70 clinically suspicious patients. In the study by Moossa [1], out of 238 patients with clinically suggestive symptoms of pancreatic cancer, only 102 cases could eventually be confirmed.

All these facts underline the importance of the awareness, by the general practitioner and the clinician in community hospitals, of the possibility of dealing with pancreatic cancer, although clinical symptoms and physical examination are not able to reveal clearly at first sight a pancreatic neoplasia. This general recommendation should be followed especially in patients over 40 years with obstructive jaundice, recurrent attacks of pancreatitis, recent weight loss of unknown origin, chronic abdominal discomfort, recent onset of diabetes mellitus, and unexplained pain located at the upper abdomen or lumbar back.

After pancreatic cancer has been suspected, further investigations have to be performed by a combination of imaging techniques [6, 7, 8] and biochemical function tests. Availability of such methods depends on the facilities of the physician responsible for the medical treatment of the patient. Thus a rational selection of the different diagnostic procedures is mandatory, based on the sensitivity, specificity, predictive values, accuracy, and cost of each method.

The most frequent diagnostic modalities used by the general practitioner or the clinician for the initial evaluation of patients with clinical symptoms of pancreatic cancer or unclear abdominal discomfort are barium upper gastrointestinal series, laboratory function tests, and ultrasonography. Barium upper gastrointestinal series were frequently used in the past in patients with clinical suspicion of pancretic cancer, since the presence of indirect signs such as widening of the duodenum or the "inverted 3" were associated with pancreatic tumors of large size. However, the current development and widespread use of more accurate methods for the diagnosis of the disease have decreased the use of this technique. Laboratory findings are of relative importance in the diagnosis of pancreatic cancer. Serum bilirubin and alkaline phosophatase levels are usually elevated in patients with cancer of the head of the pancreas, but tumors located at the body and tail do not produce biochemical abnormalities until metastases have developed. However, laboratory investigation is of great help in finding out the metabolic and nutritional status of the patient. Evaluation of the size and structure of the pancreatic gland and the morphology of the bile and pancreatic ducts are essential in order to identify pancreatic lesions. Ultrasonography (Figs. 1, 2) should be the initial radiological method for examining the pan-

Fig. 1. Ultrasonography. Focal hypoechoic mass at the head of the pancreas. (Courtesy of R. Gilabert)

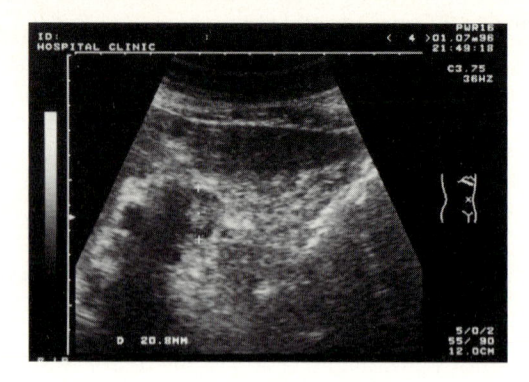

creas, the neighboring organs, and the abdominal cavity. Nevertheless, in 15%–20% of cases the examination is useless due to interferences of bowel gas or fat in the obese patient [1]. This method is able to demonstrate tumors over 2 cm in size – in most cases as an hypoechoic mass relative to the normal parenchyma – dilation of the bile duct (more than 7–8 mm in diameter), dilation of the pancreatic duct (more than 2–3 mm in diameter), retroperitoneal lymph node enlargement, liver metastases, and ascites. In the jaundiced patient, this method shows high accuracy in distinguishing the obstructive or nonobstructive origin of the disease. Sensitivity and specificity of ultrasonography in pancreatic cancer reaches values of 80%–90% when performed by an experienced radiologist.

Once clinical suspicion is supported by ultrasonography findings, the next step to follow in the algorithm of the diagnosis is confirmation of the presence of a mass in the pancreas and, if positive, staging of [9] the tumor with a series of investigations in specialized centers to determine which tumors are potentially resectable, which cannot be resected but are still localized, and which have distant metastases. Patients with tumors in any of these categories will be offered the most appropriate medical and surgical alternative.

Fig. 2. Ultrasonography. Marked dilatation of the common bile duct due to a distal obstruction by a pancreatic tumor. (Courtesy of R. Gilabert)

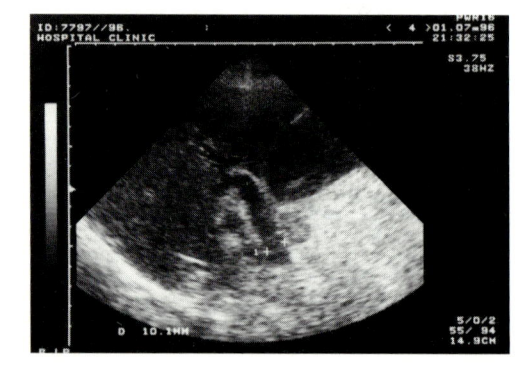

Fig. 3. Dynamic computed tomography showing a tumor at the head and body of the pancreas, vascular involvement, and liver metastases. (Courtesy of C. Ayuso)

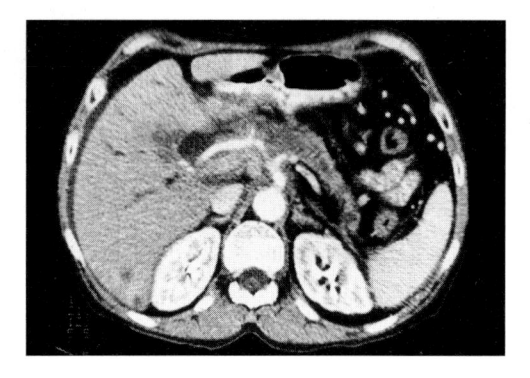

Dynamic computed tomography (Fig. 3) and spiral computed tomography (CT) (Fig. 4) are the most efficient radiological methods providing knowledge on the location, size and extrapancreatic invasion of the tumor and the presence of enlarged lymph nodes and liver metastases. Furthermore, these methods provide information on the potential resectability of the tumor.

Patients with a positive clinical suspicion but with doubtful findings on CT should be examined with endoscopic retrograde cholangiopancreatography (ERCP), which allows direct observation of the ampullary region, cytologic examination of samples of aspirated pancreatic juice, and a pancreatogram (Fig. 5). This exploration is very useful in the diagnosis of small tumors in the pancreatic duct.

The question of biopsy of the tumor is open to controversy [10] because of the risk of sowing neoplastic cells intraperitoneally or along the tract of the needle. This method should therefore be performed in patients with unresectable lesions, who can benefit from palliative measures.

Tumor markers have been proposed as useful parameters for diagnosis and follow-up of pancreatic carcinoma. The most extensive tumor markers have been Ca 19-9, carcinoembryonic antigen (CEA), C-50, Ca 12-5, immunoreactive elastase levels, and the ratio of testosterone to dihydrotestosterone. Unfortunately, none of these markers is reliable enough to be used in screening programs [3].

Fig. 4. Angiographic computed tomography. Three-dimensional reconstruction of the vascularity of the pancreas allows demonstration of vascular integrity without tumor invasion. (Courtesy of C. Ayuso)

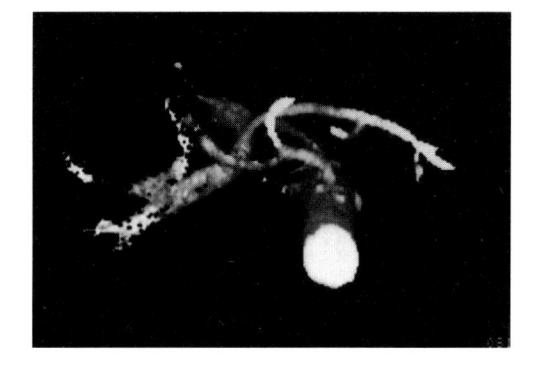

Fig. 5. Endoscopic retrograde cholangio-pancreatography (ERCP) showing dilatation of the common bile and pancreatic ducts and complete interruption of the contrast along the pancreatic duct due to a pancreatic cancer. (Courtesy of J.M. Bordas)

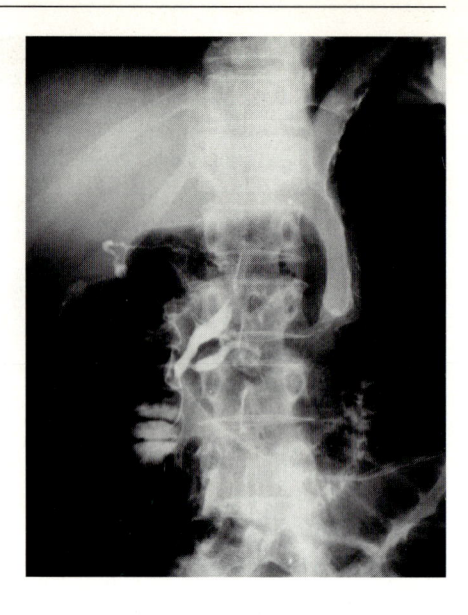

Major vascular involvement is a frequent cause of preclusive curative resection of the tumor. Therefore, angiography (Fig. 6) may play an important role in the preoperative assessment of carcinoma of the pancreas [11] in terms of resectability. However, with the increasing refinements of spiral CT, angiography is best used in selected cases to obtain accurate information on the length and circular extension of the vascular involvement in order to decide on resection of the segment of the portal vein.

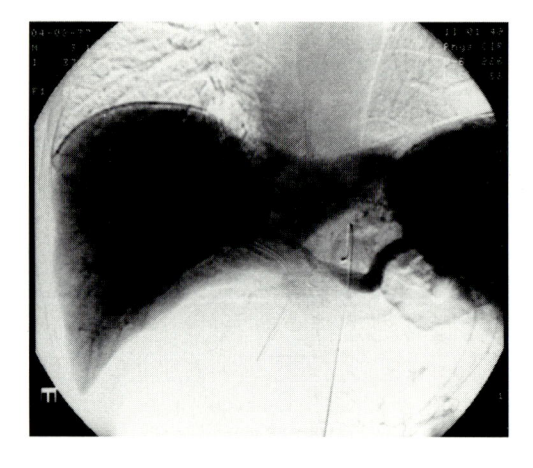

Endoscopic ultrasonography (Fig. 7) obtains direct images of the pancreatic area through the wall of the stomach and is increasingly incorporated in staging pancreatic cancer [12, 13] with the possibility of diagnosing tumors smaller than 2 cm and providing better lymph node staging. Laparoscopy and laparos-

Fig. 6. Arteriography. Portogram showing bilateral narrowing along the portal vein. (Courtesy of J. Muntañá))

Fig. 7. Endoscopic ultrasonography. Hypoechoic lesion located at the pancreatic head. (Courtesy of J.M. Bordas and A. Ginés)

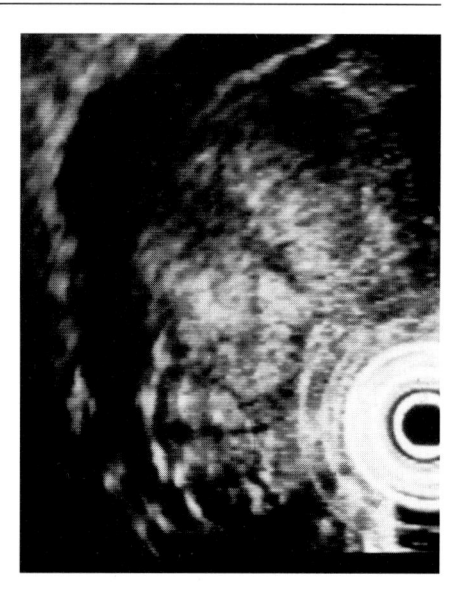

copic ultrasound have recently been successfully applied in the staging of pancreatic cancer [14, 15]. This method provides direct visualization of the abdominal cavity and allows detection of hepatic and peritoneal nodules measuring less than 2 cm in diameter, as was demonstrated by Warshaw [16] in approximately 40% of patients in whom other preoperative diagnostic methods failed to demonstrate extrapancreatic involvement. Furthermore, laparoscopic ultrasound enables evaluation of vascular involvement of the tumor. Both reasons constitute the basis of the rapid incorporation of this technique into the most recent protocols of staging of patients with pancreatic carcinoma. In this sense, CT scan, angiography, and laparoscopy must be considered complementary, since they assess different limits of resectability. This approach has made it possible to increase the resection rate to as high as 78%.

In summary, pancreatic cancer is recognized as the most lethal of all cancers, and when diagnosed, it is usually too far advanced for surgical cure. At the time of diagnosis, the tumor is confined to the pancreas in less than 10% of patients, 40% have locally advanced disease, and more than 50% of patients have distant spread.

Currently, the majority of patients with pancreatic cancer are identified on the basis of their symptoms: pain, jaundice, or both are present in over 90% of cases.

A wide variety of tumor markers has been proposed for use in diagnosis, and the most extensively studied marker is Ca 19-9 with a sensitivity of over 90% but a low specificity of approximately 75%.

Assessment of tumor resectability is essential for planing surgical resection. Tumors less than 3 cm in diameter have a more favorable prognosis. Although important advances have been made in radiologic diagnosis by ultrasound,

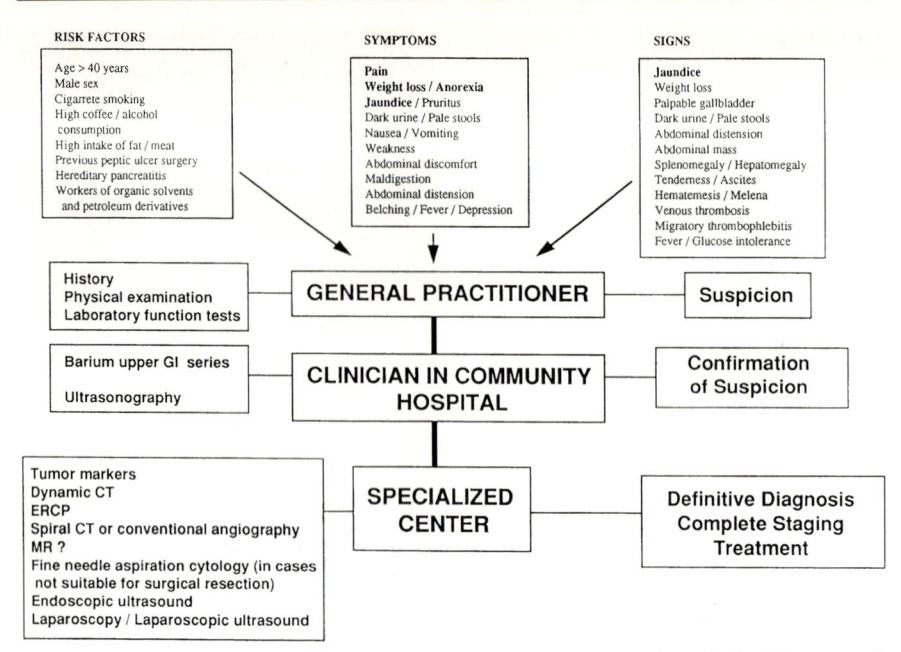

RISK FACTORS	SYMPTOMS	SIGNS
Age > 40 years Male sex Cigarrete smoking High coffee / alcohol consumption High intake of fat / meat Previous peptic ulcer surgery Hereditary pancreatitis Workers of organic solvents and petroleum derivatives	Pain Weight loss / Anorexia Jaundice / Pruritus Dark urine / Pale stools Nausea / Vomiting Weakness Abdominal discomfort Maldigestion Abdominal distension Belching / Fever / Depression	Jaundice Weight loss Palpable gallbladder Dark urine / Pale stools Abdominal distension Abdominal mass Splenomegaly / Hepatomegaly Tenderness / Ascites Hematemesis / Melena Venous thrombosis Migratory thrombophlebitis Fever / Glucose intolerance

History Physical examination Laboratory function tests	**GENERAL PRACTITIONER**	Suspicion
Barium upper GI series Ultrasonography	**CLINICIAN IN COMMUNITY HOSPITAL**	Confirmation of Suspicion
Tumor markers Dynamic CT ERCP Spiral CT or conventional angiography MR ? Fine needle aspiration cytology (in cases not suitable for surgical resection) Endoscopic ultrasound Laparoscopy / Laparoscopic ultrasound	**SPECIALIZED CENTER**	Definitive Diagnosis Complete Staging Treatment

Fig. 8. Integrated diagnostic guidelines to pancreatic cancer. *GI*, gastrointestinal; *CT*, computed tomography; *ERCP*, endoscopic retrograde cholangiopancreatography; *MR*, magnetic resonance

computed tomography, endoscopic retrograde cholangiography, and magnetic resonance, endosonography is more accurate in detecting tumors less than 3 cm in diameter with a sensitivity of approximately 93%. In addition, endoscopic ultrasonography allows distinction of focal pancreatitis and pancreatic carcinoma. The application of three-dimensional spiral computed tomography angiography may in future replace conventional angiography in accurate diagnosis of tumor invasion of the portal vein. With the advent of laparoscopy and laparoscopic ultrasound, pancreatic tumor staging has clearly improved, allowing detection of peritoneal and liver metastases not seen with other methods.

We believe that suspicion of pancreatic cancer by the general practitioner should be reinforced in community hospitals by the use of ultrasonography and confirmed in referral medical centers by more specific and sensitive imaging techniques and other diagnostic modalities, such as laparoscopic ultrasound in tumors potentially curative by surgical resection (Fig. 8).

References

1. Moossa AR, Gamagami RA (1995) Diagnosis and staging of pancreatic neoplasms. Surg Clin North Am 75: 871–890
2. Lillemoe KD (1995) Current management of pancreatic carcinoma. Ann Surg 221: 133–148
3. Warshaw AL, Fernández del Castillo C (1992) Pancreatic carcinoma. N Engl J Med 326: 455–465
4. Falconer JS, Fearon KCH, Plester CE, et al (1994) Cytokines, the acute-phase response, and resting energy expenditure in cachectic patients with pancreatic cancer. Ann Surg 219: 325–331
5. DiMagno EP, Malagelada JR, Taylor WF, et al (1977) A prospective comparison of current diagnostic tests for pancreatic cancer. N Engl J Med 297: 737–740
6. Brambs HJ, Claussen CD (1993) Pancreatic and ampullary carcinoma. Ultrasound, Computed Tomography, Magnetic Resonance imaging and Angiography. Endoscopy 25: 58–68
7. Müller MF, Meyenberger C, Bertschinger P, et al (1994) Pancreatic tumors: evaluation with endoscopic US, CT, and MR imaging. Radiology 190: 745–751
8. Marty O, Aubertin J-M, Bouillot J-L, et al (1995) Comparison prospective de l'échoendoscopie et de la tomodensitométrie dans le bilan d'extension loco-régionale de tumeurs malignes ampullaires et pancréatiques vérifieés chirurgicalement. Gastroenterol Clin Biol 19: 197–203
9. Karl RC, Carey LC (1993) Impact of staging on treatment of pancreatic and ampullary cancer. Endoscopy 25: 69–74
10. Warshaw AL (1991) Implications of peritoneal cytology for staging of early pancreatic cancer. Am J Surg 161: 26–30
11. Mori M, Mimura H (1995) Role of angiography in carcinoma of the pancreas as a preoperative assessment. Hepato-Gastroenterology 42: 752–763
12. Palazzo L, Roseau G, Gayet B, et al (1993) Endoscopic ultrasonography in the diagnosis and staging of pancreatic adenocarcinoma. Endoscopy 25: 143–150
13. Rösch T, Braig C, Gain T, et al (1992) Staging of pancreatic and ampullary carcinoma by endoscopic ultrasonography. Gastroenterology 102: 188–199
14. John TG, Greig JD, Carter DC, et al (1995) Carcinoma of the pancreatic head and periampullary region. Tumor staging with laparoscopy and laparoscopic ultrasonography. Ann Surg 221: 156–164
15. Conlon KC, Dougherty E, Klimstra D, et al (1996) The value of minimal access surgery in the staging of patients with potentially resectable peripancreatic malignancy. Ann Surg 223: 134–140
16. Warshaw AL, Gu Z, Wittenberg J, et al (1990) Preoperative staging and assessment of resectability of pancreatic cancer. Arch Surg 125: 230–233.

Subject Index

A
acidic fibroblast growth factor (aFGF) 415
acidosis 98
acinar cell
– carcinoma 398
– necrosis 17
– damage 14
adenocarcinoma 344, 397
aFGF (*see* acidic fibroblast growth factor)
alanine aminotransferase (ALT) 74
alcohol 94
– consumption 161
alcoholic chronic pancreatitis 291
alcoholics, chronic 152
alcoholism 73, 75
alkaline phosphatase (ALP) 74
ALP (*see* alkaline phosphatase)
ALT (*see* alanine aminotransferase)
amphiregulin 413
ampullar tumors 347
amylase 74, 98, 121, 272, 285
– secretion 262
anaplastic carcinoma 397
anastomotic ulceration 323
angiography 226, 432, 433
anti-BGA antibody 335
anti-insulin 335
antiproteases 111
antithrombin III 137
α_1-antitrypsin 120, 124, 273
APACHE II Score 120
arginine 87
ascites 228, 350
aspartate aminotransferase (AST) 74
aspiration cytology 395
assays 235
AST (*see* aspartate aminotransferase)
autodigestion 95

B
bacteriological study 144
basal lamina 156
basic fibroblast growth factor (bFGF) 415
betacellulin 413
bFGF (*see* basic fibroblast growth factor)
bicarbonate, output 249

bile reflux 14
biliary tract (*see also* common bile duct) 46, 143
– disease 74
– imaging procedures 75, 76
bilirubin 74
biopsy 225
bleeding 186, 225
BOP (*see* N-nitrosobis(2-oxopropyl)amine)
breath tests 261-269
– [^{14}C]breath test 262
– cholesteryl-octanoate breath test 265
– hiolein breath test 266, 268
– mixed triglyceride breath test 263, 264
– [^{13}C]Starch breath test 262
– [^{14}C]triglyceride breath test 262-264
– [^{13}C]triolein breath test 263
– H$_2$ breath test 262

C
C peptide 304
c-erbB2 412
c-erbB3 412
c-erbB4 412
c-ki-ras mutation 336
c-Kis-*ras* oncogene 336
C-reactive protein (CRP) 23, 93, 98, 114, 122, 135, 142
CA 19-9 200, 390
caerulein-induced pancreatitis 297
calcification 190, 195, 197, 199, 224, 354
calcitonin gene-related peptide 321
calcium 98
calculi 224
Cambridge Classification 4, 203
cancer (*see* carcinoma)
carbohydrate-deficient transferrin (CDT) 58, 75
carboxylic ester hydrolase (CEH) 122
carcinoma (cancer; *see also* tumor) 185, 187, 195, 197-200, 224, 291-300, 333, 343, 350, 359, 363, 371, 411, 427
– acinar cell 398
– adenocarcinoma 344, 397, 427
– anaplastic 397
– barium upper gastrointestinal series 429

- ERCP guided puncture   364
- features   350
- induction   334
- Ki *ras* mutations   365
- mucinous cystadeno-carcinoma   350, 366
- pancreatic (*see* pancreatic cancer)
- pancreatic juice cytology   363
CCK (*see* cholecystokinin)
CDT (*see* carbohydrate-deficient transferrin)
CEH (*see* carboxylic ester hydrolase)
celiac sprue   280
cerulein   249
cholangiopancreatography   57-64
cholangitis   144, 227
cholecystectomy   60
cholecystokinin (CCK)   233
choledochal cyst   197
cholestasis   168
cholesterol
- esterase   265
- lipase   265
cholesteryl-octanoate breath test   265
chymotrypsin   253, 285
cirrhosis   227
clinical decision making   127
coagulation   111, 136
collagen   291
common bile duct stenosis   321
complement   98, 111, 123
complications, local   144
computed tomography (CT)   29, 37, 39, 75, 76, 104, 142, 189, 207
- ascites   350
- contrast-enhanced   121, 126
- conventional technique   350
- diagnostic features of pancreatic cancer   350
- dilated pancreaticoduodenal vein   351
- dynamic   431, 433
- endocrine tumors   350
- findings in chronic pancreatitis   189
- high-speed spiral acquisition   349
- lymph node metastases   350
- mucinous cystadeno-carcinoma   350
- nonresectability   350
- pancreatic cancer   350
- sensitivity   192
- specificity   192
- spiral technique   350, 431, 434
- thrombotic lesions of the portal vein   351
- two-or three-dimensional reformation   352
corn starch   262
Courvoisier's sign   428
creatinine   101
CRP (*see* C-reactive protein)
CT (*see* computed tomography)
CT-angiography   352
Cullen sign   98
cystadenocarcinoma, mucinous   350, 366
cystic

- cavities   185
- fibrosis   267, 269, 280
- fluid collections   191
- infection   186
- neoplasm   354, 399
- tumors   345
cystojejunostomy   326
cysts   185, 229
cytogenetic analysis   335
cytokines   111, 123
cytology   197, 199, 395-400
- acinar cells   396
- ductal cells   396
- islet cells   396
- normal pancreas   396
- pancreatitis   396

D
decompression of the
- common bile duct   323
- duodenum   323
- main pancreatic duct   323
- major vessels   323
densification, pulmonary   101
desmoplastic reaction   300
diabetes mellitus   205, 226, 303, 333, 428, 429
diagnosis of chronic pancreatitis   253-258
diagnostic tests, evaluation   69
digestive enzymes   94
DNA sequencing   336
L-DOPA   405
double duct   200
DPDP   353
drainage   227, 325
duct(s)   224
- calcification   211
- changes in   155
- common bile
- - decompression   323
- - stenosis   321
- drainage   215-221
- grossly dilated   185
- main bile   185
- main pancreatic   183, 190
- obstruction   161
ductal adenocarcinoma   427
duodenal
- intubation   249
- stenosis   321
duodenocystostomy   134
duodenum-preserving pancreatic head resection   322, 323
duplex sonography   225
dynamic computed tomography   431, 433

E
echogenicity   183, 185
edematous   273
effusion, pleural   101

Subject Index

EGD (*see* esophago-gastro-duodenoscopy)
EGF (*see* epidermal growth factor)
EGFR (*see* epidermal growth factor receptor)
elastase   98, 121, 273
embolization   226
endocrine pancreatic
– function   87-89, 303-308, 322
– insufficiency   161, 169, 176
endocrine tumors   350
endoscopic
– pancreatic sphincterotomy   58, 61, 216
– retrograde cholangiopancreatography (ERCP)   73, 144, 195-197, 207, 208, 224, 250, 359, 431
– ultrasonography (EUS)   29, 76, 184, 195, 207, 224, 343, 346, 432
endothelial cells   111
enzyme(s)   249
– intrapancreatic   244
– linked immunoabsorbant assay technique   287
– replacement therapy   267
– secretion   250
– substitution therapy   234
epidermal growth factor (EGF)   411
– receptor (EGFR)   299
ERCP (*see* endoscopic retrograde cholangiopancreatography)
ERP (*see* pancreatography)
esophago-gastro-duodenoscopy (EGD)   225
EUS (*see* endoscopic ultrasonography)
evocation-test   272
exocrine pancreas, secretory capacity   258
exocrine pancreatic
– function   81-84, 322
– insufficiency   161, 169, 176, 261, 264, 265, 268
– secretion, negative feedback regulation   235
exogenous hormones   249
extracellular matrix   291
extracorporeal shock wave lithotripsy   218, 219

F

F ratio   279
fat
– fecal   280
– necrosis   15
FDG   404
fecal
– fat   280
– nitrogen   280
– tests   277-288
– water   280
fibrinolysis   111, 136
fibroblast proliferation   297
fibronectin   291
fibrosis   151
– cystic   267, 269, 280

– pancreatic   294
fine-needle aspiration   53-55, 144
fistula   168, 228
fluorescein dilaurate   253
FNB (*see* percutaneous fine-needle biopsy)
free radicals   161
function tests   205
– direct   249-252
– indirect   253
– – staging of pancreatic disease   256
– oral   253
functional reserve capacity   268

G

gallbladder
– contraction   236, 237
– function   236
gallstones   73
gamma glutamyl transferase (γ-GT)   74
gastric
– dumping   322
– emptying, delayed   323
gastrointestinal neoplasm   377
Gd-DTPA   353
gene mutations   417
genetic factors   161
Glasgow score system   120
glial growth factors   413
glucagon   87, 306
glucose   98
glutathione   94
graft thrombosis   135
Grey-Turner sign   98
groove pancreatitis   205
growth factors receptors   412

H

hamsters   334
HB-EGF   413
hematocrit   98
hemostasis   226
hepatic detoxification   162
heregulin   413
hiolein   266
– breath test   266, 268
[^{123}I]HIPDM   401
histopathological changes   162
hPASP   122
HTP (*see* hydroxytryptophan)
hydroxyproline   297
hydroxytryptophan (HTP)   405
hyperamylasemia   71
hyperdiploid/pseudotetraploid   335
hyperglycemia   87
hyperparathyroidism   229
hypertension, portal   168
hypoxemia   98

I

IL-6 95, 98, 113, 123, 136
IL-8 95, 136
immune dysfunction 94
immunoglobulins 156
immunoreactive
- enzyme estimation 277
- lipase 287
- trypsin 272
indirect pancreatic function tests 253
- staging of pancreatic disease 256
infection 226
- cystic 186
inflammation
- acute 294
- chronic 154, 321
inflammatory
- bowel disease 280
- cells 95
- diseases 292
- mass of the head of the pancreas 321, 325
infrared spectroscopy 277
insulin 87, 304, 337
insulin-like growth-factor (IGF)-1 338
insulinomas 355
- gastrinomas 345
interdigestive cycling 238
interstitial connective tissue 293
„intestinal housekeeper" 241
intrapancreatic enzymes 244
ischemia 95
islet amyloid polypeptide 338
islets 333
isoamylase 71, 273
isotope ratio mass spectrometry 268

J

jaundice 205, 428, 429, 433

K

K-*ras* mutations 392, 399, 418
kallikrein 136
kallikrein-kinin 111
Kausch-Whipple procedure 325
keratinozyte growth factor (KGF) 416
KGF (*see* keratinozyte growth factor)
Ki-ras 200
Kjeldahl method 277

L

L/A ratio 74
lactoferrin 9, 156
laminin 291
Langerhans's islets 87
laparoscopic ultrasound (LUS) 371-377
laparoscopy 371-377, 433, 434
- ultrasonography 433, 434
lipase 71, 74, 121, 250, 262, 264, 272, 285

lithostathine 8, 162
liver
- function 98
- metastases 372, 428, 431, 434
local complications 144
Lundh test 283
LUS (*see* laparoscopic ultrasound)
lymph node metastases 350
lymphocytes 111, 155

M

α_2-macroglobulin 98, 111, 120, 124
macrophages 110
magnetic resonance angiography 356
magnetic resonance cholangiography 356
- HASTE 356
- RARE 356
- ultrafast echo planar techniques 356
magnetic resonance cholangiopancreatography (MRCP) 76, 209, 225
magnetic resonance imaging (MRI) 29, 137, 195, 209, 434
- breathhold modalities 349
- calcifications 354
- cystic neoplasm 354
- fat suppression FLASH two-dimensional sequence 354
- insulinomas 355
- pancreatic tumor 353
- phased array technique 349, 353
- stationary dynamic imaging 354
- tumor signs
- - direct 353
- - indirect 353
- ultrafast sequences 349, 353
- *Zollinger-Ellison* syndrome 354
main pancreatic duct, dilatation 325
malabsorption 277
malignancy 226
malignant intrainsular ductal structures 337
markers of necrosis
- sensitivity 109
- specifity 109
Marseille classification 4, 204
- revised 5
matrix metalloproteinases (MMP) 291
- MMP-1 (interstitial collagenase) 292
- MMP-3 (stromelysin) 292
- MMP-2 (72-kDa collagenase type IV) 292
- MMP-9 (92-kDa collagenase type IV) 292
meal, standardized 249
mean corpuscular volume (MCV) 75
met-enkephalin 242
metabolites, toxic 162
metastases
- liver 372, 428, 431, 434
- lymph node 350
- peritoneal 374

Subject Index

methalbumin 98
methemalbumin 109, 120
mice, transgenic 152
microlithiasis 76
mixed triglyceride breath test 263, 264
MMP (see matrix metalloproteinases)
molecular markers 389
monoclonal antibodies 401
mortality 322, 324
motilin 238
motor activity of the upper gut 238
MR (see magnetic resonance)
MRCP (see magnetic resonance cholangio-pancreatography)
MRI (see magnetic resonance imaging)
mucinous
- cystadenocarcinoma 350, 366
- ductal ectasia, pancreatography 365
multifactorial score system 119
multiorgan failure 93, 111, 144
mycobacterium 18

N

NBT-PABA (bentiromide) 253, 254, 258
- meta-analysis 255
- serum test 206, 255
NDF (see neu differentiation factor)
near-infrared reflectance analysis (NIRA) 278, 282
necrosis 14, 16, 17, 40, 41
- acinar cell 17
- fat 15
- infection 97, 101, 104, 105
- markers 109
- pancreatic 15, 59, 109, 142
- - infected 49-55
- patterns 14f.
- periductal 17
- type 1 necrosis pattern 14, 16
necrotizing pancreatitis 273
neoplasm (see also carcinoma) 225
- cystic 354, 399
- gastrointestinal 377
neopterin 98
nerves, damages 156
neu differentiation factor (NDF) 413
neural microenvironment 242
neuroendocrine tumors 398
neuropeptide Y 321
neutrophils 110, 156
nicotine abuse 161
NIRA (see near-infrared reflectance analysis)
nitrogen 282
- fecal 280
N-nitrosobis(2-oxopropyl)amine (BOP) 333
nociception 242
nondispersive isotope-selective infrared spectrometry 268

O

obstruction 226
[^{13}C]octanoate 264
[^{13}C]octanoyl monoglyceride 264
octeotride 403
Opie's theory 14
opoids, endogenous 242
oral pancreatic function test 253
organ system failure 101, 103, 104
oxidative stress 162
oxygen free radicals 110

P

p53
- antibodies 391
- gene mutation 391
- mutations 417
pain 161, 173, 176-178, 215-221, 223, 242, 321, 322, 324, 427-429, 433
- abdominal 166
- chronic 156
platelet-derived growth factors (PDGF) 417
- receptors 417
pancreas
- divisum 62, 197, 229
- kidney transplantation 131
- left resection 326
- necrosis 15
- size 190
- specific protein (PSP) 72
pancreatectomy 228
pancreatic
- cancer (see also carcinoma) 291-300, 333, 350, 353, 371, 411, 427
- - adenocarcinoma 344
- - barium upper gastrointestinal series 429
- - biopsy 431
- - depression 429
- - diagnostic guidelines 427
- - early diagnosis 428
- - pancreatitis 428, 429
- - resectability 428, 431-433
- - risk factors 427
- - staging 430, 432, 434
- - surgery 427
- - vascular involvement 432, 433
- cytology 395
- duct, main 183
- ductal carcinogenesis 337
- enzyme 69, 121, 271
- fibrosis 294
- fistula 168
- function, endocrine 303-308
- function tests 205
- - direct 249-252
- insufficiency 233, 249, 271
- isoamylase 273
- juice
- - cytology 363

- - lactoferrin   9
- - lithostathine   8
- - protein plugs   8
- - tumor antigens   364
- margin   190
- necrosis   15, 59, 109, 142
- - infected   49-55
- parenchyma   190
- - resection   223
- polypeptide   238, 306
- pseudocysts   196, 326, 397
- regeneration   297
- ribonuclease   109
- secretion   81
- steatorrhea   266, 267
- stenting   219, 220
- stimulation   249
- stone protein   162
pancreaticoduodenal vein, dilated   351
pancreaticojejunostomy   325
pancreatitis
- acute   73, 81, 87, 296
- - acinar-cell-damage   14
- - aetiology   6
- - associated condition   142
- - bile reflux   14
- - biliary etiology   46, 143
- - biological diagnosis   69
- - clinical
- - - characteristics   4-6, 21-25
- - - staging   22
- - complications   38, 97, 99–101, 105, 142
- - - vascular   45
- - computed tomography   37
- - - severity index   39
- - course   4-6
- - differential diagnosis   32
- - edematous   93
- - endoscopic ultrasound   34
- - etiologies   73
- - fluid collections   43
- - gastrointestinal tract involvement   46
- - gross pathology   15
- - histopathology   16-18
- - immunocytochemistry   18
- - morphological characteristics   4-6
- - necrosis   14, 16, 17, 40, 41
- - necrotizing   93
- - pathogenesis   14, 15
- - pathomorphology   22
- - percutaneous catheter drainage   44
- - prognosis   97-105, 109-115, 142
- - sepsis   42
- - severity   119
- - - clinical assessment   120
- - solid organ involvement   46
- - sonographic
- - - detection of complications   31
- - - signs   30
- - staging   38
- - tubular complex   17

- - ultrasonographic detection of etiology   33
- - ultrasound   29-35
- - - assessment of the severity   33
- - ultrastructure   18
- alcoholic   24, 71, 72
- caerulein-induced   297
- chronic   161-163, 195, 198-200, 223, 233, 249, 271, 294, 303, 321
- - aetiology   6
- - alcoholic   291
- - calcifying   6
- - classification   197
- - clinical characteristics   4-6
- - complications   167, 192, 213, 223
- - course   4-6, 165-169
- - diagnosis   189-193, 195-200, 253-258
- - diagnostic standards   313-320
- - endoscopic retrograde cholangiopancreatography (ERCP)   7
- - endoscopic ultrasonography (EUS)   8
- - etiology   174, 175, 223
- - inflammatory   6
- - morphologic characteristics   4-6
- - mortality   321
- - obstructive   197, 198
- - pathomorphological features   151-157
- - prognosis   169, 321
- - radiologic imaging   203-213
- - retention   197
- - segmental left   326
- - staging   189-193, 195-200
- - standards in surgical treatment   321-327
- - tumor-associated   291
- classification   3-10
- - Cambridge classification   4
- - Marseille classification   4
- - - revised   5
- - Marseille-Rome classification   5
- edematous   119
- groove   205
- infectious   15, 17
- mild   16
- necrotizing   42, 119, 273
- obstructive chronic   205
- postimplantation   132
- segmental   326
- severe   16
pancreatitis-associated peptide   98
pancreatography (ERP)   359
- differential diagnosis with chronic pancreatitis   361, 362
- double duct sign   360
- malignant stenosis   359
- necrotic cavity   360
- obstruction   359
- parenchymography   361
- tapering type   359
pancreatoscopy   197, 199
pancreolauryl test   206, 253, 254
- abnormal results   258

Subject Index

- early diagnosis of chronic pancreatitis 258
- fluorescein dilaurate 253
- limitations 258
- meta-analysis 256
- serum test 256
paradoxical enzyme activities 121
Partington-Rochelle modification 322
PCR (*see* polymerase chain reaction)
PDGF (*see* platelet-derived growth factors)
percutaneous
- catheter drainage 44
- fine-needle biopsy (FNB) 346
pericystic vascular development 186
periductal necrosis 17
perineurium 156
perioperative cytology 395
peripancreatic fatty tissue 192
peripheral blood 392
peritoneal
- lavage 376
- metastases 374
peritoneum 192
PET (*see* positron emission tomography)
phospholipase A_2 98, 114, 120, 125, 273
- type I 125
- type II 125
plasma cells 155
plasma proteinase inhibitors 124
platelets 111
pleural effusion 63
PLT (*see* pancreolauryl)
PMN 93
- elastase 113, 124
polymerase chain reaction (PCR) 336
polymorphonuclear (PMN) elastase 120, 142
polypeptide, pancreatic 238, 306
portal
- hypertension 168
- vein, thrombotic lesions 351
positron emission tomography (PET) 195
posttranslational processing 242
preoperative cytology 395
pretherapeutic staging 185
procarboxypeptidase B 122
procollagen type III peptide (PIIIP) 296
proenkephalin 242
prognostic scores 93
PROP (*see* type 1 prophospholipase A_2 activating peptide)
prophospholipase 273
protease inhibitors 94
- α_1- 98, 111
protease-antiprotease balance 125
protein plugs 8
proteolytic
- cascades 112
- systems 111
pseudoaneurysms 168
pseudocysts 59, 62, 167, 224
- pancreatic 196, 397

PSP (*see* pancreas-specific protein)
Puestrow-type drainage operation 325
pylorus-preserving partial duodenopancreatectomy 322

R

Ranson score system 120
renal failure 144
respiratory failure 144
retroperitoneal
- fasciae 192
- sarcoma 397
ribonuclease 98, 120, 273
Roux-Y reconstruction 326
rupture 226

S

SAPS (*see* Simplified Acute Physiology Score)
sarcoma, retroperitoneal 397
scintigraphy 401-406
secretin 184, 249
- cholecystokinin 206
- pancreozymin test 283
selenium-75-selen methionine 401
sepsis 42, 52, 93, 144
serum
- amylase 70, 71
- markers 389
- pancreatic enzymes 141
shock 144
shunting 227
Simplified Acute Physiology Score (SAPS) 120
somatostatin 307
- analogues 403
sonography (*see also* ultrasound) 207
sphincterotomy 73
spiral computed tomography 431, 434
spleen-preserving left resection 326
splenectomy 227
staging 22, 38, 185, 189-193, 195-200, 256, 347, 371, 430, 432, 434
standardized uptake values 404
steatorrhea 205, 235, 266, 267, 268, 277
stem cells 337
stenosis 185
stent 62
stones 185
streptozotocin 333
submandibular glands 334
substance P 321
subtraction scintigraphy 403
surgical treatment 321-327
syphilis 18

T

TAP (*see* trypsinogen activating peptide)
tapering 199, 200

TGF (see transforming growth factor)
thallium-201 403
thrombosis 225
TIMP (see tissue inhibitors of metalloproteinases)
tissue inhibitors of metalloproteinases (TIMP) 291
- TIMP-1 292
- TIMP-2 292
TNF (see tumor necrosis factor)
toxic metabolites 162
toxic-metabolic destruction 161
trace elements, lack of 161
transforming growth factor (TGF) 299
- α 152, 299, 338, 411
- β 152, 293, 414
- - receptors 414
transgenic mice 152
transplantation of islets 334
[^{14}C]triolein 262
- breath test 263
[^{14}C]tripalmitin 262
Trousseau's sign 428
trypsin 75, 121
- activity 71, 285
- immunoreactive 272
trypsinogen activating peptide (TAP) 93, 98, 110, 121, 126
tuberculosis 18
tubular complexes 157
tumor(s) (see also carcinoma) 227
- ampullar 347
- associated chronic pancreatitis 291
- cystic 345
- endocrine 350
- markers 431, 433
- neuroendocrine 398
- pancreatic 353
- signs 353
tumor-associated antigens 390
tumor necrosis factor (TNF) 95, 98
type 1 prophospholipase A$_2$ activating peptide (PROP) 121, 126

U

ulceration, anastomotic 323
ultrasonography (ultrasound) 29-35, 58, 75, 126, 142, 207, 250, 343, 379-384, 429, 430
- endoscopic 195
ultrasound guided fine-needle biopsy 346
upper gut function 233
urea 98
US (see ultrasonography)

V

van-de-Kramer method 277
vascular obstruction 321
vessels 224

W

water, fecal 280
weight loss 427-429
Whipple procedure (operation) 322, 325
white blood cells 98

Y

Y chromosome 336

Z

Zollinger-Ellison syndrome 354

Springer and the environment

At Springer we firmly believe that an international science publisher has a special obligation to the environment, and our corporate policies consistently reflect this conviction.

We also expect our business partners – paper mills, printers, packaging manufacturers, etc. – to commit themselves to using materials and production processes that do not harm the environment. The paper in this book is made from low- or no-chlorine pulp and is acid free, in conformance with international standards for paper permanency.

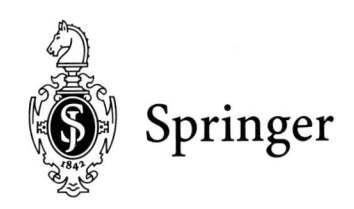

Springer

Printing: Saladruck, Berlin
Binding: Buchbinderei Lüderitz & Bauer, Berlin